Adaptive Protection of The Heart: Protecting Against Stress and Ischemic Damage

Author

Felix Z. Meerson, M.D.
Laboratory of Experimental Cardiology
Institute of General Pathology and Pathological Physiology
Soviet Academy of Medical Sciences
Moscow, U.S.S.R.

Translated from Russian by Alexander V. Galkin, Ph.D.
Moscow, U.S.S.R.

CRC Press
Boca Raton Ann Arbor Boston

Library of Congress Cataloging-in-Publication Data

Meerson, F. Z. (Feliks Zalmanovich)
Adaptive protection of the heart.

Includes biliographical references.
Includes index.
1. Heart — Adaptation. 2. Heart — Pathophysiology.
3. Stress (Physiology) 4. Coronary heart disease —
Pathogenesis. I. Title. [DNLM: 1. Adaptation,
Physiological. 2. Coronary Disease — prevention &
control. 3. Heart — physiology. 4. Stress —
physiopathology. WG 202 M495ab]
QP114.A32M4 1990 616.1′2 90-15096
ISBN 0-8493-5150-2

Direct all inquiries to CRC Press, Inc., 2000 Corporate Blvd., N.W., Boca Raton, Florida, 33431.

International Standard Book Number 0-8493-5150-2

Library of Congress Card Number 90-15096
Printed in the United States

FOREWORD

In our age of expeditious information, any book of some volume which would take a while to read is in itself somewhat antiquated; it is especially so for a treatise devoted to such a wonted problem as protecting the heart from stress and ischemia. Therefore the author feels a need to explain himself going back to the good old days when a manuscript submitted for judgment to a respectable university used to be prefaced with a brief listing of the basic propositions, ''theses'' that had not theretofore been set forth in other works. I believe that just as in the past, this enables the reader to decide whether to spend time on further reading or to make better use of it. Hence I state that this book has been written to substantiate the following ideas concerning heart damage and heart protection.

1. Stress and ischemia, and most often combinations thereof, are of paramount importance in the development of major heart diseases, and nevertheless these two factors are deeply unequal both in their place in cardiac pathology and in the extent of previous study. Indeed, genetic defects in the hepatic cholesterol-eliminating systems and excess cholesterol in food with ensuing atherogenic dyslipidemia and stenosing coronary atherosclerosis, are generally recognized as the key link in the pathogenesis of ischemic heart disease (IHD).* The position of stress in heart pathology proves to be less definite. On the one hand, an excessively long and strong stress reaction is known to provoke atherosclerosis, spasm, thrombosis, overloading of the heart, and other conditions engendering or aggravating ischemia. On the other hand, are there indeed self-contained, noncoronarogenic, not ischemia-linked, direct stress damages to the heart? What are the concrete regulatory, biochemical, morphological, and physiological substrata of such damage? Can such damage to the heart evolve because of stress disorders in other organs? Finally, what is the clinical significance of such nonischemic stress heart damages, in particular, for the pathogenesis of noncoronarogenic cardiosclerosis, arrhythmias, and sudden cardiac death? Diagnoses such as ''stress heart'' and ''stress arrhythmic heart disease'' are not found in the accepted nosology. Yet the thought that cardiac stress damage is a reality in many a patient and not at all need be associated with ischemic disease is most obviously present in the minds of more than a few cardiologists. The idea haunts the clinics and conferences. Therefore, Chapter 1 of this monograph is devoted to analyzing the noncoronarogenic stress damage to the heart, and considering their probable role in the pathogenesis of chronic stress cardiopathies, nonischemic arrhythmias, and sudden cardiac death. In other words, in this Chapter we sought to unfold the concept of ''primary stress damage of the heart'' and to bring it into use in modern cardiology.

2. The decisive role of coronary atherosclerosis in the pathogenesis of ischemic heart disease does not at present raise any doubt, but still leaves open some important questions. Thus, it has been shown that at the same degree of coronary stenosis, the clinical manifestations of IHD can be vivid — or altogether lacking. The fatal sequelae of IHD — myocardial infarction or sudden cardiac death — may occur in moderate coronary atherosclerosis that is of no such consequence for other persons. Moreover, these dramatic events happen even when the coronary arteries are intact. Facts of this kind make inevitable the question of the weight of the stress factor, first, in the pathogenesis of dangerous arrhythmias, fibrillation, and sudden cardiac death, and second, in the formation of atherosclerosis, thrombosis, and spasm, i.e., in the pathogenetic progression of the ischemic disease proper. Therefore, Chapter 2 deals consecutively with these matters, using experimental, epidemiological, and some clinical data to discriminate, on the one hand, the stress arrhythmic disease of the heart from the ischemic disease as such, and to demonstrate, on the other hand, that the two conditions are interconnected.

* References to all works used in this Foreword are given at the end of the relevant Chapters.

The notions substantiated in the first two Chapters have laid the foundation for devoting all further discourse to the problem of heart protection. In so doing, to protect the heart from stress, ischemic, and reperfusion damage, to correct the disturbances of the cardiac contractile function and electric stability in infarction, and postinfarction cardiosclerosis, we made use of a somewhat unorthodox approach, namely gradual adaptation of the organism to environmental factors, as well as biologically active substances accumulating in the organism during adaptation and taking part in heart protection.

To identify the basic issues outlined in these studies it is necessary to dwell briefly on the evolution of our views in such a general physiological problem as stress and adaptation.*

The stress reacton which we have hastily represented on the very first page as a detrimental factor, in point of fact becomes such only if exceedingly strong and protracted, but in the general biological context it is one of the greatest evolutionary achievements, an obligate link of all without exception adaptive reactions of the healthy organism. The stress, naturally and necessarily, contributes both to such primitive reactions as standing still to avoid danger and to such supreme adaptive reactions as seeking scientific truth. Thus, H. Selye, who created the concept of stress, was undoubtedly right in designating his brainchild as the general adaptive syndrome. Only in the most harsh conditions of the biological or social reality is this neurohormonal reaction inordinately amplified, changes its meaning, and turns into the common pathogenetic link of "endogenous" diseases. Indeed, now we have unambiguous proof that the excessive stress reaction is involved in the pathogenesis of duodenal and gastric ulcerous diseases, diabetes, skin, and allergic diseases, in the evolvement of immunodeficient states and escalation of blastomatous growth and, just as certainly, in the pathogenesis of arrhythmias and ischemic heart disease which we are dealing with in this book. This well-founded idea of the role of excessive stress in pathology in essence means that designing the methods for preventing stress damage is a necessary step in the prophylaxis of endogenous diseases which are a standing problem of contemporary medicine. At the same time, this idea had gathered such a psychological momentum as to prevent many researchers from appreciating the extremely important fact that animals and people become afflicted with "classical" stress diseases by far more rarely than they encounter most severe and protracted stress situations in the environment. For animals, such stress situations occur widely in the form of long periods of starvation and cold, natural calamities, and interspecific and intraspecific conflicts. For man, the qualitatively more complex, socially determined stress situations occur no less widely. Thus, in a relatively short stretch of its history, mankind went through slavery, serfdom, and World Wars, but did not (hopefully) degrade in the least. So *a living organism possesses a highly developed ability to adapt to stress situations.*

3. Mankind has survived owing to successful adaptation to stress, but only recently has it begun to study it objectively under laboratory conditions.

The basic technique used in our and other laboratories consisted of exposing animals to relatively mild and brief emotional pain or immobilization stress, to which they successfully adapted, acquiring therewith a remarkably high resistance to severe, previously lethal stress.

Such adaptation to stress further on turned out to have a notably wide and potent cross-protective effect, i.e., to enhance the resistance not only to severe stress and total stress damage of internal organs usual in such situations, but also to the lethal action of electric current, direct chemical, ischemic, and reperfusion injuries to tissues, to cold, and even to ionizing radiation. In conformity with the nature of this book, Chapter 3 deals first with the neuroendocrine mechanism of the adaptation to brief stress episodes and with its cross-protective effects, and then the main attention is focused on protecting the heart through such adaptation. Among the results, it has for the first time been found that prior adaptation to repeated short stress exposures, besides completely preventing primary stress damage to

* These matters are considered in detail in a previous monograph, Meerson, F. *Adaptation, Stress and Prophylaxis,* Springer-Verlag, Berlin, 1984.

the heart, also efficiently protects the heart from ischemic and reperfusion arrhythmias and averts animal death due to cardiac fibrillation. Further, adaptation to stress has been shown to wholly lack any anti-ischemic effect, but at the same time to significantly attenuate the necrosis upon coronary occlusion owing to its cytoprotective effect. Simultaneously, it prevents or abolishes the disorders in the electric stability of the heart in myocardial infarction and postinfarction cardiosclerosis.

It has been obvious from the very beginning that the mechanism of this generalized protective (and specifically, powerful cardioprotective) effect of adaptation deserves the most detailed study at the systemic, the organic, and the cellular levels, since stress situations are actually the most common ones in our individual lives.

4 to 5. Studies on the mechanism of the protective effect of adaptation to stress, the results of which are presented in Chapters 4 and 5, have shown that the stress reaction never occurs in isolation. In the evolution of animals and man, it came to be coupled with activation of several central and cell regulatory systems that modulate the stress reaction, restrict its duration and intensity, and that we have designated as *stress-limiting systems*. The central stress-limiting systems at the brain level are represented by an association of GABA-ergic, opioidergic, serotoninergic, dopaminergic, and parasympathetic neurons, which by their mediators control the excitation of the adrenergic neurons and the hypothalamic output of releasing factors triggering the stress reaction, and thereby limit the duration of the reaction itself. At the level of target organs operate the local stress-limiting systems, namely the antioxidant, the adenosinergic, the prostaglandin systems tempering the effect of stress hormones. Coordinated action of central and local stress-limiting systems ensures optimal modulation of the stress reaction and, in most cases, prevents stress damages to the organism.

Repeated stress exposures augment the power or the efficiency of the stress-limiting systems as manifest by enhanced biosynthesis and direct accumulation of their mediators, from opioid peptides and dopamine to prostaglandins and antioxidant factors. This and this exactly constitutes the material basis of increased direct and cross-resistance in adaptation to stress. Chapters 4 and 5 demonstrate that this novel issue has quite weighty clinical consequences.

The first one is that a genetically determined or acquired deficiency of the stress-limiting systems is a major element in evolvement of stress diseases, and in particular stress cardiac injuries, arrhythmias, and fibrillation mentioned above.

The second consequence is more optimistic, consisting of the protective benefits of adaptation which can be achieved without such drastic measures as immobilization or emotional pain stress, but using procedures like acupuncture or adaptation to other factors such as physical load or hypoxia that initially also elicit a stress reaction. Furthermore, it turned out that a protective effect in all respects similar to the adaptive one can be obtained by administration of activators, mediators of the stress-limiting systems, and their synthetic analogs. Such examples of success in the pharmacology of the stress-limiting systems are analyzed in Chapters 4 and 5.

6. Further experiments produced an unexpected result, i.e., that the protective effects of adaptation to stress are not only exhibited in the whole organism, but also in great measure retained in the isolated hearts of adapted animals, which display markedly enhanced resistance to ischemia, reperfusion injury, and high catecholamine and calcium concentrations. Analysis of this impressive cytoprotective effect of adaptation revealed that myocardial organelles and enzymic systems of adapted animals — mitochondria, sarcoplasmic reticular calcium-pumping vesicles, and creatine kinase system — are significantly more resistant to autolysis than those of controls.

There is quite a body of evidence that this phenomenon, described and examined for the first time here in Chapter 6, i.e., *adaptive stabilization of cell structures,* is associated with increased intracellular production of what is known as stress proteins, and the genetic mechanism involved requires further study.

7. The concluding Chapter concerns the use of adaptation to intermittent hypoxia in the altitude chamber, not only for heart protection from stress and ischemic damage in animals, but also for therapy and prophylaxis of some serious human diseases. The very practicability of such a clinicophysiological study stems from the general concept of environmental adaptation that has been substantiated in recent years. The gist of this concept is that stable, long-term adaptation to, let's say, physical loads, hypoxia, heat, cold, toxic agents, or novel complex situations that demand learning, cannot be provided by simple activation of the functional system mainly affected by the given factor. The principal element of stable adaptation is the enhanced expression of certain genes (and accordingly enhanced synthesis of certain nucleic acids and proteins) in the cells of the system predominating in the organismic adaptive reaction. The resulting selective activation of protein synthesis for and proliferation of just those structures that are limiting the cell function, i.e., growth of the populations of quite definite enzymes, membranes, and organelles, ultimately gives rise to the *systemic structural trace* which is the material basis of adaptation. Sometimes this trace is quite miniature and clearly demarcated. For instance, in adaptation to barbiturates and other diverse chemicals, it manifests itself as increased population and activity of the hepatic cytochrome P_{450}-linked enzymes. As a result, the organism acquires high resistance to toxic compounds and, therewith, greater capacity for oxidizing and eliminating cholesterol. In other cases, the systemic structural trace is, on the contrary, marked by a wide scope and ramified architectonics.

Adaptation to intermittent hypoxia in the altitude chamber is consistently attended with respiratory muscle hypertrophy, increased number of lung alveoli, a 1.5 to 2-fold greater coronary bed capacity, enhanced erythropoiesis and oxygen capacity, and other shifts directly testifying to a step-up in the physiological power of the oxygen-uptake systems. In recent years, it has been found that the long-term response to hypoxia is not limited to this increasing capacity of the systems responsible for oxygen uptake and transport, but is also revealed in physiologically significant changes at the regulatory level. These include growth of pyramidal neurons and altered neuroglial relations in the brain cortex; increased brain and adrenal amounts of opioid peptides and serotonin; partial atrophy of the adrenal glomerular zone and of the hypothalamic supraoptic nucleus, i.e., of the structures responsible for secretion of aldosterone and vasopressin; as well as moderate hypofunction of the thyroid gland and attenuated basal metabolism. It is easy to see that in the architectonics of this ramified, systemic, structural trace there are elements that certainly can enhance the organismic resistance not only to hypoxia, but also to other factors as well, i.e., there is a basis for the cross-protective effect of adaptation.

The contents of Chapter 7 furnishes evidence that adaptation to intermittent hypoxia not only diminishes the necrotic zone in ischemic and adrenergic cardiac injury, but also protects the heart, the liver, and other organs from stress damage, prevents stress atherogenic dyslipidemia, averts ischemic and reperfusion arrhythmias, abolishes the disturbances of cardiac electric stability in acute infarction and postinfarction cardiosclerosis, and hinders the development of hereditary hypertension in rats of the SHR line. Furthermore, such adaptation proved to be beneficial for animal behavior in extremal situations and brain resistance to hallucinogens, epileptogens, etc. So evidently, adaptation to hypoxia is highly promising in regard to therapy and prophylaxis.

Along this line, the last Chapter presents, besides the experimental data, a body of clinical testimony that this potential has been successfully deployed to lessen the risk factors of IHD, to treat the so-called idiopathic and in essence neurogenous arrhythmias, grave forms of neurasthenia, and some allergic diseases of man.

* * *

Once I. P. Pavlov wrote, "The seeking of truth by mathematical analysis and the movement of plants to light, are these not extreme links of the infinite chain of adaptations that constitutes Life on Earth''. Indeed, adaptation is an indispensable property of living matter, hence its study is one of the most far-flung — and maybe final — goals of biology. On the other hand, heart protection from stress and ischemic damage is a most actual and often dramatic everyday problem, with the clinical cardiologist devoting the better part of his abilities and time to treating advanced cases, struggling for minutes, days, months, at best, years of the patient's life. Writing a book in an attempt to bring together two such different problems, the author inevitably takes a risk of looking amateurish, and I don't think I have avoided this altogether. Nevertheless, intrusion of biological patterns of adaptation into cardiology had always seemed fruitful to me. The benefits are that such natural merging of sciences, on the one hand, allows us to use the power of controlled and rationally dosed adaptation to make the medicine really preventive, and on the other hand, may catalyze the development of novel, physiologically sound approaches in pharmacology.

PREFACE

Adaptation is a fundamental process in evolution. Dawkins has called Natural Selection the "blind watch maker" because it has no foresight, works at random, and does not plan for the future. The genetic information, in Crick's words, "needs to do something useful, or to produce other things that will be useful for jobs, to help it to survive and to produce fertile offsprings with a good chance of survival." Adaptation is a key factor in survival of the individual, therefore of the species. But adaptation does not and cannot change the genetic material. It only acts on the individual, the link in the chain of generations. But by doing so, it preserves the entire chain of generations, making possible a continuation and transmission of genetic material.

Professor Meerson has undertaken to study the physiological effects of adaptation. For many years, Professor Meerson has been interested in the physiopathology of the heart and the circulation. His work on the stages of heart failure, how the heart adapts itself to changes in load, has lead him to his various studies on the effects of adaptation. The present monumental book contains much more than the title suggests. There are detailed descriptions of the effect of stress on the heart, beginning with cardiac function, and continuing with the effect of stress on biochemical and biophysical processes, with changes occurring on the molecular level and with clinically related events. In its wide scope, it encompasses the cardioprotective effects of adaptation to stress with particular reference to adaptation of the heart to hypoxia. Here we will find a significant message: adaptation to one particular stress factor, such as intermittent hypoxia, results in profound changes of many different and seemingly unrelated functions. For example, stepwise adaptation to hypoxia alters RNA synthesis and produces changes in lung, heart, muscle, bone marrow, coronary vessels, and sympathetic neurons innervating the heart. Further, stepwise adaptation to hypoxia results in adaptational changes in the central nervous system and the spleen. It causes cessation of cardiac arrhythmias, and more generally, leads to profound changes in immune responses mediated by T-lymphocytes. The clinical ramifications of these adaptive changes are surprising: stepwise adaptation to hypoxia results in cessation of arrhythmias, diminished body weight, and increased working capacity.

What are the mechanisms which cause adaptation? Naturally, we must first consider the stimulus for adaptation, namely stress. Stress has become a much used and sometimes abused term. We speak of psychological stress, environmental stress, and physical stress. But stress can be quantitated only by its effect on the target organ. Our genetic heritage, whether expressed as personality or as physical characteristics, can become both source and target of stress. In the former, it may have very divergent effects. Stress originating from within can spark creative impulses or it can lead to destructive conflicts. Therefore, stress originating from our genetic heritage, may be both curse and privilege. Can one imagine creative activity without stress which originates from the genetic instruction inherited by our minds? Yet, predisposition of a vulnerable mind may, as stress increases, lead to physical and mental deterioration.

Meerson's thoughts are on firmer and better definable grounds: physical stress such as hypoxia, exercise, etc., force the organism to adapt itself physiologically. This certainly is of more immediate concern to the physiopathologist who is only too happy to leave behaviorism or cognitive science to others. Professor Meerson has presented us with challenging concepts which, when based on firm quantitative studies, should keep physiopathologists occupied for many years to come.

Richard J. Bing, M.D.

THE AUTHOR

Professor Felix Z. Meerson, M.D., is Chief of the Laboratory of Heart Pathophysiology, Institute of General Pathology and Pathological Physiology, Moscow, U.S.S.R.

Dr. F. Z. Meerson graduated from the 1st Moscow Medical Institute in 1949 with a degree as a physician and obtained his M.D. degree in 1958 from the Central Advanced Training Institute for Physicians in Moscow. In 1960 he became a Professor of Clinical Physiology and assumed his present position.

Dr. F. Z. Meerson is a Chairman of the Problem Committee on Pathophysiology of the adaptive processes of the Academy of Medical Sciences of the U.S.S.R., a member of the Managing Committee of the Soviet Society of Cardiologists and Soviet Society of Pathophysiologists, and a WHO expert.

Among other awards he has received the State Award of the U.S.S.R. for research in molecular cardiology in 1978 and The Gold Medal of the Exibition of Economic Achievements of the U.S.S.R. for development and grounding of the method of adaptation to hypoxia in altitude chamber for therapy and prophylaxis of human diseases. He became ''One Distinguished in Sciences of Russia'' in 1988.

Dr. F. Z. Meerson is the author of 15 books, published in the U.S.S.R., U.S., Japan, Germany and more than 500 research papers.

His current major research interests include the basic mechanisms of adaptation of the organism to environmental factors and application of the adaptation to the environmental factors for therapy and prophylaxis of human diseases.

ACKNOWLEDGMENTS

I am deeply grateful to my friends E. E. Ustinova, M. G. Pshennikova, and E. B. Manukhina for their invaluable help in manuscript preparation. The book is in large measure based on the experimental and clinicophysiological work carried out by N. A. Abdykaliev, Yu. V. Arkhipenko, L. M. Belkina, V. M. Boev, T. N. Bukina, V. I. Vovk, E. Ya. Vorontsova, L. Yu. Golubeva, V. V. Didenko, S. S. Dyusenov, Yu. N. Kopylov, V. I. Kuznetsov, A. V. Lapshin, N. P. Lyamina, E. V. Malysheva, I. Yu. Malyshev, V. V. Malyshev, E. B. Manukhina, A. A. Nikonorov, M. G. Pshennikova, T. G. Sazontova, V. A. Saltykova, V. P. Tverdokhlib, E. E. Ustinova, V. A. Frolov, A. B. Shneider, and other colleagues of mine, whose contribution is gratefully acknowledged. The book has gained much from having been translated into English by Dr. A. V. Galkin, who did not restrict himself to mere translation, but quite often acted as a scrupulous editor of matter and style.

TABLE OF CONTENTS

ABBREVIATIONS

ACTH	adrenocorticotropic hormone
ALT	alanine transaminase
AP	action potential
AP_s	systolic arterial pressure
AST	aspartate transaminase
ATPase	adenosine triphosphatase
cAMP	3′,5′-cyclic adenosine monophosphate
cAMP-PK	cAMP-dependent protein kinase
cGMP	3′,5′-cyclic guanosine monophosphate
CIC	circulating immune complexes
CM	calmodulin
CNS	central nervous system
CP	creatine phosphate
CPK	creatine phosphokinase
DAG	diacylglycerol
dopa	dihydroxyphenylalanine
E	epinephrine
EA	electroacupuncture
ECG	electrocardiogram, electrocardiography
EDRF	endothelium-derived relaxing factor
ES	extrasystole
EPS	emotional pain stress
FDA	fructose 1,6-diphosphate aldolase
GABA	gamma-aminobutyric acid
GABA-TA	GABA transaminase
GDC	glutamate decarboxylase
GHBA	gamma-hydroxybutyric acid
GPO	glutathione peroxidase
HDLP	high-density lipoproteins
HSP	heat-shock proteins
HR	heart rate
IFS	intensity of the functioning of structures
Ig	immunoglobulin(s)
IHD	ischemic heart disease
IP_3	inositol triphosphate
LCAT	lecithin: cholesterol acyltransferase
LDH	lactate dehydrogenase
LDLP	low-density lipoproteins
LPO	lipid peroxidation
MDA	malonic dialdehyde
MDH	malate dehydrogenase
NCE	negative chronotropic effect
NE	norepinephrine
OP	opioid peptide(s)
PAF	platelet activating factor
PG	prostaglandin(s)
$PIP_{(2)}$	phosphatidylinositol (di)phosphate
PK C	protein kinase C
RP	rest potential

SL	stress load
SOD	superoxide dismutase
SR	sarcoplasmic reticulum
TXA_2	thromboxane A_2
VEL	veloergometric load
VFT	ventricular fibrillation threshold
VLDLP	very-low-density lipoproteins

To the memory of my father,

who resolutely passed through those ordeals,

I dedicate this book.

Chapter 1

PRIMARY STRESS DAMAGE OF THE HEART

I. INTRODUCTION

Stress that damages the previously normal heart will be the focus of our attention in this Chapter. To assess correctly the facts bearing directly on this issue, it should be borne in mind that by no means did the stress response evolve as a detrimental reaction, but, on the contrary, it constitutes one of the evolutionary achievements, a necessary link in adaptation of the organism to the environment.

The scheme in Figure 1 illustrates the concept of the mechanism of individual adaptation established in our laboratory[1] and shows that a disturbance of homeostasis brought about by an environmental factor activates, through higher levels of regulation, the systems responsible for adaptation. This results in two chains of events: firstly (the upper part of the scheme) mobilization of the functional system specifically responsible for adaptation to the given particular factor, for example physical load, cold, or hypoxia; secondly (the lower part) a wholly nonspecific, ''ordinary'' activaton of the stress-effecting system elicited by any strong or novel stimulus.

Further on, in the cells of the functional system specifically responsible for adaptation, the enhanced physiological function turns out to be coupled with activation of the genetic apparatus: nucleic acid and protein synthesis is increased to augment the key subcellular structures limiting the cell function. Selective growth of these key structures leads to the formation of the ''systemic structural trace'' which increases the functional power of the systems responsible for adaptation and allows transformation of the initial, immediate, but unreliable adaptation into a stable and long-term one.

As this takes place, depending on the architecture of the functional system, the structural trace may be quite ramified as in adaptation to hypoxia or, conversely, relatively confined as in adaptation to chemicals when the adaptive goal is achieved mainly at the expense of elevated enzymes of the cytochrome P_{450} system in the liver and hypertrophy of this organ.[2,3]

The scheme shows that formation of the systemic structural trace and stable adaptation is potentiated by the stress reaction which plays an especially important part just at the transition from immediate to long-term adaptation. After the systemic structural trace has completely formed and become the basis of, for instance, training to physical loads, temporary connection, or enhanced resistance to hypoxia, the stable adaptation rectifies the homeostatic disturbance, with ensuing disappearance of the now needless stress reaction.

It is essential that the stress reaction not only precedes stable adaptation, but also plays a prominent role in its formation. In this context it should be remembered that the originator of the teaching on stress, Selye, with fascinating sagacity defined this link of the adaptive mechanism as the general adaptive syndrome.

At present many circumstances concerning the mechanism of stress and its adaptive and damaging effects have become clear. As regards higher animals, it is now evident that emotions are decisive in the origin of stress. According to the information theory of emotions developed by Simonov[4] they are brought about by the ''conflict'' between the actual needs of the organism (alimentary, sexual, self-preservation, self-assertion, domination) and the lack of sufficient information on whether or not these needs can be satisfied in the particular environment. This discrepancy between the need and the information necessary to fulfill it is perceived at the level of the brain neocortex and gives rise to descending cortical influences which activate the special neural apparatus of emotions: a system of nervous centers located in the area of hypothalamus, amygdaloid complex, and paleocortex. This system, according to numerous data, acts as a connecting link between the neocortex, which primarily senses

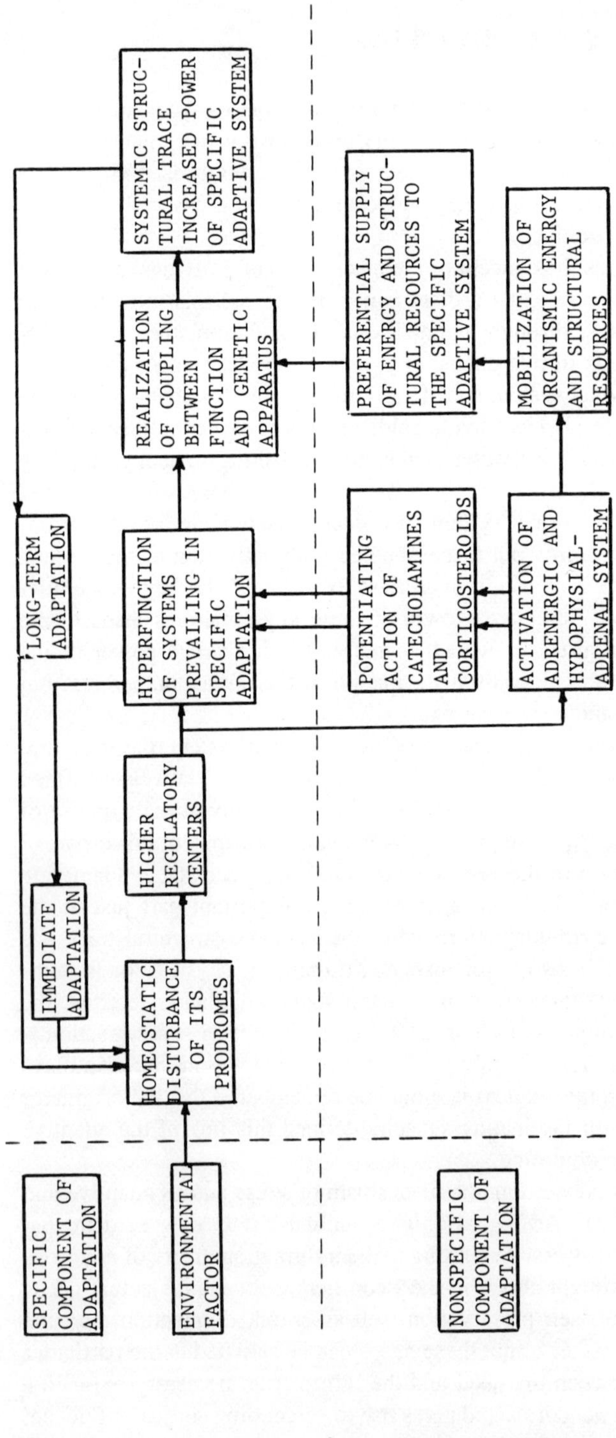

FIGURE 1. Mechanism of long-term adaptation. For explanations see text.

the information deficiency, and the centers in the hypothalamus. Excitation of the latter centers is subjectively realized as emotions of fear, anxiety, rage, pleasure, etc. In our opinion, this actuates two interconnected regulatory mechanisms which together constitute the main content of the stress reaction.

The first mechanism manifests itself as ascending activatory, mostly adrenergic influences from the emotion centers to the brain cortex, and development of diverse behavioral responses as if the organism is trying to fill in the "information gap" between the need to realize an instinct and the possibility of its realization. A relatively simple example of an emotional attempt to compensate for, to fill in the information gap is the defensive dominant formed in frightened children or in adults encountering a new and complex situation. The dominant of this kind is reflected in diverse, often exaggerated defense reactions to various and in many cases biologically insignificant environmental factors. By chance one of such reactions may turn out to be exact; in this case it is reinforced and a new environmentally adequate habit is formed: adaptation takes place.

In the more complex processes constituting the basis of human mentality, emotions, through the mobilizing adrenergic and other effects of stress, can ensure rapid and varied recombination of memorial traces preserved in the brain and thereby create new associations, some of which are reinforced by the reality and become the basis of new notions of the surrounding world. Thus Archimedes or Newton, inspired by mighty emotion, in painstaking thought, perceived fundamental physical laws behind simple things like a body immersed in water, or a falling apple. Initially, each such event comes to that in the brain of a single man and a new temporary connection is established, a new structural trace. This trace is first expressed, but in the experience of this one man, and only later, through relatively simple practices of imitation and education, becomes the property of mankind, i.e., part of the progress which is the supreme form of human adaptation. It is obvious, however, that such creative stress-based thinking, like any other stress event, is attended by great expenditures for the population, since the overwhelming majority of new associations prove to be of very modest value, or may be altogether erroneous, but nevertheless take complete possession over the person and find their imitators and followers. Ultimately, the sequelae of this sort of "creative errors" find their place in the case records of psychiatric clinics or constitute the dark pages of the history of mankind.

The second chain of events contributing to the matter of stress is directed inside the organism and is the basis of timely energy and structural provision for thinking and behavior. With all this it may become decisive for the pathology of internal organs, in particular stress damage to the heart. In this connection one should as a first approximation answer the questions, under what circumstances does the adaptive effect of stress become detrimental? what particular damages have been demonstrated in the heart? what clinical significance might these damages have?

In its general form the answer stems from the concept developed above that stress is a link in adaptation and ends as soon as adaptation is achieved (see Figure 1). Accordingly, if a functional system adequate to the environment is not formed, then the homeostatic disturbances caused by the environment in the organism persist. The stress also persists and becomes unusually long and intense. It is in this situation that stress may evoke stress diseases from duodenal ulcers and immunodeficient activation of blastomatous growth to psychic disorders and cardiac damage.

In other words, excessively intense and prolonged activation of the descending branch of the stress reaction also involves heavy costs for individuals and for the population as a whole, since the major noninfectious diseases constituting a standing medical problem are mostly elicited or aggravated by stress.

The diverse situations causing heavy and prolonged stress fraught with internal organ damage ultimately boil down to the conflict between an imperative need to immediately carry out a defense, alimentary, sexual reaction, or reflexes of "freedom" or domination, and an insurmountable ban on carrying them out. In its most elementary form this conflict is reproduced by subjecting animals to a pain or immobilization stimulant and at the same time depriving them of a possibility to evade these factors. In a qualitatively more complex form this conflict is realized when a person is under some socially determined influence jeopardizing his existence or dignity while the natural response is prohibited by other also socially determined conditions requiring self-restraint to avoid still greater dangers. The self-restraint is indeed ensured through critical exertion of the cortical inhibitory mechanisms, but as this takes place it is only the external behavioral component of the response that is suppressed or modified. Its internal vegetative component, i.e., the stress reaction with mobilization of the circulatory and respiratory functions, etc., is retained and may even turn out to be more intense and protracted than upon execution of the behavioral response. This situation, considered from various angles in the works of Pavlov, Lang, and Anokhin, is characterized in particular by the intense stress reaction manifesting itself as a manifold increase in blood catecholamine and glucocorticoid levels. It is just under such conditions that the adaptive effect of stress on internal organs becomes a damaging one and a basis of disease. We shall further consider this fatal transformation as applied to the heart.

II. CONVERSION OF THE CARDIOTROPIC ADAPTIVE EFFECT OF STRESS INTO A DETRIMENTAL ONE

In response to the emotiogenic stress situations in the environment, the brain centers determining the stress reaction evoke a significant increase in the secretion of releasing factors and hormones and in the liberation of neuromediators. The hypothalamus produces corticoliberin, somatoliberin, and other releasing factors activating the hypophysial secretion of ACTH and other tropic hormones.[5-7] There is a rise in the ''output'' of corticosteriods from the adrenal glands[5,6,8] and of catecholamines from the adrenergic terminals and adrenals.[9-11]

The release of tropic hormones, catecholamines, and corticosteriods stimulates or suppresses the secretion of hormones of the next line of regulation. Secretion is stimulated for glucagon,[12] thyroid and parathyroid hormones,[5,13,14] somatotropic hormone,[5,15] aldosterone, angiotensin, renin,[5,16,19] vasopressin,[14,16] and thyrocalcitonin,[14] and suppressed for insulin[17] and sex hormones,[18] and so on.

A detailed description of the secretion and action of hormones and mediators during stress is not the subject of this exposition, but it should be emphasized that it is just these regulatory factors that carry out the adaptive or — at excessively high concentrations — the damaging effects of stress on the heart. The general adaptive influence of stress on the heart is naturally realized during any behavioral reaction from physical work to solving mathematical problems. Analysis of the components of this phenomenon yields at least five cardiotropic adaptive effects of stress.

The first adaptive effect of stress is the potentiation of organ and tissue function through activation of the most ancient signal pathway, namely the rise in the cytoplasmic concentration of the universal mobilizer of cell function, Ca^{2+}. Penetration of Ca^{2+} into the cell, besides other factors, depends on its extracellular concentration. In the initial phase of the stress reaction a rapid rise in the blood level of the parathyroid hormone draws Ca^{2+} from the bones so that its content in the blood may increase by 40 to 50%.[14] Since there is a certain interrelation between the Ca^{2+} concentrations in the extracellular space and in the cardiomyocytes,[19] this effect may entail enhanced entry of Ca^{2+} through the potential-dependent Ca^{2+} channels and the Na^+/Ca^{2+} exchange mechanism.

On entering the cell, Ca^{2+} combining with its main intracellular receptor calmodulin (CM) passes into the active state (Ca-CM), activates the CM-dependent protein kinases (Ca-CM-PK), and thereby stimulates most intracellular processes from myofibrillar contraction and relaxation to glycolysis and lipolysis.[20]

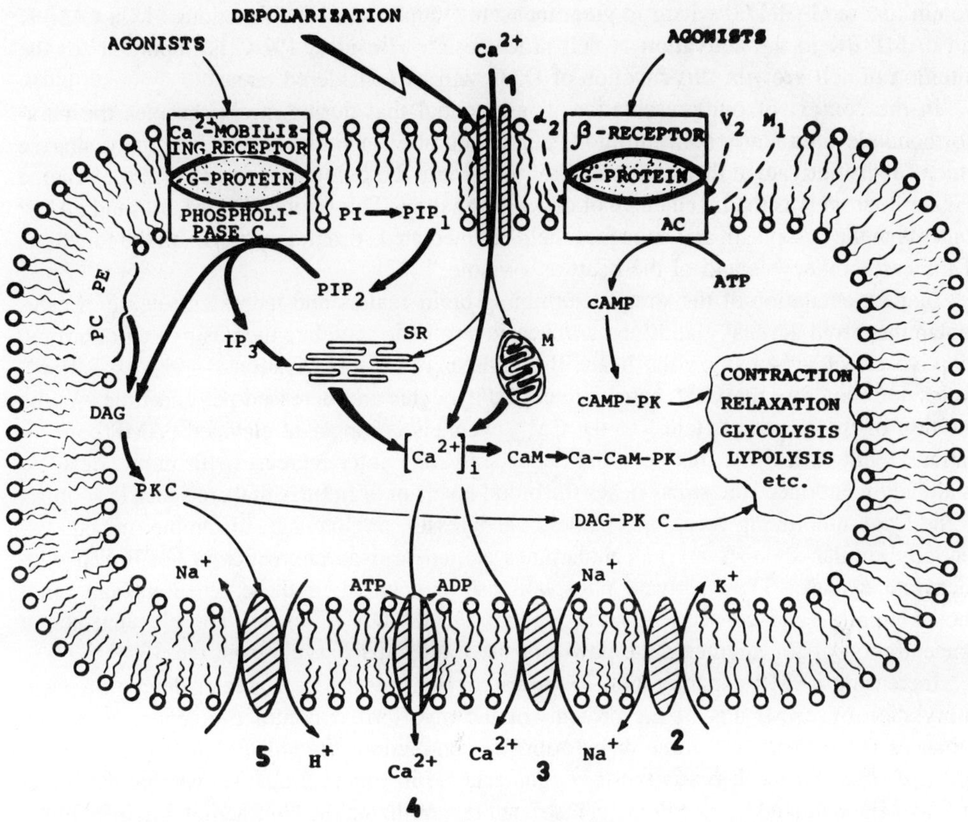

FIGURE 2. Activation of the cell regulatory mechanisms in stress. For explanations see text.

Figure 2 displays the basic regulatory mechanisms that, at the cardiomyocyte membrane level, control the Ca^{2+} entry into the cell, the changes in its sarcoplasmic content, and thus the myocardial function. Firstly, propagation of the pulse generated by the sinus node, i.e., cell membrane depolarization, entails the opening of the potential-dependent Ca^{2+} channels and Ca^{2+} entry which, until recently, has been believed to cause Ca^{2+} release from the sarcoplasmic reticulum (SR) through some as yet obscure mechanism. Secondly, as shown in Figure 2, the action of catecholamines via activation of adenylate cyclase produces cAMP, which, through the cAMP-dependent protein kinase (cAMP-PK), effects phosphorylation of the proteins of the potential-dependent Ca^{2+} channels. This prolongs their ''opened state'' during depolarization and thereby increases Ca^{2+} entry into the cell. Similarly, i.e., through cAMP-PK, cAMP potentiates the major cellular processes activated by CM. Thirdly, Figure 2 shows the comparatively recent discovery of a receptor-dependent way of Ca^{2+} mobilization from the SR.[20-22] The gist of this important mechanism is that catecholamines, vasopressin, angiotensin, and other agonists of the Ca^{2+}-mobilizing receptors activate phospholipase C coupled with these receptors in the cell membrane.[23] The enzyme hydrolyzes phosphatidyl inositol 4,5-diphosphate (PIP_2), a derivative of the minor phospholipid phosphatidyl inositol (PI) found in the interior of the membrane lipid bilayer. PIP_2 hydrolysis yields two compounds: inositol triphosphate (IP_3) and diacyl glycerol (DAG).[23,24] At a certain stage of the process, another isoenzyme of phospholipase C is activated which hydrolyzes other phospholipids — phosphatidyl choline and phosphatidyl ethanolamine — which also produce DAG.[23] IP_3 quickly reaches the SR and, acting as a ligand for a specific receptor localized therein, causes Ca^{2+} release from the SR to the sarcoplasm. DAG is a specific activator of protein kinase C (PK C) which in great measure "duplicates" the functions of Ca-CM-PK and cAMP-PK in the activation of cell processes.[20,24] Besides, PK C is important for the initiation of cell growth; this function of DAG will be considered later.

In the context of our presentation it is essential that during stress, besides the parathormone-elevated Ca^{2+} concentration, quite a number of other factors become operative which finally activate al three ways of Ca^{2+} entry into the cytoplasm depicted in the scheme (Figure 2) as well as the mechanism of cAMP formation. This augments the Ca^{2+} and cAMP contents in the cytoplasm and enhances their PK-mediated stimulatory effect on the functions of the cardiomyocytes and of the heart as a whole.

Indeed, excitation of the stress-determining brain centers and increased release of catecholamines from adrenal glands and adrenergic terminals actualize the positive chronotropic adaptive effect of stress on the heart: the number of "depolarization — repolarization" cycles and therefore the Ca^{2+} entry into cardiomyocytes are increased per unit time. As the duration of the "opened state" of the Ca^{2+} channels is longer at elevated cAMP concentrations, with each cycle this potential-dependent Ca^{2+} entry increases still more. Besides, as already mentioned, the stress raises the blood levels of hormones that are specific agonists of the Ca^{2+}-mobilizing receptors, namely vasopressin, angiotensin, histamine, et seq. Essentially similar agonists are catecholamines acting on α-adrenoreceptors not linked with adenylate cyclase. They activate phospholipase C coupled to these receptors and other phospholipases, and consequently the regulatory "IP_3-DAG" cycle. The elevated acting concentration of IP_3 augments the power of the Ca^{2+} "discharge" from the SR.[20,24]

Increasing cAMP concentration in the sarcoplasm results in a greater degree of phosphorylation by cAMP-PK of the proteins of the myofibrillar contractile apparatus, which enhances the velocity and force of myofibrillar contraction: *the positive inotropic adaptive effect of stress on the heart is realized.* The scheme in Figure 2 also shows that the effect of Ca-CM potentiated by cAMP is not restricted to mobilizing the contraction, but is involved in the *prompt energy provision* for it through activation of glycolysis. The more *stable energy supply* for enhanced function is known to be ensured as the increased ATP hydrolysis in myofibrils via the creatine kinase system stimulates the oxidative ATP resynthesis in mitochondria. It is quite important that the rising concentrations of Ca-CM and cAMP can increase the rate of transition from contraction to relaxation by activating the Ca^{2+} pumps in the SR and sarcolemma. Here, cAMP activates relaxation not only by potentiating the Ca-CM action at the level of the membrane Ca^{2+} pumps, but also at the level of myofibrils where phosphorylation of troponin I by the cAMP-PK decreases the affinity between troponin C and Ca^{2+} and thereby increases the relaxation velocity.[20] The result is *the other component of this adaptive effect of stress on the heart: activation of the relaxation process.*

Obviously the cardiotropic effect of stress, mediated by the Ca-CM signal pathway and the modulating regulatory circuits (cAMP and IP_3-DAG), may play a prominent part in the mobilization of cardiac function and therefore in the adaptation of the organism to various environmental factors.

At the same time it should be emphasized that the now well-proven stress-induced adrenergic increase of Ca^{2+} levels in cardiomyocytes[25-27] can be an adaptive factor, only provided sufficient power of the membrane calcium and sodium pumps and of the sodium-calcium exchange mechanism which, as shown in Figure 2, ensure timely removal of Ca^{2+} from the cells to the extracellular space and maintain the normal sarcoplasmic Ca^{2+} concentration that is 10,000 times less than that in plasma.[23] This evolutionarily established concentration gradient is necessary not only to preserve the role of Ca^{2+} as the prime signal controlling the cell function, but also to prevent excessive activation of Ca-dependent phospholipases and proteases, free-radical lipid oxidation, myofibrillar contracture, etc., i.e., to prevent the well-known cardiotoxic effect of calcium.[26,28]

Under congenital deficiency of the cation-pump enzymes or excessively long stress, when the amount of calcium and sodium increases in the cytoplasm, the excess of these cations first of all causes a more or less pronounced depolarization of the sarcolemma which is later manifested in a decreased rest potential, lower threshold of ventricular fibrillation, and higher probability of arrhythmias. Further buildup of Ca^{2+} leads to incomplete relaxation of myofibrils in diastole and development of the myocardial "poststress rigidity" which in principle can interfere with diastolic relaxation and hence with the Starling mechanism, thereby attenuating the cardiac contraction force. Simultaneously, the excess of calcium combined with the catecholamine action on the β-receptors may cause overmobilization and sometimes exhaustion of the glycogen reserves; excessive calcium entry into mitochondria may impair oxidative phosphorylation and thus ATP resynthesis. The result is a certain complex of disturbances to the energy supply for cardiac function.

In limited groups of cardiomyocytes the buildup of Ca^{2+} can be responsible for the "calcium triad" of damage to the cell structures comprising irreversible contractural damage of myofibrils, activation of phospholipases and proteases, and free-radical lipid oxidation. The experimental material characterizing these phenomena will be considered below. Here it is important to say that the transformation of the Ca-CM-induced adaptive mobilization of the cardiac function into the cardiomyocyte damage by excess Ca^{2+} is usually not an isolated event, but is intrinsically linked with an immoderate augmentation of the adaptive lipotropic effect of stress in biomembranes (see below). In other words, *the excess of calcium and its detrimental effect usually result from impaired functioning of the membrane-bound lipid-dependent cation pumps.*

The second adaptive effect of stress is that the "stress hormones" — catecholamines, vasopressin, and others — either through corresponding receptors or directly, affect the activity of lipases,[29,30] phospholipases,[23,29,31] and the intensity of free-radical lipid oxidation,[32,33] i.e., the main processes responsible for the renewal of the membrane lipid bilayer. The *lipotropic effect of stress* alters the structural organization, the phospholipid and fatty acid compositon of the membrane lipid bilayer, and thereby the lipid milieu of the membrane-bound functional proteins. This allows comparatively rapid changes of the activity of the main membrane proteins, i.e., vital enzymes, receptors, ionic-transport channels localized in the cell membrane (see Figure 2).

Thus, for example, catecholamines and other hormones and mediators on contact with appropriate receptors have been shown to activate the phospholipid methyl transferase methylating the membrane phospholipids surrounding the receptors. This results in phospholipid migration and decreasing viscosity (or increasing "fluidity") of the membrane.[34] Membrane "fluidity" is also increased upon phospholipid hydrolysis by phospholipase A_2 owing to the detergent action of lysophospholipids.[35,36]

Such moderate alterations of the membrane lipid bilayer promote the "mobility" of the peptide chains of the functional membrane-bound proteins and enhance their activity.

The adaptive significance of the lipotropic effect of stress appears to be great: this effect can rapidly optimize the activity of all key membrane-bound proteins and thereby the cell and whole organ function, thus facilitating the immediate adaptation of the organism to environmental factors. However, in excessively long and intense stress it is the amplification of just that very effect — overactivation of phospholipases, lipases, lipid oxidation — that causes membrane damage and acquires the key role in the transformation of the adaptive effect of stress into the detrimental one. The damaging factors here are free fatty acids accumulating from excessive triglyceride hydrolysis and from phospholipid hydrolysis by phospholipases C, A_1, and A_2, as well as lysophospholipids formed upon phospholipid cleavage by phospholipase A_2. The high fatty acid level increases the content of their long-chain derivatives acyl coenzyme A and acyl carnitine.[36,37] These compounds and lysophospholipids are amphiphiles, possessing hydrophilic (polar) and hydrophobic (nonpolar) moie-

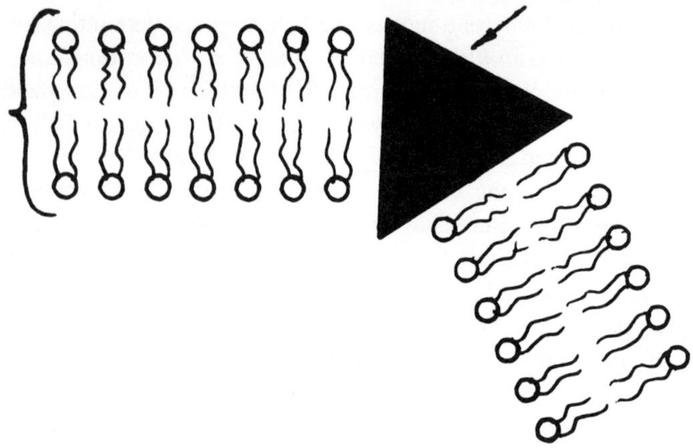

FIGURE 3. Sarcolemmal damage by lysophospholipids. For explanations see text.

ties. This feature allows them to interact with the phospholipids of the lipid bilayer and to alter its structure by penetrating into the bilayer and substituting for phospholipids. At high concentrations the amphiphiles form micelles which "break up" the membrane and ruin its integrity. The most "toxic" in this respect are lysophospholipids because of their wedge-like structure (Figure 3), and especially lysophosphatidyl choline.[31,36,38] Such action results in enhanced permeability of the cell membranes to ions and particularly to Ca^{2+}. Specifically, it has been shown that when catecholamines act on the heart, activation of phospholipase A_2 and lysophospholipid formation induce increased permeability of the cardiomyocytal SR membranes and a release of Ca^{2+} therefrom,[39] with ensuing overloading of the sarcoplasm with this cation and cell damage.[31] This mechanism appears to be also involved in the phenomenon of desensitization: a decrease in the number of operative β-adrenoreceptors in the heart under stress or excess catecholamines. Indeed, this phenomenon is prevented by phospholipase A_2 inhibitors suppressing phospholipid hydrolysis[40] and, conversely, induced by phospholipase A_2 activation.[35]

Another detrimental factor of the lipotropic effect in intense or protracted stress are the products of lipid peroxidation (see Chapter 5).

In general, the overenhancement of the stress lipotropic effect in biomembranes may lead to their damage and be involved in the inactivation of ionic channels, receptors, and especially calcium and sodium cation pumps. As applied to the heart, the latter alteration increases Ca^{2+} and Na^{+} concentrations in the sarcoplasm, decreases the membrane potential, and thereby becomes the cause of impaired electric stability of the heart, arrhythmias, and the above-considered cardiomyocyte damage by excess Ca^{2+}. In the final analysis the ionic disturbances in cardiomyocytes and their hypercalcium damage induced by the immoderate lipotropic effect apparently constitute the key link of cardiac damage in stress and the major cause of the damage to the contractile function of the heart and development of arrhythmias.

The third adaptive effect of stress is the mobilization of the energetic and structural resources of the organism as manifested by elevated blood levels of glucose, fatty acids, nucleotides, amino acids, and enhanced respiratory and circulatory functions. This effect comes to increasing the availability of oxidizable substrates, biosynthetic precursors, and oxygen for the organs performing extra work.

In assessing this adaptive effect of stress, it should be borne in mind that the chief role in mobilizing the carbohydrate reserve in the organism is played by catecholamines and glucagon which activate glycogenolysis and glycolysis via the adenylate cyclase system in the liver, the skeletal muscle, and the heart.[5,41] As this takes place, catecholamines are released at the earliest stage of the stress response, whereas glucagon is produced somewhat later[42,43] and as if it ''duplicates'' and ''backs up'' the effect of catecholamines. This last point can be of importance when the catecholamine action is not fully realized because of desensitization of β-adrenoreceptors by excess catecholamines, and the adenylate cyclase is activated through the glucagon receptors.[44] These hormones cause glucose to be supplied into the circulation directly from the carbohydrate depots of the liver and skeletal muscle. Another source of glucose comes from the effect of glucocorticoids and to some extent of the parathormone:[45] activation of proteolysis, increasing free amino acid pool, and activation of gluconeogenesis in the liver and skeletal muscle.[7,8,45] Glucocorticoids act on their receptors to stimulate at the nuclear level the synthesis of gluconeogenetic enzymes glucose 6-phosphatase, phosphoethanol pyruvate carboxykinase, etc.[7] The outcome of this activation is transamination of amino acids and production of glucose. It is in principle important that both hormonal mechanisms of glucose mobilization in stress ensure the timely supply of glucose to such vital organs as the brain and the heart. Under stress associated with acute physical load, especial significance is again acquired by the glucocorticoid-induced activation of the glucose — alanine cycle providing for glucose formation from amino acids directly in muscle tissue.[46]

Mobilization of the lipid depots in stress is chiefly ensured by catecholamines and glucagon which, through the adenylate cyclase system, activate lipases and lipoprotein lipases in the adipose tissue, the skeletal muscle, and the heart.[29,47,48] Hydrolysis of plasma triglycerides seems to involve the parathormone and vasopressin, secretion of which is substantially increased in stress.[14,49,50] The fatty acid pool thus liberated is utilized in the heart and skeletal muscle.

A peculiar role in the mobilization and utilization of the energy resources in stress is played by the well-known phenomenon that catecholamines suppress insulin secretion and stimulate glucagon secretion.[12,17] On the one hand, the increasing glucagon/insulin ratio promotes activation of gluconeogenesis in the liver; on the other hand, the decreased insulin level limits glucose utilization in the tissues. Under such conditions a certain advantage in the glucose supply is gained by the organs and tissues with adaptively enhanced blood flow, i.e., by the systems bearing the main load.

On the whole, mobilization of the energy and structural resources in stress is quite pronounced. Assessing this phenomenon, however, one should keep in mind that its adaptive role can be realized only on condition of the timely formation of a functional system responsible for adaptation which would utilize these resources to sustain the organ and tissue hyperfunction and then to form the systemic structural trace. Under conditions when the organism ''cannot find a way out'' of the situation and an environmentally adequate functional system (i.e., an adequate behavioral stereotype) is not formed, the protracted stress and attending intensive mobilization of resources cease to be an adaptive factor and entail progressive exhaustion of the organism.

Besides simple exhaustion, mobilization of the energy depots may lead to direct cardiac damage. This happens because in protracted stress the catecholamine activation of lipases and phospholipase A in the adipose tissue produces high blood levels of fatty acids and lysophospholipids, which by the mechanism considered above can alter the membrane lipid bilayer of cardiomyocytes and impair their function. The significance of this factor is directly confirmed by the experiments in which the heart was damaged by the known method of Rona et al.[51] with large doses of the β-adrenomimetic isoproterenol. The size of cardiac necroses and lethality proved to be substantially greater in animals with excess adipose tissue. Recent studies[52] using the same means of cardiac damage have shown that to a large extent the damage is effected through accumulation of the fatty acid derivative acyl carnitine, and correspondingly can be averted with an agent inhibiting carnitine synthesis, thereby precluding acyl carnitine accumulation. These facts are very important for understanding the mechanism of cardiac damage in behavioral stress, since in such cases the β-adrenergic effect on the heart, i.e., essentially the isoproterenol-like effect, has been proved to be predominant.[53]

Another possible cause of impaired cardiac function in prolonged stress is the significant decrease in the number of specific glucocorticoid receptors in the liver, which leads to attenuated hepatic synthesis of gluconeogenetic enzymes and attenuated glucose production.[7] This increases the proportion of fatty acids among the cardiac substrates and may deepen their damaging effect.

The fourth of the main adaptive effects of stress can be defined as the ''addressed transfer of the energy and structural resources from inactive systems to the functional system carrying out the adaptive reaction.''

An important factor of this selective redistribution of resources is the well-known locally originating ''working hyperemia'' in the organs of the system responsible for adaptation, with simultaneous narrowing of the vessels of ''inactive'' organs. It is indeed known that under stress induced by acute physical load the portion of the minute volume of blood flowing through the skeletal muscles increases fourfold to fivefold, whereas in the digestive organs, kidneys, and other tissues this index, conversely, decreases fivefold to sevenfold as compared to the resting state.[54] Nonanesthetized aminals under heavy behavioral stress are known to consistently develop an enhanced coronary flow.[55] This also appears to happen at the expense of other organs.

The given mechanism ensures preferential supplies of oxygen and substrates to the organs that take the main load. The leading role in carrying out this stress effect belongs to catecholamines as well as to vasopressin and angiotensin II, whose secretion is activated in stress.[14,16] These hormones narrow the vessels in those organs and tissues where this is not counteracted by the ''working'' hyperemia and mobilization of the closed (reserve) capillaries.

Some observations give grounds for thinking that the enhanced blood supply to the working organs at the expense of the ''idle'' ones does not exhaust the problem of the radical redistribution of resources in stress. Thus it has been noted that after surgical aortic ostial stenosis in rabbits, when the stress elevation of blood glucocorticoids activates hepatic gluconeogenesis and causes an almost complete involution of the thymus, this ''catabolic effect'' of stress in no way hinders the immense activation of nucleic acid and protein synthesis in the myocardium, and the cardiac mass in operated animals may increase by 80%.[56] Such facts prompt an idea that, besides the flow redistribution, the organs with enhanced function become less sensitive to glucocorticoids and are therefore capable of activating their nucleic acid and protein synthesis in proportion to the enhanced function.[57]

Obviously, the redistribution of resources of the organism in stress, aimed at priority supplies to the system responsible for adaptation, regardless of its mechanism is an adaptive phenomenon.

Yet in an excessively pronounced stress reaction this may be attended by functional disturbances in and even damage to other systems not involved in the given adaptive reaction; for instance, ischemic ulceration of the gastrointestinal tract under heavy physical loads,[58] etc. A conversion of the redistributive effect from an adaptive to a detrimental one at the cardiac level seems hardly probable at first glance; indeed, behavioral stress studies with intact animals have shown that the β-adrenergic effect of catecholamines prevails, and owing to the vasodilatory action of cAMP ensures dilation of the coronary vessels and myocardial hyperemia even in pronounced stress.[55,59] However, prolonged stress and high blood concentrations of epinephrine, vasopressin, and histamine may cause partial desensitization of β-adrenoreceptors and a coronary spasm developing under the action of these agonists on the Ca^{2+}-mobilizing receptors (see Figure 2).

Such a coronary spasm has been experimentally demonstrated with vasopressin[50] and has also been observed in apparently healthy persons under stress.[60]

Another way in which the effect of resource redistribution may turn into the effect of cardiac damage is that a drastic striction of the vessels of internal organs, in particular liver and pancreas, may cause a deep functional disturbance in these organs. The resulting seepage of trypsin into the blood from the pancreas[61] and impaired cholesterol oxidation in the liver[62] can in their turn directly damage the myocardium or be conducive to atherosclerosis as will be shown further.

The fifth adaptive effect of stress worth attention is that upon a single sufficiently heavy exposure to stress the above-mentioned "catabolic phase" of the stress response is followed by a much longer "anabolic phase". It manifests itself, in particular, as a generalized activation of nucleic acid and protein synthesis in different organs.[63] Such activation can promote the formation of systemic structural traces and development of stable adaptation to most various environmental factors. Thus, for example, it speeds up elaboration and fixation of temporary connections in the brain or provides for a more efficient response of immunocompetent organs to a foreign antigen.[63] To explain this adaptive effect of stress one should bear in mind the dynamics of hormonal shifts in stress and the function of the above-mentioned IP_3-DAG link in the regulation of cell processes. It has been shown that as the stress response develops, the initially elevated catecholamine and glucocorticoid concentrations decline with a concurrent rise in the levels of other hormones and specifically thyrocalcitonin, which restricts catecholamine and glucocorticoid secretion, causes deposition of Ca^{2+}, and normalizes its concentration in the blood, thus acting as an "antipode" of the parathormone[14,64] and as one of the stress-limiting mechanisms which will later be considered in more detail. Simultaneously, secretion is enhanced for hormones of direct anabolic action: somatotropic hormone, insulin, as well as thyroxin, which is known to promote the biosynthesis of mitochondrial structures.

Clearly, the action of these hormones on the cell can be of importance in the development of the anabolic phase of the stress response and in the growth of particular cellular structures that had taken the main load during the mobilization of the cell function.

Recent data give grounds for believing that a substantial part in the "delayed" anabolic effect of stress is played by DAG, shown above to be produced on phospholipid hydrolysis when agonists of the Ca^{2+}-mobilizing receptors act on the cell (see Figure 2). DAG has been found to be a messenger which in the cells of different animals, by agency of PK C, activates the Na^+/H^+ exchange mechanism in the plasma membrane, thereby raising the cytosolic pH.[24,65] According to present-day notions, the elevation of cytosolic pH activates nucleic acid and protein synthesis to the extent of cell proliferation.[20,24,65] Thus, DAG is one of the main intracellular signals relaying information from the cell surface to the nucleus and playing a key role in cell growth initiation. It is conceivable that the stress-activated regulatory circuit

$$\text{DAG} \rightarrow \text{PKC} \rightarrow \begin{matrix}\text{Na}^+/\text{H}^+\\ \text{exchanger}\end{matrix} \rightarrow \begin{matrix}\text{elevated}\\ \text{pH}\end{matrix} \rightarrow \begin{matrix}\text{cell}\\ \text{nucleus}\end{matrix}$$

is involved in the delayed adaptive anabolic phase of the stress response. Moreover, it cannot be excluded that this regulatory mechanism ensures the coupling between the extent of function and the growth of cell structures at any load on the organ, e.g., in the development of cardiac hypertrophy caused by valvular diseases or hypertension as well as by repeated stress situations. In the general case, excessive stress activation of this regulatory circuit, combined with the stress immunodeficiency, may contribute to the oncogenic effect of stress.

As applied to the heart, of great interest is the possible role that the excessive activation of the cardiomyocyte genetic apparatus through this regulatory circuit may play in the evolvement of myocardial hypertrophy induced by catecholamines, and especially in the pathogenesis of incurable idiopathic cardiomegalies whose nature is obscure.

In assessing the transformation of the adaptive effects of stress on the heart into the detrimental effects, it should not be forgotten that we are dealing with a vitally important organ. Considering that all animal or human beings many times in their lifespan encounter grave, almost hopeless stress situations, one must admit that if all such basically possible transformations were actualized, then the mammals and specifically Homo sapiens *should have long vanished off the face of the earth. In reality, a primary stress death from damage to the heart or other organs is a far rarer occurrence than the most severe and protracted stress situations. Most humans and animals experiencing such situations do not die and either do not fall ill at all or recover, i.e., the stress reaction and the effects of stress factors in the cells happen to be opportunely limited.* Accordingly limited are the stress damages themselves. With the heart, for instance, even in the most severe stress it goes no further than a total but transitory impairment of the whole organ, and death of only separate cardiomyocyte groups with ensuing microfocal cardiosclerosis.[66] This means that the organism possesses potent mechanisms ensuring adaptation to stress situations. We shall further show that this is provided for by important features inherent in the very design of the stress reaction as well as by the modulatory stress-limiting systems linked with this reaction and restricting its intensity and duration. In this chapter, basing on the above concept of the transformation of the adaptive cardiotropic effects of stress into the detrimental ones, we shall concentrate on the cardiac stress damage as such.

Before proceeding to a systematic consideration of the functional, metabolic, and structural disorders of the heart under the damaging effect of stress, we should first deal with two essential points. *The first one is to draw a clear discriminating line between the cardial component of the stress response of a healthy organism and the genuine stress damage to the heart; the second is to demonstrate experimentally the very phenomenon of the transition of the stress effect from adaptive to detrimental, i.e., to prove the real existence of what we have been so liberally postulating.*

Differentiating the cardial component of the stress response from cardiac stress damage, we shall not delve into the rather complicated question of to what extent the stress situations causing human disease can be reproduced in animals. There seem to be sufficient grounds for the generally established opinion of researchers that such situations can be approximately simulated mainly in the mentioned conflict between a ''need'' to carry out a defense reaction and a ''ban'' on this reaction. In the course of such simulation studies it very soon became clear that the extent of stress and ensuing damage substantially increase if the basic elementary conflict is overlaid with additional inputs potentiating the activation of the emotional apparatus. Such additional inputs are introduction of signals notifying of an inevitable pain shock, and delivery of shocks at random and not too short intervals, engendering the expectation of pain associated with anxiety and fear. Of similar significance is the creation of additional conflicts: delivery of pain stimulation in response to a conditioned alimentary reaction or to a reaction by which the animal previously managed to avoid danger. The importance of these additional emotiogenic factors in the stress damage to internal organs has been first proved with ulcerous lesions of the gastric mucosa, which are the most convincing, visible, and reliably measurable stress damages.

Most clearly, the role of additional emotiogenic factors has been assessed in the studies where the stress intensity was judged from the decline in brain catecholamines and the stress damage from the area of the ulcerous lesions of the gastric mucosa developing in stress because of arteriolar spasm.[67] In the experiments of all researchers the introduction of emotiogenic factors further reduced the catecholamine concentration in the brain and appreciably expanded the ulceration area.[68,69]

The comparatively easy induction of stress ulcers in the gastric mucosa make it in most cases clear enough whether the gastric stress damage has occurred or not. The heart does not usually develop macroscopically observable necroses even in quite serious stress situations. Therefore the question of the presence or absence of a stress damage proves much more complicated. Indeed, the mobilization of cardiac function is an indispensable link in the defensive, aggressive, sexual reactions in animals and in the major socially determined reactions in humans. It can be envisaged that in the basic conflict between these vital reactions and bans on their realization, i.e., in intense and protracted stress, the cardiovascular component of the reaction is not simply sustained despite the lack of reactions as such, but can be attended by myocardial damage. However, there is a far way to go from this assumption to the actual proof of stress damage to the cardiac muscle. This is so because, unlike the stomach where the ulcers are well seen, the heart provides much less definite indications of the damage to its structures. The changes in its performance even under heavy stress exposures often manifest themselves as quite normal phenomena like tachycardia or bradycardia. The numerous studies revealing such changes mean much for evaluating the cardial component of the behavioral reactions,[70-72] but do not per se solve the question of whether or not the heart is damaged by stress. Electrocardiographic shifts, even when there are stress disturbances to cardiac metabolism and structure, may be relatively small owing to a diffuse pattern of damage. The alterations of the contractile function are not infrequently limited to its mobilization. Thus, Randall et al.[73] used catheterization to study the contractile function of the left ventricle in nonanesthetized primates placed in a classical stress situation: a great "urge" for a defense reaction was created (an audio stimulus followed by electric pain stimulation) while the reaction itself was precluded by fixation. The response to the conditional audio stimulus was manifest in the rise of systolic pressure, higher contraction velocity, and tachycardia. Denervation experiments showed that this cardial component of the organismic reaction was determined mainly by excitation of the sympathic cardiac innervation and to a much lesser extent by catecholamines in the circulating blood. Obviously these and numerous similar data sufficiently characterize the cardiac contractile function in stress conditions, but do not answer the question of whether or not the stress causes damage to the myocardium.

Later, the role of emotional stress was quite definitely proved in the studies by Miller and Malov.[74] There the stress situation was created for rats by electric pain stimulation through the chamber floor. Myocardial damage revealed itself in the pronounced leakage of enzymes from isolated hearts of stressed animals and in enhanced myocardial incorporation of technetium-labeled pyrophosphate routinely used to diagnose myocardial infarction. Upon administration of nembutal the same "dosage" of electric stimulation produced no cardiac damage. Thus, in a sufficiently long and intense stress we observe not merely an inclusion of the cardial component into the reaction, but genuine cardiac damage, caused not at all by such physical factors as electricity, mechanical pressure, etc., but by pain and impossibility to escape it, i.e., by an emotional factor.

The other point of interest — the transformation of the adaptive effect of stress into the detrimental one — was dealt with in our studies of the contractile function in isolated hearts taken from animals subjected to emotional pain stress (EPS) in the anxiety neurosis model according to Desiderato et al.[75] The duration of exposure to stress was varied to discern the phenomenon of transformation.

In the EPS model, male rats were starved for 1 d and then put into a special chamber in which electric current (4 mA) could be passed through the floor. The rats could avoid electric pain stimulation only by going to a platform in the center of the chamber. Consequently, the conditioned defense reflex of avoidance was developed quickly: the animals were constantly on the platform. Afterwards, short strong currents (6 mA for 2 s) were passed through the floor of the platform at random intervals for 6 h. The main features of this EPS model consist in the conflict between the conditioned reflex of avoiding the current by going to the platform and the unconditioned pain stimulation on the platform, attended by tense and fearful expectation of pain because electric shocks on the platform occurred at random intervals.

This EPS strongly activated the hypophysial-adrenal and adrenergic systems, as shown by a threefold to fourfold increase in the amount of corticosteroids in the adrenal cortex, plasma, and cardiac muscle. Simultaneously, the amount of catecholamines decreased in the hypothalamus and the striate body as well as in the executive organs: cardiac muscle and small intestine (Table 1). This well-known phenomenon is due to the fact that in stress the release of catecholamines into the blood and their utilization in the target organs considerably outstrips their resynthesis. Subsequent restoration of the catecholamine content, as follows from Table 1, is much sooner achieved in the sympathoadrenal system itself (i.e., in the hypothalamus and the adrenal glands) than in the target organs where the norepinephrine concentration is still depressed 5 d after the stress exposure. In whole, the restoration process is conditioned by the poststress activation of catecholamine biosynthesis.[76] Accordingly, Table 2 shows that after EPS the auricles increase ^{3}H-norephinephrine synthesis from ^{3}H-tyrosine by 40% over the control. Conversely, the neuronal uptake of ^{3}H-norepinephrine declines by 42% immediately after EPS and remains at that level for 1 d. This apparently provides for increased mediator concentration in the synaptic spaces, i.e., for enhanced adrenergic effect.

It should be noted that the activation of the adrenergic and hypophysial-adrenal system in EPS consistently leads to stress damages. In our experiments, as in the experiments of other researchers, the gastric mucosa rapidly developed ulcerous lesions typical of stress. Thus, these experiments reproduced a serious detrimental stress situation.

In these experiments the hearts were obtained under urethane anesthesia 2 h after the end of the stress exposure and studied for their contractile function in isovolumic conditions according to Fallen et al.[77] After a 60-min perfusion of the heart under normal oxygenation, the oxygenated and glucose-containing Krebs-Henseleit solution was replaced with the non-oxygenated and glucose-lacking one. This hypoxic exposure lasted 20 min and was followed by reoxygenation. The coronary flow was assessed as the amount of liquid passing through the coronary bed per unit time.

As follows from the data of Table 3, under aerobic conditions the hearts of animals subjected to short-term stress do not differ from the controls in the developed and diastolic pressure, but the pressure drop rate and the coronary flow increase by about 40%. On the contrary, the cardiac muscle of animals exposed to prolonged stress exhibits a depressed contractile function, with the developed pressure and the pressure buildup and drop rates decreased roughly by one third. The diastolic pressure, which in the given experimental conditions reflects the dynamics of the diastolic myocardial tension, proved to be 2.5 times higher.

It is evident in Table 3 that the major difference between the effects of short and long stress reveals itself in myocardial hypoxia. Thus, under hypoxic conditions the contractile function and coronary flow parameters in the hearts of animals subjected to a short stress exceeded the controls, while the hypoxic contracture was abated by a factor of 2.6.

During reoxygenation all the myocardial contraction and relaxation parameters in animals exposed to a short stress were completely restored within the first minute, and the hypoxic contracture disappeared. In the control animals at the same stage of reoxygenation the developed pressure and the pressure buildup and drop rates remained diminished by more than half.

The reaction to hypoxia in animals that had undergone a long stress was marked by a decline in the basic contraction and relaxation parameters as in controls, but the hypoxic contracture at 20 min of hypoxia was more pronounced. During reoxygenation the hypoxic

TABLE 1
Norepinephrine Content (ng/g) in Rat Tissues Upon Emotional Pain Stress (EPS)

Conditions	Myocardium	Small intestine	Hypothalamus	Striate body	Adrenal gland
Control	1117 ± 8	732 ± 42	900 ± 43	244 ± 38	157 285 ± 14 213
During EPS	864 ± 45[a]	477 ± 32[a]	688 ± 61[a]	167 ± 32	133 692 ± 12 082
After EPS					
2 h	841 ± 31[a]	434 ± 31[a]	633 ± 72[a]	—	109 622 ± 10 372[a]
24 h	616 ± 81[a]	415 ± 61[a]	757 ± 49	166 ± 41	242 747 ± 26 754[a]
2 d	658 ± 41[a]	574 ± 42[a]	786 ± 138	218 ± 23	199 695 ± 22 758
5 d	924 ± 49	616 ± 49	823 ± 108	204 ± 39	157 319 ± 15 029
10 d	—	694 ± 68	834 ± 52	251 ± 18	143 547 ± 14 384

[a] $p < 0.01$.

TABLE 2
Uptake and Synthesis of ^{3}H-Norepinephrine (cpm/g) in Auricles Upon EPS

	Uptake	Synthesis
Control	90 031 ± 6470 (n = 15)	7155 ± 677 (n = 12)
During stress	52 227 ± 13 541[a] (n = 10)	9772 ± 1182[b] (n = 6)
After stress		
2 h	—	9590 ± 579 (n = 6)
24 h	54 064 ± 6011[c] (n = 9)	9555 ± 1119[c] (n = 6)

[a] $p < 0.02$.
[b] $p < 0.05$.
[c] $p < 0.01$.

contracture, as indicated by the diastolic pressure, disappeared much more slowly in long-stressed than in control animals. Thus, a brief exposure to stress enhances the resistance of the cardiac contractile function to hypoxia, whereas prolonged stress produces an opposite effect.

The data in Table 4 show the release of creatine phosphokinase from the isolated heart into the perfusate under aerobic, hypoxic, and reoxygenation conditions. As follows from Table 4, the loss of the enzyme by the heart is minimal under normal oxygenation and increases in hypoxia. During reoxygenation still more enzyme is released into the perfusate. Notably, in both hypoxia and reoxygenation the enzyme leakage from the hearts of animals subjected to a short stress is 36 and 26% lower as compared to the controls, whereas with the hearts of animals subjected to a long stress it is, conversely, almost twice as high.

The loss of enzymes by the cardiac muscle results from energy-deficient damage to the cardiomyocyte sarcolemmal membrane and correlates quantitatively with the decline in myocardial ATP.[78] Therefore, the data obtained testify that a preliminary short exposure to stress attenuates the hypoxic damage to the membrane apparatus of cardiomyocytes, while a long one aggravates it.

By and large, the results of the experiment show that an intense but brief EPS exposure elicits quite stable alterations in the cardiac muscle, which are retained when the organ is separated from the neurohumoral influences of the whole organism. If the stress is protracted

TABLE 3
Effects of Short and Long EPS on Myocardial Resistance to Hypoxia and Reoxygenation

Indices	Series	Aerobic	Hypoxia 20 min	Reoxygenation 1 min
Developed pressure mmHg	Control	100.3 ± 4.1	22.9 ± 1.4	53.5 ± 5.1
	1h EPS	102.2 ± 3.9	38.6 ± 2.1[a]	100.9 ± 6.9[a]
	6 h EPS	68.4 ± 4.9[a]	14.9 ± 1.2[a]	44.6 ± 3.8
Diastolic pressure mmHg	Control	4.3 ± 1.3	40.3 ± 3.2	20.3 ± 2.5
	1 h EPS	4.4 ± 2.1	15.0 ± 2.4[a]	6.1 ± 1.4[a]
	6 h EPS	8.1 ± 0.8[a]	48.5 ± 3.5[a]	32.6 ± 6.7[a]
Max pressure buildup rate mmHg/s	Control	1900 ± 89	400 ± 27	875 ± 69
	1 h EPS	2150 ± 120	875 ± 92[a]	2016 ± 190[a]
	6 h EPS	1380 ± 110[a]	286 ± 92[a]	586 ± 80[a]
Max pressure drop rate mmHg/s	Control	1000 ± 84	188 ± 22	538 ± 55
	1 h EPS	1451 ± 120[a]	550 ± 20[a]	1125 ± 108[a]
	6 h EPS	840 ± 45[a]	126 ± 12[a]	375 ± 108[a]
Coronary flow ml/min	Control	8.0 ± 1.4	6.0 ± 0.8	6.5 ± 0.5
	1 h EPS	11.0 ± 1.2	11.3 ± 1.1[a]	11.2 ± 0.7[a]
	6 h EPS	7.5 ± 0.6	4.9 ± 0.3	6.5 ± 0.8

Note: Control (n = 12), 1 h EPS (n = 9), 6 h EPS (n = 12).

[a] Difference from control significant at $p < 0.05$.

TABLE 4
Effects of Short and Long EPS on The Leakage of Myocardial Creatine Phosphokinase into the Perfusate in Hypoxia and Reoxygenation

Series	CPK activity in the perfusate (IU/l)		
	Perfusion 90 min	Hypoxia 20 min	Reoxygenation 2 min
Control (n = 10)	9.8 ± 0.9	34.0 ± 2.4	49.5 ± 2.8
1 h EPS (n = 18)	10.0 ± 0.9	21.5 ± 3.5[a]	29.6 ± 3.9[a]
6 h EPS (n = 17)	12.4 ± 1.2	72.9 ± 5.0[a]	87.3 ± 4.1[a]

[a] $p < 0.05$.

(duration increased sixfold) these positive changes are completely abolished, displaced by the decreasing resistance of the heart to hypoxia.

Thus, these experiments made it possible to observe directly how the adaptive effect of stress turns into the detrimental one. The significance of this phenomenon for pathology in general, and cardiac pathology specifically, cannot be overemphasized; we therefore thought it worthwhile to verify it using a basically different technique which allows the cardiac contractile function under isotonic conditions (and primarily the cardiac resistance to the contractural and arrhythmogenic action of excess Ca^{2+}) to be compared upon brief and prolonged exposures to stress created with the same method of Desiderato et al.[75]

The curves in Figure 4 depict a typical experiment with heart perfusion according to Langendorf. Here it should be borne in mind that the upper outline of the mechanogram corresponds to maximal relaxation and the lower to maximal contraction of the isotonic heart. It can be seen that at normal Ca^{2+} concentration the 1-h stress, unlike the 6-h one, slightly increases the amplitude and velocities of contraction and relaxation. An immense difference between the 1- and 6-h stresses is observed under Ca^{2+} loading. After the 1-h stress, contracture and extrasystoles are virtually absent in contrast to the control; there is

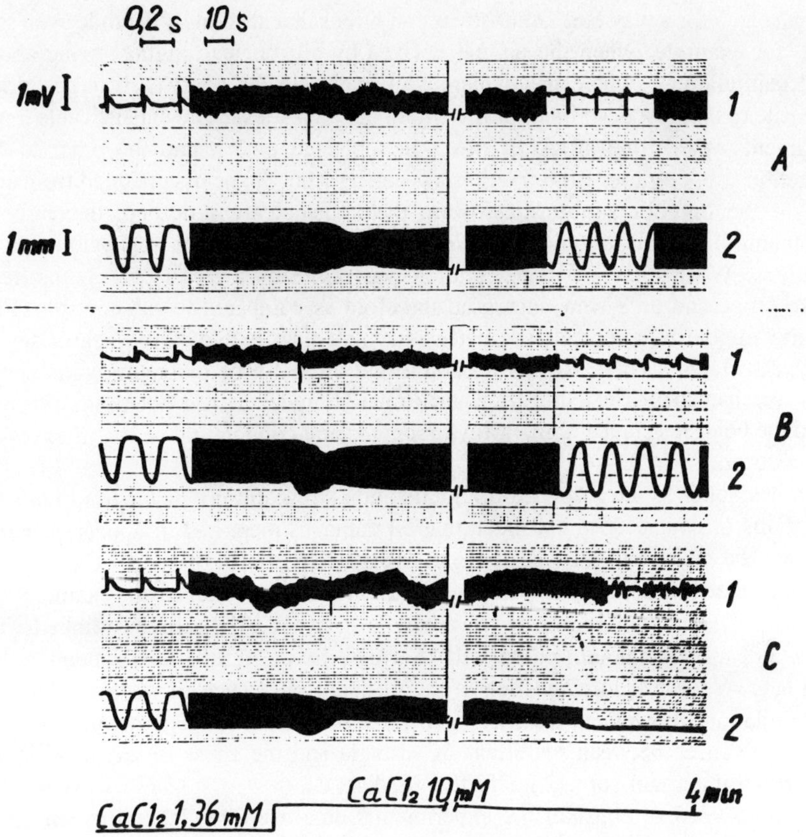

FIGURE 4. Effect of an increase of calcium concentration from 1.36 to 10 m*M* on the function of isolated hearts from control rats (A) and rats subjected to a 1-h (B) and a 6-h (C) EPS. 1, ECG; 2, mechanogram of the isotonic heart. For explanations see text.

also no cardiac fibrillation. Contrariwise, after the 6-h stress the scope (percent of initial contraction amplitude) and area (the product of scope by duration, percent of the contraction area) of contracture are about twice those in the control; there are numerous extrasystoles, and at the third minute of exposure to Ca^{2+} irreversible cardiac fibrillation develops.

This result provides unequivocal evidence that a short stress, through its adaptive effects described earlier, enhances the cardiac muscle resistance to Ca^{2+} overloads. A long stress, because of the detrimental shifts also described earlier, entails an opposite result, reducing the efficiency of the membrane calcium-transporting mechanisms and ultimately decreasing the resistance of the heart to the contractural and arrhythmogenic action of excess Ca^{2+}.

Here we must underline the significance of this phenomenon at the level of the whole organism, where the damaging effect of excess Ca^{2+} is the common final link of the pathogenetic chain in most various cardiac conditions from ischemic disease to hereditary cardiopathies and, as we shall see, a key link in the pathogenesis of primary stress damage to the heart.

The adaptive effect of stress on the heart and its transformation into the detrimental effect constitute an important reality for the cardiologist.

However, notwithstanding the elegance and instructiveness of this concept, the most recent experiments in our laboratory show that it pertains to the ''stress of struggle'', the one most widely represented in nature and experiment, when animals or people finding themselves in a difficult, hazardous, or even injurious situation can carry out some active reactions in search for a way out. Other stress conditions that absolutely exclude even seeking an escape, for example, when the animal is fixed by all four extremities, bring about the "stress of capitulation" where the dynamics of events in the heart is different, and in a sense opposite to that just described for the emotional pain stress. The data in Table 5 present the experiments where one group of rats was subjected to 2 h and the other to 6 h of immobilization stress by four-limb fixation. As can be seen, the hearts obtained from animals after 2 h of the immobilization stress were distinguished by a definite decrease in the contraction amplitude and in the contraction and relaxation velocities at physiological Ca^{2+} concentrations. When the Ca^{2+} concentration was raised by a factor of 7.3, the maximal contracture scope and area were increased threefold as compared to the controls. Finally, at the fourth minute of hypercalcium perfusion more than half of these hearts developed ventricular fibrillation. There is thus no doubt that after 2 h of the capitulation stress the membrane mechanisms of calcium transport in cardiomyocytes had been quite deeply impaired and the heart resistance to the arrhythmogenic and contractural action of excess Ca^{2+} had been reduced.

The hearts obtained after the 6-h immobilization stress did not differ from the controls (Table 5). This of course does not mean that all damages there had disappeared, but demonstrates that the decline in the resistance to the adverse effects of excess Ca^{2+} had worn off in animals that had capitulated long before their hearts were taken for examination.

That such dynamics of the heart resistance to excess Ca^{2+} is directly linked with the performance of the SR calcium pump will be shown by the results of biochemical studies presented later. Yet the whole question of the mechanism of such immediate adaptation to forced capitulation, as well as the more general issue of the neurohumoral, cellular, and molecular differences between the stress of struggle and the stress of capitulation are, in our opinion, an important subject for further studies.

Hereinafter we shall consider the experimental data from this laboratory on the stress damages to the contractile function, electric stability, ionic transport, and energy metabolism constituting the basis of the primary cardiac stress damage. Then, using clinical data we shall assess the significance of such damage from the clinical point of view.

III. STRESS DAMAGES TO THE CARDIAC FUNCTION

The studies conducted for the last 15 years in our laboratory show that even upon prolonged and heavy stress or administration of a large dose of the synthetic β-adrenoreceptor agonist isoproterenol, in conditions of the whole organism the disturbances of cardiac contractile function prove to be moderate and may often be only demonstrable with such special techniques as imposing a maximal load on the heart by aortic clamping, imposing a high contraction frequency, etc. At the same time with the isolated heart these disturbances, which in the whole organism would have been masked owing to the regulatory mobilization of compensating factors, can be revealed definitely enough.

In accordance with this, we shall now consider the disturbances of the contractile function of the isolated right auricle and ventricular papillary muscle caused by prolonged (6 h) EPS.

The atrial contractility and elasticity were studied in isometric spontaneous contractions with the use of a DMP-4F Physiograph, Narco Biosystems, U.S. The auricle was placed in a constant-temperature (34°C)) bath with oxygenated Krebs-Henseleit solution (95% O_2/5% CO_2) where the auricle itself was fixed immovably while the top of the auricula was attached to an F-50 myograph coupled with a spring micrometer. The auricle was left to contract spontaneously for 40 to 50 min and then gradually stretched with the micrometer to a length at which it developed the maximal systolic contraction force (T_{max}), i.e., to the maximal physiological length (L_{max}). The changes in length were recorded for each 100-mg increment of the stretching load. The load (mg) corresponding to L_{max} was taken as the maximal tension at rest (T_r).

TABLE 5
Effect of the Duration of Immobilization Stress on the Indices of Contractility, Arrhythmias, and Contracture of Isolated Hearts at a 7.3-Fold Increase of the Ca^{2+} Concentration in the Perfusing Solution

Series	Heart rate	Contraction amplitude (mm)	Contraction velocity (mm/s)	Relaxation velocity (mm/s)	Contracture %		Extra systoles	Ventricular fibrillation (cases)
					Scope	Area		
Control (n = 15)	274 ± 8	2.60 ± 0.08	51.0 ± 2.8	57.6 ± 3.0	21 ± 4	10.0 ± 1.8	5 ± 2	0
2-h stress (n = 11)	269 ± 8	2.07 ± 0.16 $p < 0.01$[a]	42.8 ± 3.4	46.8 ± 4.2 $p < 0.05$[a]	59 ± 17 $p < 0.05$[a]	35.8 ± 10.1 $p < 0.02$[a]	7 ± 3	6 (54.5%) $p < 0.05$[b]
6-h stress (n = 8)	272 ± 6	2.66 ± 0.14	54.6 ± 3.6	64.6 ± 3.8	18 ± 6	9.4 ± 3.9	3 ± 2	0

[a] Student's criterion.
[b] X^2 Criterion with the Yate's correction.

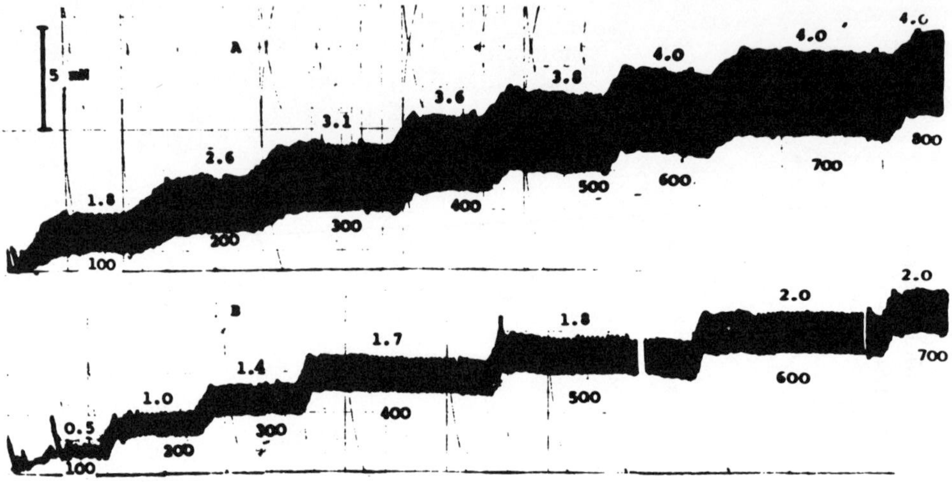

FIGURE 5. Mechanograms of the isometrically contracting right auricles from (A) control and (B) EPS animals. The numbers above the tracing denote the developed force in mN; the numbers below the tracing denote the muscle-stretching load in mg.

The mechanograms in Figure 5 present a typical experiment and provide an estimate of the depression of the myocardial contraction force in animals subjected to stress.

Atrial extensibility was judged from the "load — length" dependence in the course of extension to L_{maz}. Atrial contractility was judged from the maximal contraction force (mN), frequency of spontaneous atrial contractions (min^{-1}), and the integrative index "maximal intensity of functioning of structures" calculated as the ratio of the product of T_{max} and contraction frequency to the atrial mass and expressed in mN/mg·min. The state of the self-regulatory mechanism of myocardial contractility was assessed by the dependences "load — force" and "length — force" (the Frank-Starling dependence) and by the index $\Delta T/\Delta L$ (mN/mm). The $\Delta T/\Delta L$ index denotes the increment of atrial contraction force in response to each 1-mm increment of atrial length during stretching, and reflects the "functional value" of the extension of the auricle by 1 mm. This index, together with the Starling curve, characterizes the realization of the Frank-Starling mechanism.

The curves in Figure 6 show that auricles of the animals that have undergone EPS exhibit lower extensibility and contraction force. The decreased myocardial extensibility would impede the elongation of cardiomyocyte sarcomeres in diastole and therefore restrict the realization of the Frank-Starling mechanism. Indeed, it is evident from Figure 6 that the auricles of rats exposed to EPS when stretched develop about half the contraction force than do the controls. Thus, obviously, one of the causes of the poststress depression of the atrial contractile function is the lesser extensibility that handicaps the Frank-Starling mechanism (Figure 6D).

The two basic facts established in these studies, namely the decreased atrial extensibility and the depressed Starling curve, give grounds for believing that one of the main causes of impaired cardiac contractile function in stress is the upset of the myocardial self-regulatory mechanisms. Reduced myocardial extensibility may hinder optimal sarcomere elongation in diastole, decrease the diastolic volume, increase the diastolic pressure, and interfere with ventricular filling; combines with the lesser specific increase in force per unit muscle length, all this can apparently impair the pump function of the heart in whole.

The data presented pertain to the myocardium of the auricles, so to prove the validity of the above assertion it was necessary to check whether or not the poststress reduction of extensibility and the attending depression of contractility also occur in the myocardium of

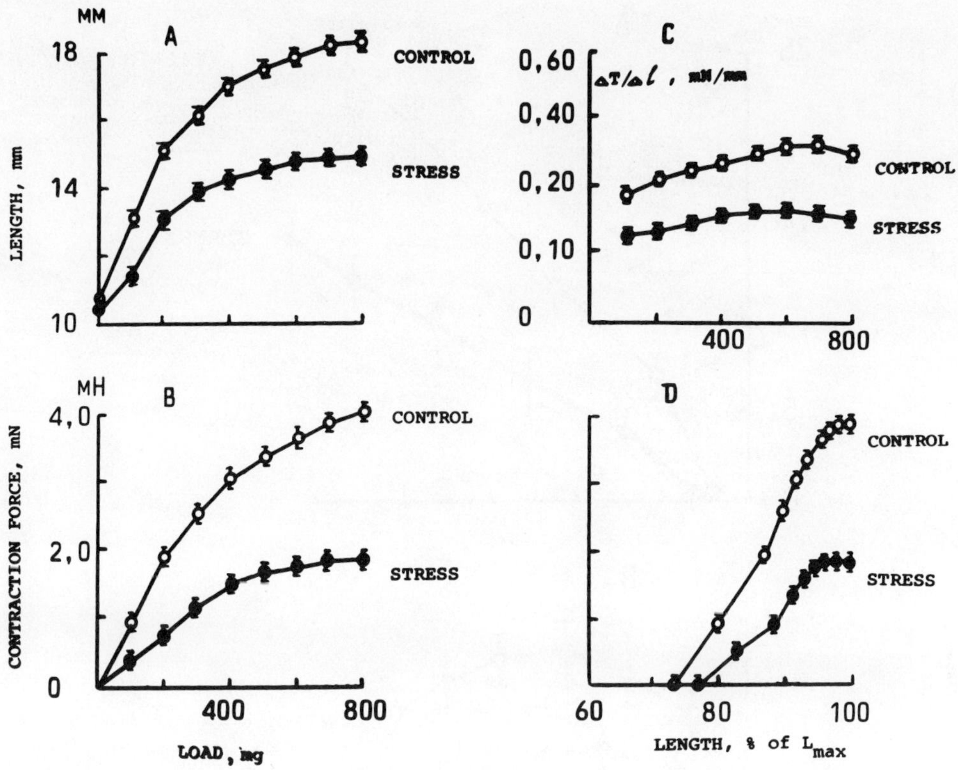

FIGURE 6. Effect of EPS on the rat right atrial extensibility and contraction force. The stress can be seen to depress (A) atrial extensibility, (B) contraction force at equal stretching load, (C) increment of force per unit increment of atrial length ($\Delta T/\Delta L$), and (D) the Starling curve.

the ventricles which are central in the pump function of the heart. To this end, in the next series of experiments we studied the effect of EPS on the extensibility and contractile function of the left ventricular posterior papillary muscle.

The relevant results are represented by curves in Figure 7 and testify that the alterations caused by EPS in the left ventricular myocardium are similar to those in the auricles. It is shown that in rats subjected to EPS the elongation of the papillary muscle under a similar load is 1.5 to 2 times less than in controls. Reduced extensibility of the ventricular myocardium combines with depressed contraction amplitude. Thus, in EPS rats the amplitude of isotonic contractions of the papillary muscle is on average 18 to 24% lower compared to the control ($p < 0.01$).

The data obtained provide evidence that reduced extensibility and hampered operation of the Frank-Starling mechanism constitute a typical manifestation of the poststress damage to both atrial and ventricular myocardium, and allow one to think that these alterations may be involved in the impairment of the pump function of the heart.

In further studies it was deemed important to elucidate the extent to which the stress damage to the elasticity and contractility of the atrial myocardium was reversible. The experiments showed that both the poststress myocardial rigidity and the reduction in its contractile force were transitory: they were most pronounced 2 h after the end of stress, still definite but much abated in 1 d, and not observable in 3 d.

Prior administration of the α-adrenoblocker phentolamine to animals proved to have no effect on the development of the complex of myocardial functional disorders typical of stress. By contrast, administration of the β-adrenoblocker propranolol completely abolished the upset of extensibility and contractile function. The curves in Figure 8 reflect this protective

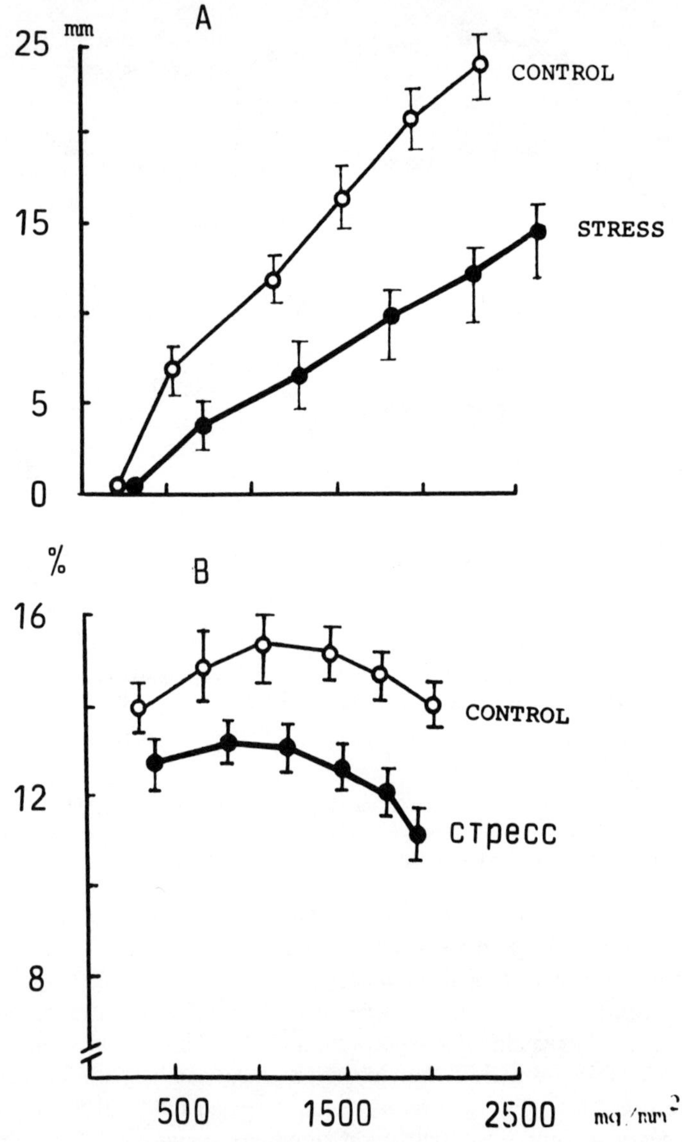

FIGURE 7. Effect of stress on the (A) extensibility and (B) contraction amplitude of the left ventricular papillary muscle. The abscissa is the load in mg/mm^2; the ordinates are (A) increase in muscle length (length at the 250 mg/mm^2 load taken as 100%); (B) contraction amplitude in mm.

effect of the β-blocker and indicate that the discovered phenomenon of stress rigidity is due precisely to the excessive β-adrenergic action of surplus catecholamines.

The question of how this action leads to the observed impairment of extensibility and contractility is rather complicated. Discussing it we should bear in mind that in accordance with the present day notions of cardiac contractility[79] the physiological extensibility of the myocardium and the realization of the Frank-Starling mechanism are in great measure determined by the state of the relaxation mechanism. The "residual" actomyosin bridges retained in the sarcolemma during diastole can affect the tension of rest. Obviously the increasing number of residual bridges, whatever their cause, may promote the "internal shortening" of myofibrils and reduce myocardial extensibility. The process of relaxation

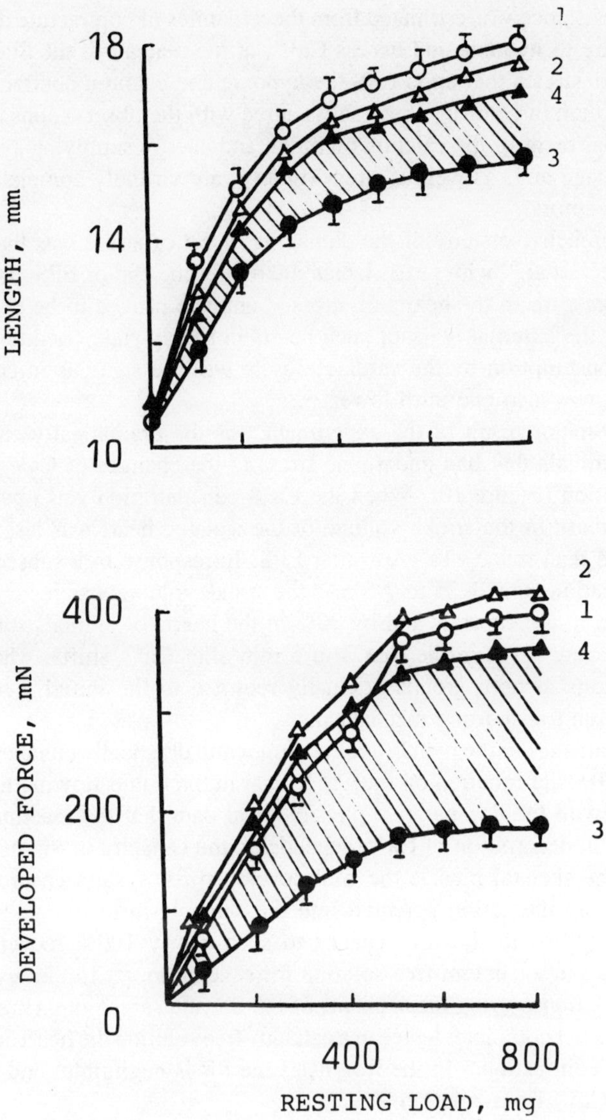

FIGURE 8. Effect of stress and propranolol of the rat right atrial (A) extensibility and (B) contraction force. The abscissa is the load at rest in mg; the ordinates are (A) atrial length in mm, (B) developed force in mN. 1, Control; 2, propranolol; 3, stress; 4, propranolol plus stress.

and dissociation of the actomyosin bridges formed in systole is known to be provided for by two major factors: (1) energy supply to the myofibrils, comprising ATP synthesis by the mitochondrial and glycolytic systems, energy transfer through the creatine kinase system, and ATP resynthesis in the contractile apparatus;[80] and (2) prompt removal of Ca^{2+} from this apparatus, performed by the calcium pumps of the sarcolemma and SR. The two factors are inseparable since the calcium pumps need ATP.

It will be further shown that both the calcium pump operation and the myocardial energetics are impaired in stress. While studying the myocardial stress rigidity we tried to make a rough assessment of these factors, and to this end compared the influence of EPS on the development of calcium and hypoxic contracture.

Myocardial resistance was estimated from the dynamics of contracture development after the end of exposure to hypoxia and excess Ca^{2+}, at the plateau of the Starling curve.

Figure 9 demonstrates that upon EPS the hypoxic and calcium contractures are reliably more pronounced than in control. These shifts agree with the observations (to be considered below) of the impairment of the calcium pumping and energy supplying systems in primary cardiac stress damage and, as well as stress rigidity, are virtually completely prevented by blocking the β-receptors.

A more comprehensive study of the damaging effect of stress was then carried out by the method of Neely et al.[81] with hearts isolated 2 h after the end of EPS. The stroke volume and the systolic pressure in the hearts of stressed animals proved to be decreased by 10 to 20%. As a result, the external work of such hearts in steady-state conditions was one third lower. Oxygen consumption by the cardiac muscle was the same as in control, hence the cardiac efficiency was also one third lower.

However, the major result of the experiment was the dramatically enhanced response of the hearts of animals that had undergone stress to the changes of Ca^{2+} concentration in the perfusing solution (Figure 10). When the Ca^{2+} concentration was lowered from 2.5 to 1.25 m*M* the decrease in the stroke volume of the isolated heart was less than 40% in the controls, but more than twice was great after EPS. In response to a subsequent increase of the Ca^{2+} concentration from 1.25 to 7.5 m*M* the stroke volume was restored by 20 to 30% of the initial value in the controls and by 70% in the hearts of animals subjected to stress. These alterations were vivid in the first 3 to 5 min after Ca^{2+} shifts, whereas further on, the cardiac functions in both groups gradually returned to the initial levels owing to the adaptation of the ion transporting mechanisms.

Thus, stress damages to the membrane calcium pump drastically enhance the dependence of the cardiac contractile function on the Ca^{2+} level in the liquid flowing through the heart. This is in accord with the comparative physiological data that the reaction of muscle to a changing external concentration of Ca^{2+} depends on the capacity of the mechanisms for its transport. So in the skeletal muscle the well-developed SR system ensures that almost all Ca^{2+} released during the action potential into the sarcoplasm to initiate myofibrillar contraction is then returned to the SR. Thanks to such nearly 100% recycling, the skeletal muscle can contract in a calcium-free solution for several hours. In the myocardial cells of mammals the Ca^{2+} transporting mechanisms of the SR and sarcolemma are not so powerful and the recycling is not complete, hence in a calcium-free solution the heart ceases functioning after a few dozen contractions. In the frog heart the SR is negligible, and it stops instantly upon removal of Ca^{2+} from solution.[82]

Taken together, the available facts evidence that the greater dependence of the cardiac function on the external Ca^{2+} *concentration in animals that have undergone stress results from impaired membrane transport of* Ca^{2+}.

The results of experiments on the papillary muscle of animals subjected to EPS are in accord with this conclusion and, besides, furnish some additional information on the primary stress damage to myocardial contractility.[83]

The contractile function of the isolated left ventricular papillary muscle was studied under electric pacing of its isotonic contractions at an optimal load providing maximal physiological length, in the Krebs-Henseleit solution with 95% O_2/5% CO_2 at 29 ± 1°C. At imposed contraction frequency the amplitude and the velocity of contraction and relaxation of the papillary muscle from animals that had undergone stress proved to be decreased 2 to 3-fold.

The experiments were mostly aimed at elucidating the effect of stress on the response of papillary muscle to the shifts of Ca^{2+}, Na^+, and H^+ concentrations in the perfusing solution.

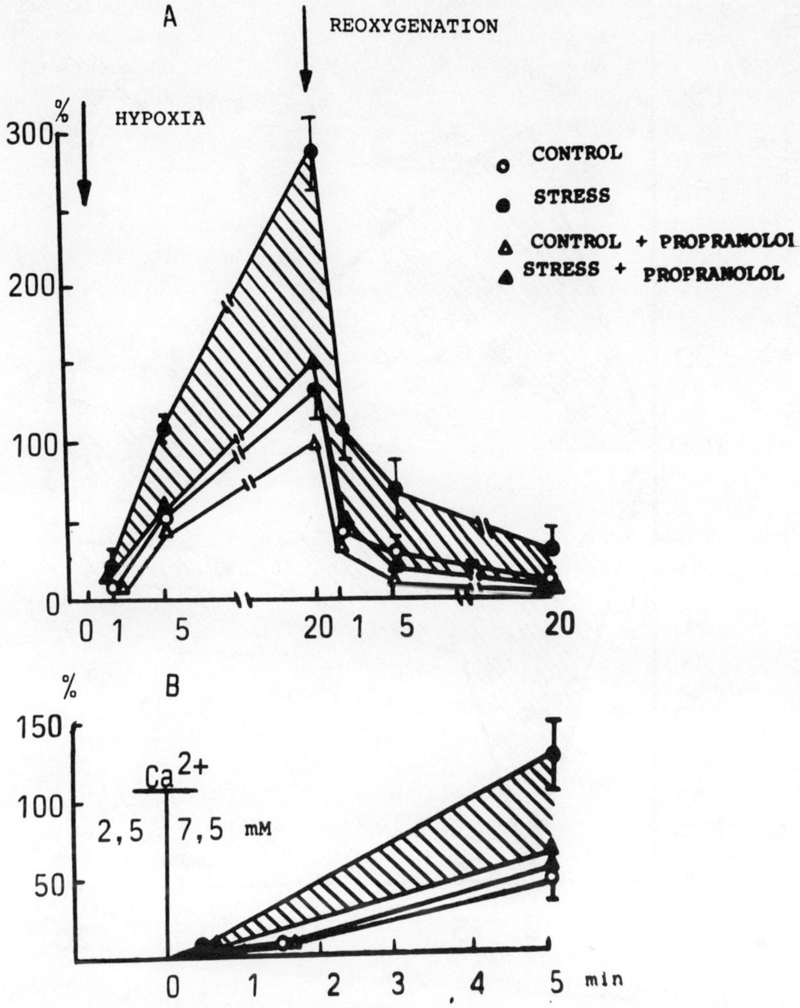

FIGURE 9. Effect of stress and propranolol on the contracture caused by (A) hypoxia and (B) increased Ca^{2+} concentration. The abscissa is time in min; the ordinate is the contracture index (ratio of the increment in tension of rest to the initial developed tension, percent).

It has been shown that upon stress the depressed myocardial contractility is accompanied with its higher sensitivity to the changes in extracellular concentrations of Ca^{2+} as well as of the natural antagonists of this cation, Na^+ and H^+, which are known to compete with Ca^{2+} for the binding sites in the sarcolemmal structures and to be, at increasing concentrations, capable of displacing Ca^{2+} from these binding sites and thereby reducing the contractile function of the carcdiac muscle.[84,85]

Figure 11 presents the results of studying the negative inotropic effect of Ca^{2+} antagonists — Na^+ and H^+ — after stress. Increasing the H^+ concentration (lowering the pH from 7.4 to 6.85) or the Na^+ concentration (adding sodium chloride to 165 m*M*) in the Krebs-Henseleit solution flowing around the papillary muscle elicits a typical decrease in the myocardial contractile indices (the negative chronotropic effect due to competitive displacement of Ca^{2+} by these cations). The stress potentiates this effect considerably, as seen in Figure 11: excess Na^+ or H^+ depresses the myocardial contractile function approximately twice more in animals that have undergone stress than in the controls.

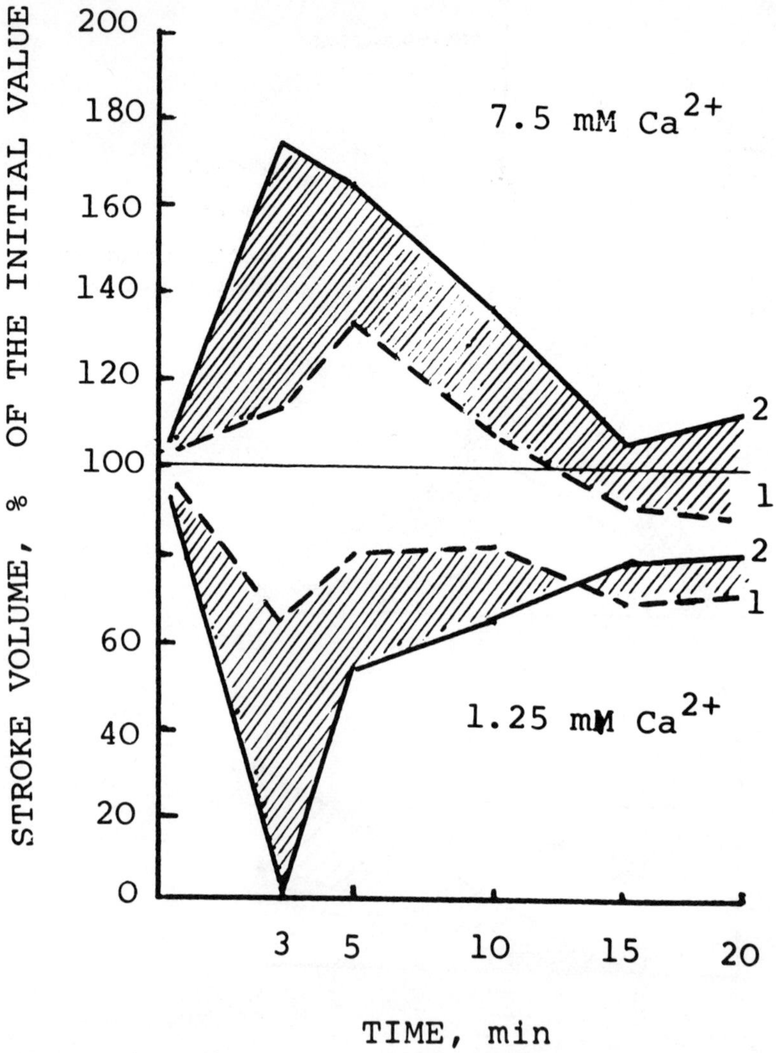

FIGURE 10. Dynamics of the response of isolated working hearts from (1) control and (2) stress animals to the changes of calcium concentration in the perfusing solution. The abscissa is time in min; the ordinate is the stroke volume, percent of initial. The shaded zone reflects the effect of stress. (A), Response to an increase from 1.25 to 7.5 m*M* Ca^{2+}; (B), response to a decrease from 2.5 to 1.25 m*M* Ca^{2+}.

In assessing the results of these experiments, it should be emphasized that the cationic tests for the Ca^{2+} binding and transporting ability of the membrane apparatus to a certain extent mimic the cationic disturbances in the myocardium typical both of maximal physical loads (where they limit the enhancement of cardiac function)[86] and of cardiovascular diseases.[87,88] In particular, the experimentally created excess of H^+ (lowered pH) in the extracellular space mimics the condition attending many diseases including ischemic heart damage, namely metabolic acidosis in which excessive amounts of HCO_3^- and H^+ ions appear in the blood and pass through the membranes into the cells.[85] The lower myocardial resistance to excess Ca^{2+} and Na^+ in stress, as will be shown in Section VII, is caused by the impaired performance of the calcium and sodium membrane pumps in the cardiomyocytes. By analogy it can be thought that the lower resistance of myocardial contractility to excess protons is caused by impaired performance of the sarcolemmal Na^+-H^+ pump responsible for timely removal of H^+ from the sarcoplasm.

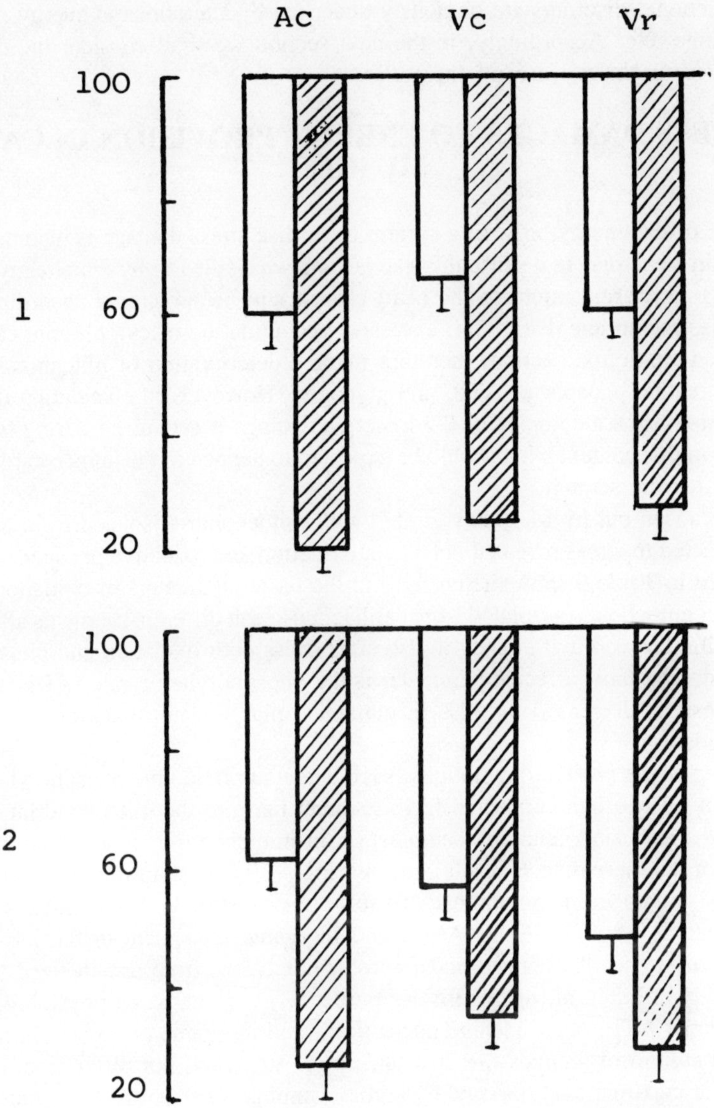

FIGURE 11. Effect of stress on the inotropic response of the papillary muscle to shifts in Na^+ and H^+ concentrations. The ordinate is the relative contractile indices, with 100% assigned to those at physiological ion levels. Ac, Contraction amplitude; Vc, contraction velocity; Vr, relaxation velocity. Empty columns, control; shaded columns, stress. 1, Increase of Na^+ concentration to 165 m*M*. 2, Decrease of pH to 6.85.

In the aggregate, there is unequivocal evidence that a single, long enough stress impairs the contractile function of the cardiac muscle, gives rise to a peculiar syndrome of myocardial stress rigidity, decreases the force, amplitude, and velocity of myocardial contractions, depresses the Starling curve, and drastically upsets the resistance of cardiac function to deviations from ionic homeostasis in the milieu. Special studies concerned with the effect of stress on the cardiac papillary muscle hypertrophied because of aortic stenosis have shown that the myocardial contractile function, already initially reduced under such conditions, is further depressed by stress to a critical level that may predetermine cardiac insufficiency.[83] Thus, *in certain circumstances the stress-induced depression of the contractile function may be involved in the development of heart failure.*

Such functional disorders are obviously underlied by alterations in energy metabolism, cation exchange, etc. Accordingly, in the next section we shall consider the disturbances caused by stress in the myocardial energetics.

IV. STRESS DAMAGES TO ENERGY PROVISION IN CARDIAC MUSCLE

The state of the energy-providing system in cardiac stress damage is incomparably less studied than in ischemia. In a sense this gap is somewhat filled in by the already mentioned data on the β-adrenergic injury to the heart caused with isoproterenol according to Rona, where, besides membrane disruption, excessive accumulation of cytoplasmic calcium, and its pronounced cardiotoxic action, there are marked deterioration of mitochondria and exhaustion of creatine phosphate, ATP, and glycogen. However, in elucidating the question of to what extent such a complex of β-adrenergic damage is actualized during true stress in animals, and in this context what should be expected to happen in the human cardiac muscle, we had to start from scratch.

A work carried out by Malyshev et al.[89] with mitochondria isolated from the hearts of animals subjected to stress revealed defects in oxidation and oxidative phosphorylation. The data presented in Table 6 show the changes in the basic parameters of oxidation and phosphorylation in mitochondria isolated from cardiac muscle at different moments after exposure to stress. It can be seen that already in 2 h after stress both oxidation and phosphorylation are depressed. The most affected parameter is the phosphorylation rate (ADP/t), which, in 2 d after stress, is decreased by 50% in glutamate plus malate oxidation and by 47% in succinate oxidation.

According to the present day notions, such defects in oxidative phosphorylation can be brought about by two interconnected factors: direct harm to the mitochondrial membranes by the "lipid triad" and calcium accumulation in mitochondria. It was important to find out whether or not these defects result in decreasing ATP concentration in the working heart at relative rest and under maximum load. To solve this question L. Yu. Golubeva determined the concentrations of ATP, ADP, AMP, and inorganic phosphate in the left ventricular myocardium of the hearts obtained under aerobic conditions from anesthetized animals and instantly frozen in liquid nitrogen with the Wollenberger forceps. At physiological rest the concentrations of ATP, other adenine nucleotides, and inorganic phosphate in the left ventricular myocardium of animals that had undergone stress did not differ from those in the control, and at maximal load imposed by aortic clamping for 90 s the ATP content declined also to the control level.

Hence it follows that the above-described defects in oxidation and phosphorylation in the cardiac mitochondria from stressed animals do not, however, affect the overall ATP content in the myocardium. This apparent discrepancy between the *in vitro* and *in vivo* data may have several explanations. Thus it is possible that the damage to the mitochondrial membrane lipid bilayer by lipid peroxidation and related processes is limited *in vivo* by natural antioxidants, but highly pronounced in isolation.

The works of Jacobus[90] and Saks et al.[91] allow one to think that the defects in oxidative ATP resynthesis revealed upon isolation of myocardial mitochondria from stressed animals are, under conditions of the whole organism, not sufficient to decrease the overall ATP level, but they attenuate the creatine phosphate (CP) content and hinder the transport of energy-rich phosphate groups from mitochondria to myofibrils and sarcolemmal and SR membranes, which in principle may impair myofibrillar contraction and relaxation.

In this connection, together with L. Yu. Golubeva, we have specially determined the CP content and creatine phosphokinase (CPK) activity in the hearts of animals subjected to EPS.

TABLE 6
Oxidation and Phosphorylation in Animal Cardiac Mitochondria Upon EPS

Time after EPS (h)	V_3	V_4	V_3/V_4	ADP/O	ADP/t
			Glutamate + Malate		
Control	173 ± 12	48 ± 5.9	3.95 ± 0.3	2.9 ± 0.2	469 ± 20
2	123 ± 5.2[a]	38 ± 1.1	3.20 ± 0.1[b]	2.4 ± 0.2	301 ± 30[c]
24	133 ± 9.2[b]	55 ± 3.0	2.45 ± 0.1[c]	2.0 ± 0.1[a]	275 ± 29[c]
45	104 ± 4.5[c]	42 ± 4.2	2.40 ± 0.2[c]	2.0 ± 0.1[a]	234 ± 11[c]
72	154 ± 6.1	58 ± 4.6	2.70 ± 0.2[a]	2.6 ± 0.2	434 ± 44
96	171 ± 7.8	39 ± 2.6	4.00 ± 0.3	2.5 ± 0.2	422 ± 48
			Succinate		
Control	251 ± 17	88 ± 5.7	2.85 ± 0.2	2.0 ± 0.2	524 ± 38
2	226 ± 8	75 ± 4.8	2.90 ± 0.2	1.7 ± 0.1	413 ± 27[b]
24	215 ± 20	118 ± 9.6[b]	1.85 ± 0.2[a]	1.4 ± 0.2[b]	323 ± 27
45	189 ± 13[a]	102 ± 9.8	1.80 ± 0.1[c]	1.3 ± 0.2[b]	280 ± 24[c]
72	241 ± 15	107 ± 11	2.25 ± 0.2	1.9 ± 0.2	469 ± 32
96	218 ± 20	98 ± 5.1	2.20 ± 0.2	2.0 ± 0.2	439 ± 32

Note: V_3, Respiration rate (natoms 0/min per mg protein) upon ADP addition; V_4, same after ADP exhaustion; V_3/V_4, respiratory control ratio; ADP/O, phosphorylation ratio; ADP/t, phosphorylation rate (nmol ADP/min/mg protein).

The data in Table 7 demonstrate that prolonged EPS did not affect the myocardial content of adenine nucleotides, whereas the CP content fell by one third while the total CPK proved to be almost 40% lower. It also follows from Table 7 that the decline in CPK activity in myocardial tissue was only in small measure due to its decrease in the postmitochondrial supernatant, which was just 12%. In essence this fact means that we observed the loss of CPK associated with mitochondria. A rough calculation shows that in the control the activity of structure-bound CPK (difference between total and postmitochondrial CPK) amounted to some 45% of the total, which agrees with the data of other works,[93] whereas after stress its portion decreases by a factor of 2.5. Stress is known to activate lipid peroxidation, lipases and phospholipases, impair mitochondrial function, damaging thus the cardiomyocyte membranes and promoting the leakage of CPK and other membrane-bound enzymes.[1] It can be thought that mitochondrial and other membranes damaged by stress (as compared to the control) more readily lose CPK during standard treatment, and the enzyme goes into the soluble fraction. Of course this suggestion must be verified by assaying CPK in mitochondria and determining the isoenzyme spectrum in the cytosolic fraction. Thus, in stress the disturbances in the CPK system occur earlier than direct damage to ATP resynthesis. Such impaired transport of high-energy phosphates may contribute to the depression of cardiac contraction and relaxation in stress.

This suggestion is in accord with the results of a recent study of Kupriyanov et al.,[94] who have shown that in the course of recuperation from transitory intoxication with deoxyglucose the heart can function at quite low ATP concentrations, but its functional level correlates with a high enough concentration of CP in cardiomyocytes. In another work the same group[95] made a detailed study of the function of isolated hearts from animals who had been fed guanidine propionate, an inhibitor of creatine transport into cardiomyocytes, to depress the myocardial CP level. It turned out that at normal ATP, but lowered CP content, the cardiac contractile function was impaired, and mainly affected were the relaxation velocity

TABLE 7
Effect of EPS on Myocardial Energy Metabolism

	Metabolite content (μmol/g tissue)				Creatine phosphokinase activity (nmol/min·g tissue)	
	ATP	ADP	AMP	CP	Total	Postmitochondrial supernatant
Control (n = 15)	5.4 ± 0.15	1.2 ± 0.09	0.43 ± 0.04	8.8 ± 0.20	959 ± 39	537 ± 14
Stress (n = 10)	5.1 ± 0.11	1.0 ± 0.20	0.50 ± 0.03	6.0 ± 0.20	566 ± 18	473 ± 12
Reliability				$p < 0.05$	$p < 0.01$	$p < 0.05$

and myocardial extensibility, i.e., the situation was familar to the one that several years before we had described in hearts exposed to stress.[1] In other words, the decreasing CP content at normal ATP content that we have found upon exposure to stress may be essential to the described impairment of myocardial extensibility in stress — the phenomenon of stress rigidity and corresponding disturbances of the contractile function.

The disorders in glycogen metabolism in EPS that we have found further are likely to play a no less important part in these phenomena. Table 8 presents the data that we have obtained with Golubeva and Pavlova on the effects of stress on phosphorylase activity and glycogen content and synthesis in the cardiac muscle.

It follows that stress caused activation of phosphorylase and an almost twofold decrease in the glycogen concentration. This consumption of the cardiac glycogen reserve was not accompanied by activation of glycogen synthesis: its specific radioactivity did not change, and the rate of glycogen synthesis (judged from total radioactivity) per unit cardiac mass was almost twice lower. This shift was apparently due to the marked decrease in the glycogen content and accordingly in the number of glycogen granules or glycosomes which harbor both hydrolysis and biosynthesis of this polysaccharide; a similar phenomenon had been earlier shown in liver upon pain stress.[96] Activation of phosphorylase to mobilize glycogen is well known as one of the first results of the β-adrenergic effect in stress, with the phosphorylase A/A + B ratio[97] and the decline in myocardial glycogen[98] being proportionate to the probability of arrhythmias and cardiac fibrillation. This fact was quite consistently observed in our experiments. Table 9 presents analogous data, with the difference that glycogen and lactate were determined in the left ventricular myocardium both at physiological rest and maximum load imposed by aortic clamping for 90 s.

It can be seen that stress decreases the glycogen content almost by half. With the maximum cardiac load further reducing it by 120 to 130 mg in both poststress and control animals, after 90 s of aortic clamping the myocardial glycogen content in poststress animals proves to be 2.2 times lower than in controls. This is direct evidence that a longer loading or hypoxia would sooner exhaust the myocardial glycogen reserve after stress. Such a depletion of the endogenous glycolytic substrate should not and does not tell on the dynamics of the overall myocardial ATP level, since even with glucose as the sole substrate the portion of glycolytic ATP in its overall resynthesis is small, about 1/20 of the total amount of ATP produced by oxidative phosphorylation in mitochondria. In point of fact, besides carbohydrates mitochondria utilize fatty acids as well as pyruvate and lactate from the blood; accordingly, the contribution of glycolytic phosphorylation to the energy provision for the heart working in aerobic conditions would be still smaller. Nevertheless, it has been definitely shown that blocking the glycolysis with low doses of monoiodoacetate or 2-deoxyglucose impairs the cardiac contractile function despite unlimited supplies of oxygen and pyruvate, the end produce of glycolysis.[99] There is thus no doubt that glycolysis, on the one hand, provides an insignificant portion of ATP used by the cell, but on the other constitutes an indispensable link in the mechanism of energy supplies for the cardiac contractile function.

TABLE 8
Effect of EPS on Phosphorylase Activation and Glycogen Content and Biosynthesis in the Rat Myocardium

	Phosphorylase A/A+B ratio	Glycogen content (mg/g tissue)	^{14}C incorporation into glycogen, cpm: Specific per mg glycogen	^{14}C incorporation into glycogen, cpm: Total per g tissue
Control (n = 10)	0.43 ± 0.03	6.40 ± 0.31	205 ± 22	1310 ± 201
EPS (n = 10)	0.61 ± 0.04	3.60 ± 0.23	215 ± 17	776 ± 95
	$p < 0.01$	$p < 0.01$		$p < 0.01$

TABLE 9
Effect of EPS on Myocardial Glycogen and Lactate at Physiological Rest and Maximal Cardiac Load

	Control		EPS	
Indices	Rest	Load	Rest	Load
Glycogen (mg/100 g)	640 ± 31 (n = 9)	519 ± 18 (n = 7)	360 ± 23[a] (n = 17)	288 ± 27[a] (n = 10)
Lactate (μmol/100 g)	88 ± 19 (n = 7)	548 ± 34 (n = 13)	105 ± 12 (n = 8)	638 ± 50 (n = 8)

[a] Difference from control significant at $p < 0.01$.

This has prompted a suggestion that the small amount of ATP formed in glycolysis is a unique, irreplaceable source of energy for a certain vital function of the muscle cell. The suggestion is favored by several facts.

1. Blocking the glycolysis with monoiodoacetate consistently impairs myocardial relaxation, eliciting cardiac contracture.[100] In this connection an idea has been put forth that glycolysis generates the ATP fraction used for the operation of the SR calcium pump, i.e., for removal of Ca^{2+} from myofibrils to allow diastolic relaxation.
2. The multienzyme glycolytic system is for the most part localized on the SR membranes[101] and, accordingly, muscles with more developed SR always possess a more powerful glycolytic system as, in particular, do skeletal muscle compared to the cardiac muscle. Substantial amounts of glycogen — the main cell glycolytic substrate — are found along the longitudinal SR, i.e., in immediate proximity to the calcium pump.[102]
3. The processes of glycogenolysis-glycolysis and Ca^{2+} removal from the sarcoplasm are regulatively dependent on the sarcoplasmic Ca^{2+} content. Indeed, a rise in Ca^{2+} and active calmodulin during excitation simultaneously causes phosphorylation of phosphorylase B to phosphorylase A (activation of glycolysis) and phosphorylation of the sarcolemmal and SR phospholambam (activation of the calcium pump and relaxation).

It is thus quite probable that the portion of ATP produced in glycolysis is used by the calcium pump ATPase to ensure relaxation. These facts of course do not exhaust the problem, but they are in line with the hypothesis that the comparatively small amount of glycolytic ATP is a unique, indispensable source of energy for a certain vital physiological operation, namely for the relaxation process.[103,104]

This issue has been confirmed and developed in later studies. The most demonstrative result has been obtained by Bricknell et al.,[105] who studied the role of glycolysis in the energy provision for membrane Ca^{2+} transport with a model of cardiac contracture developing in prolonged myocardial ischemic hypoxia. This contracture, being an energy-deficient muscle-relaxation disorder, results not from simple lack of ATP in the contractile apparatus, but precisely from the ATP-deficient interruption of the membrane pump responsible for Ca^{2+} removal from the myofibrillar troponin complexes.[106,107] To collate the roles of the mitochondrial and the glycolytic ATP in the calcium pump function, the authors have studied the development of contracture (1) under blocked glycolysis and intact oxidative phosphorylation and mitochondrial ATP transport, and (2) under operative glycolysis and blocked mitochondrial ATP transport. The scheme in Figure 12 shows that in the first series glycolysis was switched off by removing glucose from the perfusing solution and adding glycolytic inhibitors — monoiodoacetate or deoxyglucose; simultaneously, acetate was added as a substrate to maintain oxidative phosphorylation. In the second series the glucose concentration was normal, glycolysis proceeded freely, oxidative phosphorylation also was not specially blocked, but translocation of mitochondrial ATP to the perimyofibrillar space was inhibited with atractyloside (Figure 12B).

In both series the isolated heart was first allowed to function aerobically, then it was stopped with KCl, and myocardial ischemia was created by reducing the perfusing flow to 1 to 0.5 ml/min. The oxidative phosphorylation which is the main source of total myocardial ATP under such conditions was similarly attenuated in both series, and accordingly the ATP level was also approximately the same. However, despite the same ATP concentration the state of relaxation in ischemia proved quite different. With blocked glycolysis and intact oxidative phosphorylation, in 100 min after the onset of ischemia a pronounced contracture developed, with the indices of tension at rest approximating those of systolic tension in aerobic conditions prior to cardiac arrest. With intact glycolysis in the cardiac muscle, no appreciable contracture developed. These data fit into the hypothesis of the prime importance of the glycolytic ATP for the relaxation process. They allow one to think that the decline in myocardial glycogen reserve in poststress animals observed in our studies and the attending disturbances in glycolysis and glycogen resynthesis may be involved in the stress disorders of myocardial contraction and relaxation, and first of all in the above phenomenon of myocardial stress rigidity and its decreased resistance to hypoxia and excess calcium. To test this suggestion, we made a study of the effects of high glucose concentrations and of a cofactor of glycogen resynthesis, uridine, on the extensibility and contractility of the myocardium from animals subjected to a 6-h EPS.

In Figure 13, the curves on the left reflect the stress-induced defects in extensibility and contractile function described earlier, and on the right the effects of a fourfold increase (from 2.5 to 10 m*M*) of the glucose concentration in the perfusing solution. Analysis of the curves demonstrates that such a rise in glucose practically restores the stress-impaired extensibility and contraction force of the auricle. A similar effect is observed with the left ventricular papillary muscle. In considering this protective effect of glucose on the stress damage to the cardiac contractile functions it should be borne in mind that administration of glucose into the coronary bed enhances the glycogen content, aerobic and anaerobic glycolysis, creatine kinase activity, and macroergic phosphate content in the ischemic myocardium.[108] Concurrently, the loss of myocardial calcium is diminished and the ischemic disturbances in the cardiomyocyte electric activity (shortening and step-down of the action potential, arrhythmias) are prevented.[109] In our experiments the excess of glucose could also normalize the glycolytic process, restore the flux of glycolytic ATP to the membrane calcium pump, and thereby abolish the excess of myofibrillar Ca^{2+} and myocardial stress rigidity.

The fact that the declining glycogen content and its impaired resynthesis in stress are associated with relaxation and contraction defects substantiates the use of some cofactor of glycogen resynthesis to restore its content and metabolism in cardiomyocytes and to restore therewith myocardial relaxation. In our experiments use was made for this purpose of the nucleoside uridine. The first step in glycogen synthesis is known to be impossible without

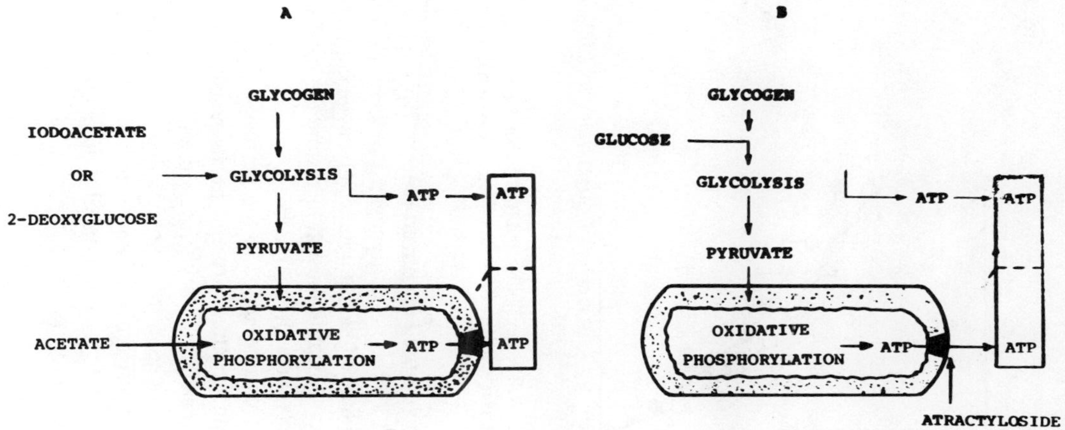

FIGURE 12. Scheme for comparative assessment of the effect of blocking (A) glycolysis and (B) mitochondrial ATP translocation on the development of ischemic contracture. For explanations see text. (After Bricknell, O. L., Daries, P. S., and Opie, L. H., *J. Mol. Cell. Cardiol.*, 13, 941, 1981. With permission.)

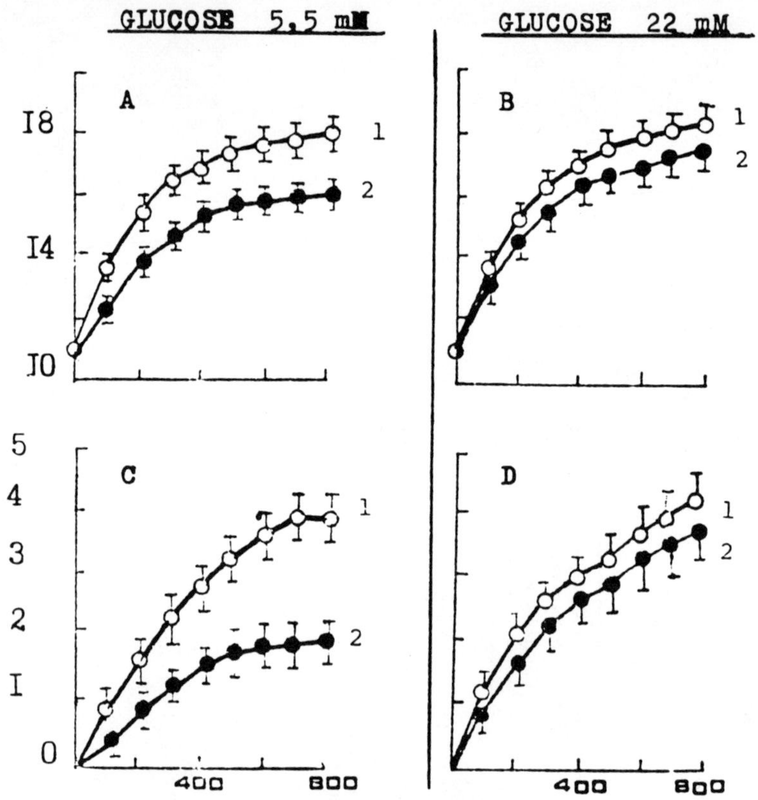

FIGURE 13. Effect of increased glucose concentration on the (A,B) extensibility and (C,D) contractile function of auricles from rats subjected to EPS. The abscissa is the load at rest in mg; the ordinates are (A,B) atrial length in mm, (C,D) contraction force in mN. 1, Control; 2, EPS.

uridine phosphorylated to uridine triphosphate, which is used to convert glucose 1-phosphate to UDP-glucose, the direct substrate for glycogen synthesis by glycogen synthase. In full conformity with this, uridine has been proved to enhance glucose uptake, glycogen content, and renewal of the ATP microstores in the aerobic myocardium, and to restore the cardiac function, glycogen, and adenine nucleotide contents under hypoxia.[110]

Basing on this, we have studied the effects of uridine added to the perfusing solution on the stress defects of myocardial extensibility and contractility and on its resistance to hypoxia and excess Ca^{2+}. The experiments were carried out with isolated auricles at 5.5 m*M* glucose. Half of both control and poststress auricles were supplemented with uridine at 2×10^{-5} *M*. Figure 14 shows that in our experiments uridine acted identically to quadrupled glucose: it did not affect the atrial extensibility and contractility in controls, but completely abolished the defects in extensibility and most of the depression of contractile function after stress.

Figure 15 depicts the effects of uridine on atrial hypercalcium contracture. It can be seen that a threefold rise in Ca^{2+} elicited a significant increase in the tension of rest, i.e., contracture which was reliably more pronounced in poststress than in control auricles. In the presence of uridine the contracture was much smaller: the resistance of the myocardial relaxation process to excess Ca^{2+} was markedly enhanced by the cofactor of glycogen resynthesis. As this took place, an apparently paradoxical phenomenon was observed: in the poststress auricles the protective effect of uridine was greater than in controls. Indeed, the hypercalcium contracture assayed as the absolute tension in these experiments was quite reliably reduced by uridine in the poststress auricles, whereas with the controls its effect did not reach statistical significance. As a result, the contracture in the presence of uridine

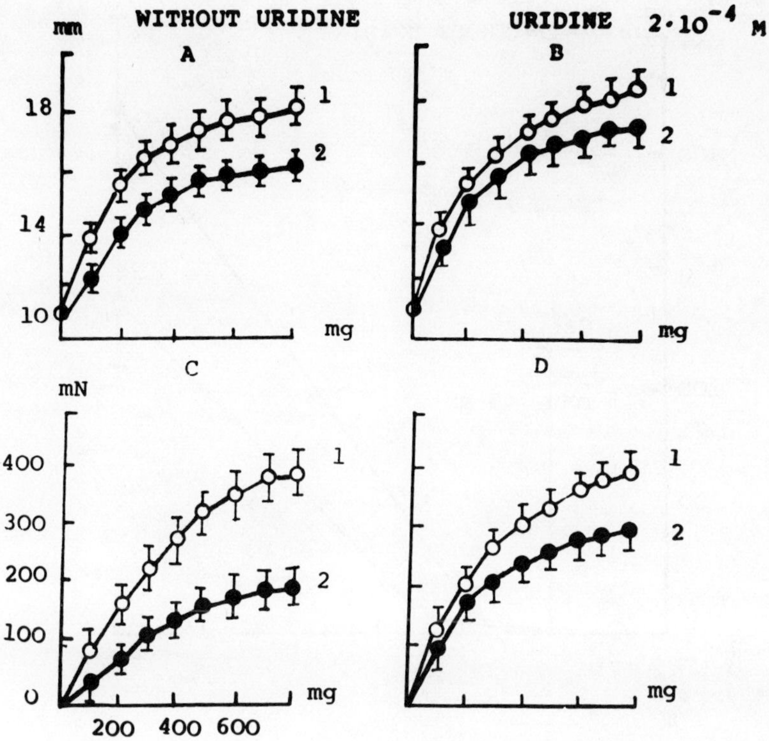

FIGURE 14. Effect of uridine on the (A,B) extensibility and (C,D) contractile function of auricles from rats subjected to EPS. The abscissa is the load at rest in mg; the ordinates are (A,B) atrial length in mm, (C,D) contraction force in mN. 1, Control; 2, EPS.

proved to be more pronounced in the control than in the poststress auricles. Such potentiation of the uridine effect by stress may be because the glycogen deficit caused by stress enhances the sensitivity of the glycogen-synthesizing system to excess uridine. A certain role may also be played by an increased uridine permeation through stress-damaged cardiomyocyte membranes.

On the whole, the above gives grounds for thinking that stress induces quite pronounced defects in the creatine kinase and glycolytic systems which may be involved in the stress disturbances to the electric stability and contractile function of the heart, most likely through upsetting the energy provision for the cardiomyocyte calcium pump.

In this context note should be made of some points of interest for clinical cardiology. The first one is that the stress-induced hindrance to myocardial extensibility is not only a marker of impaired relaxation, but may also interfere with cardiac filling and pump function, i.e., decrease its stroke volume and output. It cannot be excluded that such phenomena contribute to the evolvement of collaptoid stress conditions.

The second point is that stress-induced glycolytic defects revealed in the myocardium and the ensuing functional alterations must be most pronounced in those parts of the heart whose energy supplies are most dependent on glycolysis. Undoubtedly such a part is the cardiac conductive system whose cells have much fewer mitochondria than the cells of contractile myocardium. This system must to the largest extent suffer from repeated stress situations inevitably encountered in one's life. In full conformity with this suggestion is the fact that right and then left bundle-branch blockade of the bundle of His may develop very early in practically healthy persons and is often regarded as a hallmark of age wearing of the heart.

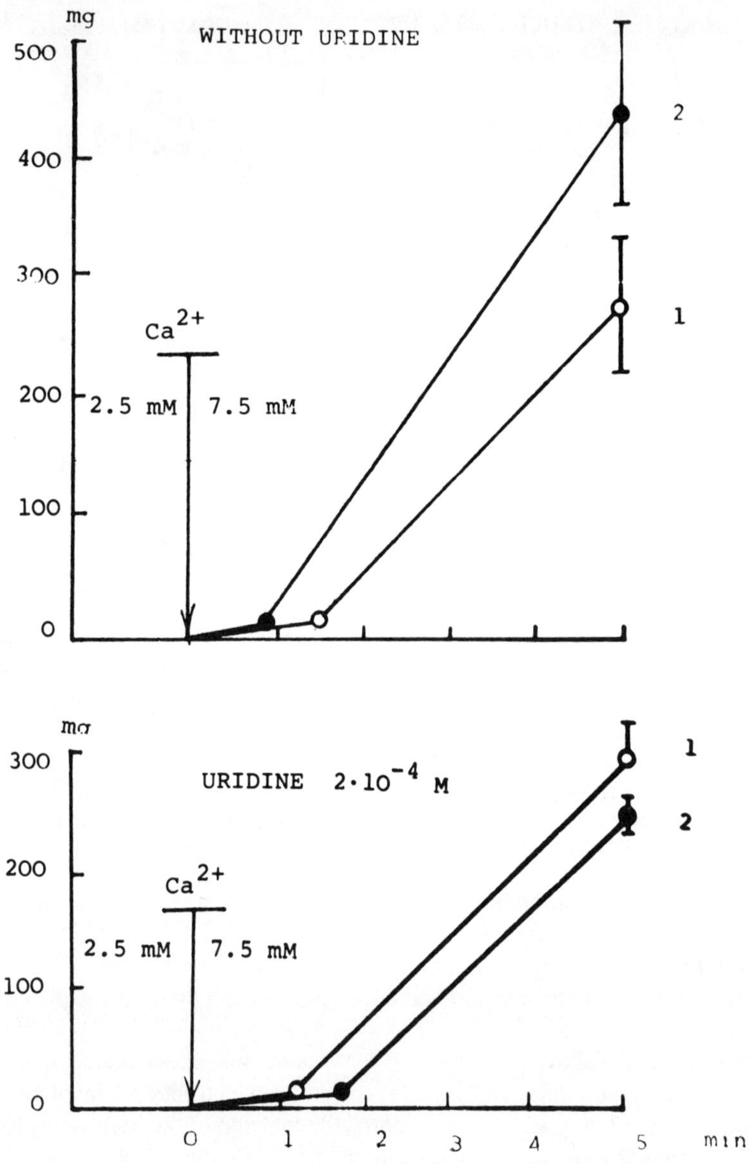

FIGURE 15. Effect of uridine on the calcium contracture in auricles from rats subjected to EPS. The abscissa is time in min; the ordinate is the increment in tension of rest in mg. 1, Control; 2, EPS.

Finally, the third point is that the stress alterations in the myocardial cell are not at all limited to the disturbances in the contractile function and energy metabolism considered above, but are much more deep. This is evidenced by our finding, of some years ago, of the stress damage and subsequent repair of nuclear DNA in the cardiac muscle, and structural damage to the myocardium.

V. MYOCARDIAL DNA INJURY AND OUTBURST OF ITS REPARATIVE SYNTHESIS IN STRESS

Activation of lipid peroxidation (LPO), lipases, phospholipases, and consequent membrane damage considered above must naturally lead to the injury to main cell structures in the cardiac muscle. Indeed, such a transitory injury to proteins and nucleic acids has been found to occur in a 6-h EPS.[111]

It has been found that stress substantially decreased the half-life of ribosomal RNA and increased the percentage of RNA replaced within 1 d in the internal organs. This complex of changes directly testifying to enhanced breakdown of RNA was clearly pronounced in the cardiac muscle: the half-life was decreased by about one fourth and the portion of replaced RNA increased by one third. Further, the half-life of the total myocardial protein after stress proved to be decreased by more than one third. Thus, stress brings about significant acceleration of RNA and protein breakdown.

Taking this into account, we studied the influence of stress on the apparatus which is central for the cell formation and at the same time the most conservative and protected from deterioration, namely on the DNA of the cell nuclei.

We reasoned from the fact that, e.g., in radiation sickness the accumulation of free-radical LPO products in the cell is accompanied by injury to the DNA helix. A similar phenomenon could well happen in LPO activation by stress. On this basis we [112] conducted the experiments aimed at evaluating the polymeric state and reparative synthesis of DNA in cardiac muscle cells after EPS.

Stress causes partial depolymerization of myocardial DNA, most probably because of single-strand nicks. In most of the myocardial cells that continue functioning after the exposure to stress, these DNA nicks are rapidly repaired.

Further studies demonstrated that such changes —DNA damage and subsequent repair — upon stress are found not only in the heart, but also in kidneys, liver, brain, and other organs.[113]

Considering the biological significance of this phenomenon and its role as a marker of organ stress damage, we further made a more comprehensive study of it by comparing the effects of stress on DNA replication and repair in nuclei and mitochondria of heart and liver, and by elucidating the dependence of the stress injury to DNA (as judged from the outburst of its reparative synthesis) on the cardiac function.[114]

First, the effect of a 6-h EPS was compared on the replicative and reparative synthesis of DNA in the heart and the liver. In the control the replication rate was approximately twice lower in cardiac than in hepatic nuclei. EPS greatly accelerates nuclear DNA replication in the heart cells; this increse is observable 4 to 6 h after the end of stress and reaches its maximum in 10 to 12 h, with the replication rate exceeding the control by a factor of 3.5. After 22 to 24 h and later the replication in cardiac cells returns to the initial level. In the hepatic nuclei the pattern is quite different, with EPS decreasing the replication rate about by half for 48 h after stress and still by some 20% after 72 h.

The next series concerned reparative DNA synthesis in cardiac and hepatic nuclei on the background of hydroxyurea, which is known to inhibit nuclear DNA replication, but to have almost no effect on its reparative synthesis.[115,116] In our experiments hydroxyurea suppressed DNA synthesis by 88% in the cardiac and by 89% in the hepatic nuclei. These results are comparable with the data obtained for other cells.[117,118] DNA synthesis taking place in the presence of hydroxyurea apparently reflects the reparative synthesis.

As can be seen in Figure 16, the rate of DNA synthesis in both cardiac and hepatic cells is significantly increased upon EPS — the outburst of DNA repair (testifying to its damage) is realized to the most. Notably, the reparative synthesis is activated in cardiac cells on the background of enhanced, while in hepatic cells, of suppressed replication.

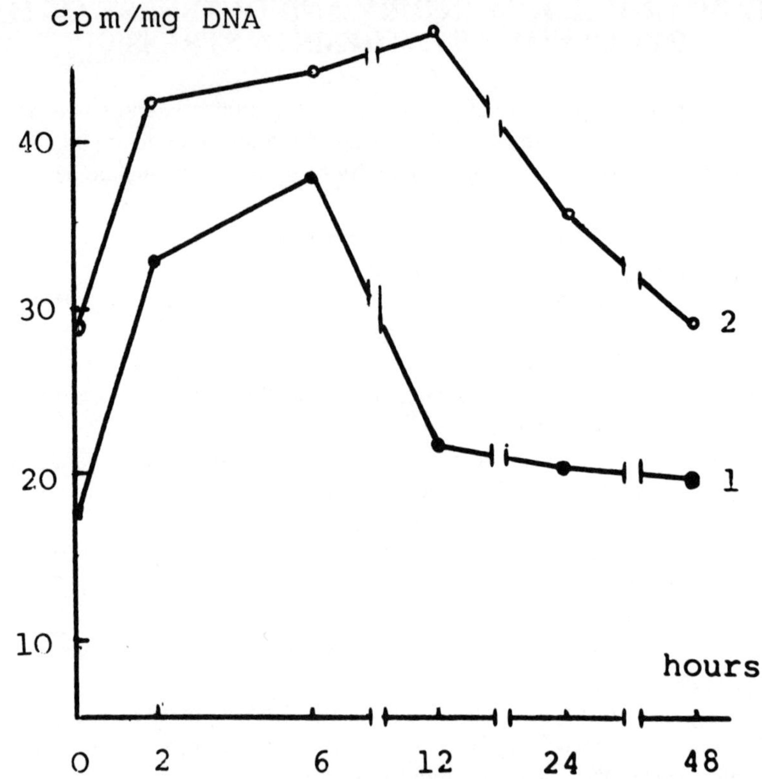

FIGURE 16. Effect of EPS on reparative DNA synthesis in (1) cardiac and (2) hepatic nuclei. The abscissa is time after EPS in hours, the ordinate is ^{3}H-thymidine incorporation in cpm/mg DNA.

Then DNA synthesis was studied in cardiac and hepatic mitochondria. In agreement with the known data,[119] the specific radioactivity of pulse-labeled mitochondrial DNA exceeded that of nuclear DNA. The high rate of precursor incorporation into mitochondrial DNA is held to reflect its replicative synthesis.[120] Hydroxyurea, the inhibitor of nuclear DNA replication, proved to have no effect on the mitochondrial process. EPS does not affect mitochondrial DNA replication in the heart and substantially suppresses it in the liver, as shown in Figure 17.[114]

Thus, under the influence of EPS the two different systems of DNA synthesis in two vital organs — the heart and the liver — change in different ways. In the heart the rates of nuclear DNA replication and repair increase, while those of mitochondrial DNA synthesis remain the same. In the liver the rates of nuclear and mitochondrial DNA replication decrease, while the nuclear repair rate increases as well.

It is essential that *by the criterion of suppressed DNA replication the liver proved to be a more stress-sensitive organ than the heart,* and we shall further see that this is not a stray occurrence, since many organs are damaged by stress not at all less than the cardiac muscle.

In studying the second question of interest, and namely how the myocardial function affects the DNA resistance to stress injury, i.e., the extent of its repair, we made use of operative (surgical) stress.

Preliminary experiments showed that operative stress caused by laparotomy entails an outburst of reparative synthesis in the myocardial nuclei as consistently as EPS. However, if the operation ends in coarctation of aorta with resulting compensatory heart hyperfunction, there is no outburst of DNA synthesis in the myocardium. This prompted an idea that the enhanced function somehow stabilizes the DNA structure, preventing its injury and correspondingly its repair.[121]

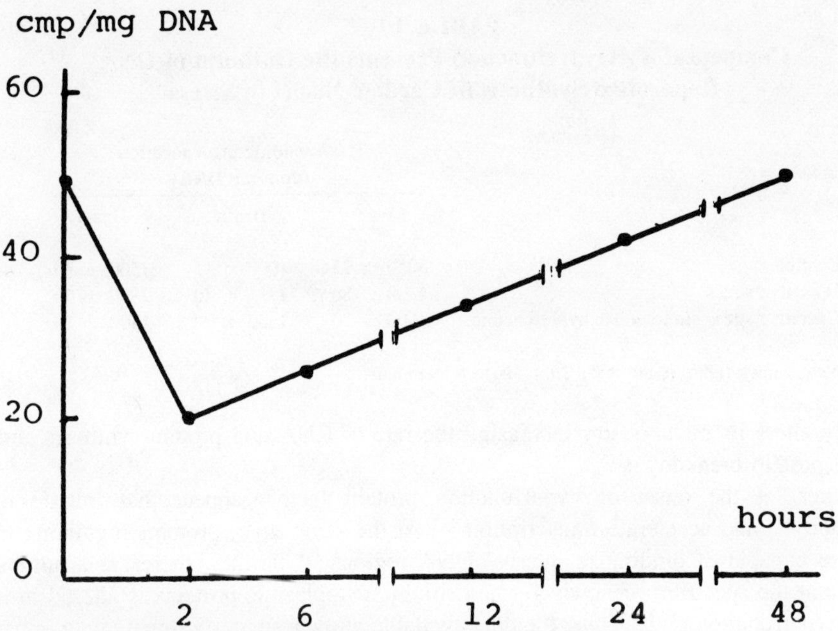

FIGURE 17. Effect of EPS on DNA synthesis in liver mitochondria. The abscissa is time after EPS in hours, the ordinate is ^{3}H-thymidine incorporation in cpm/mg DNA.

To check this suggestion, it was important to find out whether the ''stabilizing effect'' of myocardial hyperfunction is realized only locally in the cardiac cell nuclei or if it also encompasses other internal organs where DNA repair is also enhanced in stress.[122,123] To this end, the influence of operation without coarctation of aorta and of a similar operation ending in coarctation of aorta and compensatory heart hyperfunction was studied on the DNA repair rate in the cell nuclei of the heart, the liver, and the brain.[114]

The data presented in Table 10 allow a comparison of the rates of reparative nuclear DNA synthesis in hepatic, cardiac, and brain cells both at rest and after operative stress. It can be seen that the greatest reparative ability is found in the liver and the smallest in the brain, with the heart being intermediate in this respect. Both kinds of operation, without and with aortic coarctation, cause an outburst of DNA repair in hepatic and brain cells. Another thing is found in the heart. The operation without coarctation, i.e., operative stress, causes an outburst of DNA repair in the heart like in other internal organs. However, upon aortic coarctation with ensuing myocardial hyperfunction, there is no outburst of repair. *Hence, the DNA injury by operative stress does not occur under compensatory hyperfunction of the cardiac muscle. This protective effect is local and does not expand on other organs.*

In eukaryotic cells the DNA injuries can be repaired by two means: excision and postreplicative repair. The latter is inhibited by hydroxyurea.[124] Therefore, *in our experiments we were only dealing with excision repair*. In mammals there are two ways of this, the sort and the long one. In the first, three to seven nucleotides are eliminated from DNA and the process is completed within an hour. In the second, several dozen nucleotides are removed and the process lasts 20 to 24 h and longer.[125]

After operative stress, the enhancement of reparative synthesis in cardiac, hepatic, and brain cells is quite definite after 24 h. Thus, under the given conditions the excision repair proceeds via the long way.

A principal question is why no acceleration of DNA reparative synthesis is observed upon operative stress in the cardiac muscle performing compensatory hyperfunction. In discussing this question, one should keep in mind the following. Organ hyperfunction

TABLE 10
Compensatory Hyperfunction Prevents the Outburst of DNA Reparative Synthesis in Cardiac Nuclei in Stress

	^{3}H-Thymidine incorporation (dpm/mg DNA)		
	Liver	Brain	Heart
Control	3050 ± 25	1000 ± 15	1500 ± 80
Operative stress	4300 ± 80	1315 ± 40	2900 ± 50
Operative stress with cardiac hyperfunction	4600 ± 70	1350 ± 20	1400 ± 20

Note: Each figure is the mean from six to ten animals.

markedly alters its metabolism, increasing the rate of RNA and protein synthesis and decreasing protein breakdown.[124]

Further, at the onset of hyperfunction protein factors appear that initiate organ hypertrophy[126] and accelerate transcription.[127] At the same time, proteins regulating translation are capable of binding to internal DNA regions.[128] Further, there are a number of reports that the spectrum of newly formed soluble cytoplasmic proteins is altered in myocardial hyperfunction.[124,129] Thus, the data available allow a suggestion that under enhanced function in myocardial cells some proteins accumulate to stabilize the DNA structure and prevent it from the damaging action of stress.

By and large, *there is no doubt that the metabolic effects of myocardial hyperfunction prevent the stress-induced damage to cardiac DNA. The stabilizing effect of cardiac hyperfunction on the DNA template is local and does not cover other internal organs.*

VI. EXTRACARDIAC DAMAGES IN STRESS AND THEIR POSSIBLE CONTRIBUTION TO IMPAIRMENT OF CARDIAC FUNCTION

The stress reaction is a generalized phenomenon, and accordingly not only the heart, but the whole organism may become the target of excessive stress reaction. In the process, damage to the respiratory apparatus controlling blood oxygen tension, to the liver predetermining the cholesterol level, to the pancreas that may release trypsin, can in a most direct way tell on the status of the heart and indirectly contribute to its damage by stress. Here we shall consider such possibilities as applied to the respiratory system, where in our opinion there are sufficient grounds for introducing the term ''stress lung'', and more briefly as applied to the liver and the pancreas.

It is known that the respiratory system has vast functional reserves and, by adjusting the pulmonary ventilation and oxygen transport and utilization, ensures the energy balance in various ambient conditions. Further, it has been shown that exposure to stress is accompanied by mobilization of the respiratory apparatus.[130-132] The resistance of the respiratory system to heavy stress has not been studied until recently. Yet the stress damage to the respiratory system may be essential for the impairment of its function in most various conditions and diseases caused by stress situations.

In accordance with this, we studied the influence of severe immobilization stress on pulmonary ventilation, oxygen diffusion from air to blood, blood transport of respiratory gases, and O_2 consumption by tissues.

The control animals were first anesthetized and then fixed by four limbs in the supine position, whereas the ''stressed'' animals were kept in this fixed position for 6 h before anesthesia. Then a standard acute test was performed in both groups under anesthesia. As a result, all the disturbances described below were observed only in animals subjected to immobilization without anesthesia, i.e., indeed subjected to stress. This important experimental detail indicates that it is not immobiization as such and not the procedures of the acute test carried out under anesthesia, but just the stress reaction evoked by immobilization that damages the organism in whole and the respiratory system in particular.

The data presented in Table 11 show that a 6-h immobilization stress substantially alters the basic parameters of oxygen transport in the organism and circulation. Thus the alveolar ventilation in animals subjected to stress proved to be decreased by half, yet the oxygen tension in the alveolar air remained at the normal level. Such a relation of these parameters is usually due to attenuated O_2 consumption by the organism.[133] However, a study of the P_{O_2} cascade revealed that at the same partial oxygen pressure in the alveolar gas mixture in stress and control, the O_2 tension in arterial blood running off the lungs in stresss animals is lowered by 26.5 hPa (20 mmHg column). Such stress-induced arterial hypoxemia may result from hindered oxygen diffusion from the alveoli to the lung capillaries and some other factors to be considered below.

Notably, such hypoxemia is not attended with lowered mean P_{O_2} in the blood of tissue capillaries and mixed venous blood. This at first glance paradoxical fact should be due to decreased oxygen consumption by tissues.

Furthermore, Table 11 shows that in animals that have undergone immobilization stress the minute blood volume is decreased by 45%.

Taken together, these data mean that *the drop in arterial O_2 tension and in the minute volume in stress diminish the O_2 supply to tissues by a factor of about 2.5. However, this does not decrease the O_2 tension* in the tissue capillaries and in the mixed venous blood, since the O_2 consumption by tissues and the whole organism is diminished to the same extent.

Despite the maintained balance between oxygen supply to and consumption in tissues, Table 12 demonstrates that the lactate content in blood is almost twice as high in poststress animals, and the pH is lowered by 0.25 in the arterial and mixed venous blood with an attending fall in bicarbonates and aggravated deficit of bases at a practically normal CO_2 tension in the arterial blood. In other words, the given stress exposure elicits decompensated metabolic acidosis in rats. To appreciate this phenomenon, one should take account of an important index — the ratio of supplied to consumed oxygen which usually varies between 3 and 4 in the control and regularly decreases in various types of hypoxia. The secondary tissue hypoxia, due to insufficient oxygen supply to the cells and attended with lactate accumulation and metabolic acidosis, has been shown[134] to set in only after this index falls to 2.0 to 1.5. In the present study there was no reliable decrease in this index upon immobilization stress (see Table 11), hence there was no deficit of O_2 due to its inadequate supply to the cells. Therefore, in stress the excess of lactic acid and acidosis are not the result of secondary tissue hypoxia. The most plausible cause of these shifts is the depressed tissue respiration and oxygen utilization by mitochondria and marked activation of glycolysis with associated mobilization of the glycogen reserves in liver, heart, and other organs.[135] Under suppressed mitochondrial respiration the surplus pyruvate formed in glycolysis cannot be used by the respiratory chain, is converted to lactate, and goes into the blood. Such an interpretation is supported by the fact that the plasma from animals subjected to immobilization stress shows a threefold elevation of malonic dialdehyde, an intermediate product of lipid peroxidation; the latter is known to be activated in stress and to play an important role in cell membrane damage.

It is essential that as a result of stress damage to tissue respiration the overall energy consumption by the organism (calculated from oxygen consumption, respiratory quotient, lactate content, and coefficient of Margariya) decreases by 50%, with the portion of energy derived from anaerobic processes involving lactate accumulation increasing from 6 to 20%.

TABLE 11
Effect of Immobilization Stress on the Main Parameters of Oxygen Transport in the Organism

Indices	Control	Stress
Alveolar ventilation		
$\dot{V}_A$, ml/min·100 g	47.3 ± 3.5	23.2 ± 2.3[a]
Oxygen tension (mmHg/in.)		
Alveolar air, P_{AO_2}	105 ± 3	104 ± 2
Arterial blood, P_{aO_2}	87.1 ± 1.5	67.1 ± 5.6[b]
Mixed venous blood, P_{vO_2}	37.5 ± 1.4	34.1 ± 3.2
Tissue capillary blood, P_{TO_2}	50.3 ± 1.1	46.0 ± 3.4
Hemoglobin, C_{Hb}, g/l	126 ± 3	115 ± 4[c]
Circulation minute volume		
$\dot{Q}$, ml/min·100 g	48.8 ± 5.4	26.7 ± 5.0[b]
Oxygen transport rate by		
Arterial blood, $\dot{V}_{aO_2}$, ml/min·100 g	8.21 ± 0.71	3.33 ± 0.57[a]
Oxygen consumption rate		
$\dot{V}_{O_2}$, ml/min·100 g	2.57 ± 0.29	1.13 ± 0.11[a]
Ratio of oxygen arterial transport and consumption $\dot{V}_{aO_2}/\dot{V}_{O_2}$	3.21 ± 0.18	2.80 ± 0.26

[a] $p < 0.001$.
[b] $p < 0.01$.
[c] $p < 0.05$.

TABLE 12
Effect of Immobilization Stress on the Acid-Base Equilibrium, Lactic Acid, and Malonic Dialdehyde Content in Blood

Indices	Control	Stress
Arterial blood pH	7.39 ± 0.01	7.14 ± 0.02[a]
Mixed venous blood pH	7.35 ± 0.01	7.10 ± 0.02[a]
CO_2 tension in arterial blood, P_{aCO_2} (mmHg)	36.0 ± 2.7	34.8 ± 3.3
True arterial bicarbonate AB (mmol/l)	21.4 ± 1.6	11.6 ± 1.2[a]
Buffer bases of arterial blood BB (mmol/l)	44.8 ± 1.5	30.8 ± 1.2[a]
Normal buffer bases NBB (mmol/l)	47.0 ± 0.3	46.5 ± 0.2
Buffer base shift in arterial blood, BE (mmol/l)	−2.5 ± 1.3	−15.7 ± 1.2[a]
Lactic acid, C_L (mmol/l)	2.8 ± 0.5	5.0 ± 0.3[a]
Malonic dialdehyde, C_M (mmol/l)	1.26 ± 0.06	4.28 ± 1.28[b]

[a] $p < 0.001$.
[b] $p < 0.01$.

In the aggregate, the above provides evidence that *stress damage elicits a peculiar hypoxic condition having features of hypoxic (arterial hypoxemia), hemic (decreased hemoglobin concentration), circulatory (smaller minute volume), and primary tissue (impaired tissue consumption of O_2 and activated glycolysis) hypoxia.*

The above data per se do not yet point to the damage to respiratory organs and circulation and may create an illusion that the observed depression of these functions results from lowered basal metabolism. Actually the situation is different. Cardiac and vascular disorders in stress are now well known, while stress damage to the respiratory apparatus and the lungs proper have been reported only in a few works.[130,131] We have obtained unambiguous evidence to such disturbances in breathing either air or a hypoxic mixture enriched in carbon dioxide: upon stress, despite the low blood P_{O_2} and marked acidosis, the respiration rate and volume are both decreased.

The disorders in external respiration and in its response to changing oxygen parameters and carbon dioxide tension in blood are usually explained by brain hypoxia.[130] However, in the present case the respiration regulatory disorders cannot be simply attributed to a decreased oxygen supply to the brain. As already mentioned, the secondary tissue hypoxia (which develops when the oxygen delivery is inadequate to the tissue demand) is only weakly pronounced upon stress. Moreover, the comparison of the extent of arterial hypoxemia (decreased supply of O_2 to the tissue capillaries) found in this study with the well-known hypoxic hypoxia caused by inspiring oxygen-depleted mixtures[134] demonstrates that a drop in arterial oxygen tension to 80 to 90 hPa cannot by itself depress respiration. The attenuated O_2 delivery due to the lesser blood flow also does not appreciably change the P_{O_2} in the tissue capillaries of the organs well supplied with oxygen, which include the brain (see Table 11). All this prompts a suggestion that immobilization stress elicits defects of respiratory regulation which are not directly associated with the stress hypoxia.

Our study of the effect of stress on external respiration revealed that the respiration rate is lowered mainly at the expense of a substantially prolonged expiratory phase, which may indirectly point to decreased excitabiity of the respiratory center.

In elucidating the mechanism of the described hypoxemia we proceeded from the accepted concept that it may chiefly be due to three factors: increased diffusion resistance of the alveolo-capillary membranes, inadequacy of blood flow and ventilation in certain pulmonary regions, and finally anatomic bypassing.[136] All these factors result in a part of mixed venous blood going into the arterial bed without oxygenation, i.e., being shunted. It is therefore convenient to evaluate their role in arterial hypoxemia by an equivalent amount of blood discharged into the arterial bed per unit time, assuming that the P_{O_2} in this shunted flow is constant and equal to the oxygen tension in mixed venous blood. This approach has been first used by Piiper et al.,[137] who introduced the notion of an equivalent shunt in describing oxygen diffusion in the lungs. We have somewhat improved this method,[138] taking into account the nonlinearity of the hemoglobin dissociation curve, pH shifts, and a number of other factors, which allowed its use not only with hypoxic hypoxia, but with other conditions including stress.

Analysis of the data in Table 13 shows that the growth of overall pulmonary shunting and consequently arterial hypoxemia is mainly due to a more irregular distribution of ventilation and blood flow and to a greater anatomic bypassing. Thus, not only are ventilation and blood flow decreased, but their coordination in many regions of the pulmonary tissue is hampered in stress.

Another fact attracting attention in Table 13 is a marked loss in pulmonary diffusion capacity for oxygen. In our experiments, in the resting state its contribution was small; but under real conditions of active life, or in stress combined with hypoxic hypoxia or physical load, this damage may have fatal consequences.

It further follows from Table 13 that the pulmonary diffusion capacity is decreased mainly because of the membrane component, i.e., because the stress impairs the diffusion properties of the membrane separating the alveolar space from the blood. This is especially important as an indication of direct stress damage to the tissue of the pulmonary aerohematic barrier.

Thus, the complex of the stress-induced disturbances in external respiration, its regulation and biomechanics, as well as the depression of pulmonary gas exchange, among other things, are due to lung damage as such. The ''stress lung'' condition implies at least three components: upset coordination between local blood flow and ventilation; increased anatomic bypassing, i.e., direct flux of mixed venous blood into the arterial bed; and, finally, decreased pulmonary diffusion capacity, in all probability caused by direct damage to the alveolar and capillary cell membranes.

TABLE 13
Effect of Immobilization Stress on the Parameters of Blood Oxygenation in Lungs

Indices	Control	Stress
Lung diffusion capacity		
D_L (μmol/min·kPa·100 g)	221 ± 27	93 ± 27[a]
Membrane component of D_L		
D_M (μmol/min·kPa·100 g)	647 ± 30	141 ± 20[b]
Blood component of D_L		
V_c (μmol/min·kPa·100 g)	335 ± 48	269 ± 40
Equivalent shunts (% of blood flow)		
Total, E_T	7.02 ± 0.61	31.20 ± 5.80[b]
Diffusion, E_D	1.05 ± 0.02	2.13 ± 0.04[b]
Anatomical, E_A	3.00 ± 0.32	8.00 ± 0.71[b]
Due to lung inhomogeneity, E_I	2.97 ± 0.95	21.07 ± 1.60[b]

[a] $p < 0.01$.
[b] $p < 0.001$.

We have assessed this last component by direct electron-microscopic examination of lungs from animals that had undergone stress.[138]

Immobilization stress has been found to evoke drastic ultrastructural alterations in the lungs, most pronounced in the aerohematic barrier (AHB).

In the electron microscope, lung tissues from stress animals reveal substantial seepage of blood liquid and erythrocytes into the alveolar lumen, i.e., development of an edematous-hemorrhagic syndrome (Figure 18A).

Simultaneously, in the alveolar epithelium stress induces regions of total edema of type I pneumocytes with velum-like protuberances (Figure 18B), testifying to increased hydration of the lung tissue. Rather often seen were regions of complete destruction of the alveolar epithelium (Figure 18C). The interstitial layer also displayed regions of thickening, which indicated enhanced liquid accumulation (Figure 18D)

Significantly altered was also the lung capillary endothelium, where regions of subendothelial edema were not infrequently found as pockets peeling off the endothelium (Figure 19A).

Another electron-microscopically revealed manifestation of the reaction to stress damage is the marked enhancement of pinocytosis, especially pronounced in the lung capillary endothelium (Figure 19B). In occasional regions of cytoplasmic veils, particularly of endothelial cells, there was ''excessive vesiculation[139] with the number of vesicles per 1 μm along the barrier amounting to 35 and more (compared to the normal 5 to 10) (Figure 19B). The micropinocytotic vesiscles were from 0.06 to 0.15 μm in diameter. In some cases they fused to form larger vacuole-like structures. Such pinocytotic activation probably reflects enhanced transport of structural and energetic provisions from the circulatory bed and cell endoplasmic reticula to the injured alveolar epithelium with a view to subsequent repair.

The mentioned alterations in the alveolar apparatus are accompanied by substantial thickening of the AHB at the expense of all its layers: lung capillary endothelium, interstitial layer, and alveolar epithelium. In sum, the AHB thickness is augmented about threefold. Such pronounced thickening of the AHB has not been reported in pathological conditions studied heretofore, including hypoxic cell injury.[140] We are inclined to explain this by excessive hydration of the AHB structures. Thus, stress elicits pulmonary tissue edema which in some regions results in intra-alveolar edema.

It is interesting that the AHB edema is accompanied by formation of peculiar ''clefts'' in both endothelial and epithelial layers comparable in size to and sometimes exceeding the barrier thickness (Figure 19C). The barrier itself in such localities becomes thinner, which may to some extent facilitate O_2 transfer from air to blood. Such a structural response is considered typical of hypoxic exposure.[141]

A fact worth attention is the practically complete lack of both intracellular (reserve) and extracellular (active) surfactant in the lungs of stress animals, which indicates depression of the pulmonary surfactant system. This appears to be only natural in view of intimate interrelation between the number and activity of pulmonary β-adrenoreceptors on the type II pneumocytes, and pulmonary surfactant synthesis and secretion.[142] Since stress (including immobilization) decreases the number of β-adrenoreceptors in a number of organs and tissues,[143,144] and supposedly in the lungs as well, the loss of total surfactant becomes more explicable.

One should also note an appreciable increase in the amount of primary and secondary lysosomes in pulmonary cells (Figure 19D).

In whole, the ultrastructural alterations that we have observed in lungs after a single heavy stress exposure comprise edema and marked thickening of the AHB in all its components, edematous-hemorrhagic syndrome and injury to the alveolar epithelium, and defects in the pulmonary surfactant system. This complex of alterations combines with the pulmonary functional disorders described above, which in whole we designate as "stress lung", is very likely to hinder oxygen transport from the alveoli to the pulmonary capillaries. It is therefore plausible that the stress damage can substantially disturb the external respiration and cause hypoxemia, which in its turn can promote cardiac damage or handicap its function. However, in our version of stress — the immobilization "stress of capitulation" — this element should not be overestimated, since such impeded oxygen supply in animals that had undergone stress was concurrent with another quite important event, namely a direct decrease in the oxygen consumption by the organism, which could to some extent limit the immediate hypoxic injury to tissues and specifically to the myocardium. More important is the observed lowering of the blood pH, which may depress the cardiac contractile function mainly because of calcium displacement from the sarcolemmal and myofibrillar binding sites. Finally, the greatest danger in our opinion comes from possible infection of the lungs profoundly damaged by stress and formation of a sort of vicious circle in the cardiorespiratory system.

Stress damages to the liver and prevention thereof will be further considered in detail in connection with the role of stress in evolvement of atherogenic dyslipidemia and coronary atherosclerosis (see Chapter 2). Here it should be noted that stress (and in particular the EPS used by us) consistently causes damage to hepatic cells manifesting itself as a drastic rise in the plasma level of the liver-specific enzyme fructose 1-phosphate aldolase. This damage results in great measure from activation of hepatic free-radical peroxidation as manifest by a markedly increased content of malonic dialdehyde and inactivation of superoxide dismutase. The most essential thing is that the stress damage encompasses the cytochrome P_{450} system and, affecting its important member cholesterol 7-α-hydroxylase, hinders cholesterol oxidation to bile acids.[145]

This results in a higher plasma content of low-density beta-lipoproteins and a lower content of alpha-lipoproteins. The atherogenicity index is substantially enhanced.[146] The significance of stress atherogenic dyslipoproteinemia in coronary atherosclerosis and ensuing ischemic heart damage at present raises no doubts and will be considered in Chapter 2 devoted to the place of stress in the evolvement of ischemic disease. Here it is essential that hypercholesterolemia, caused by various and in particular alimentary factors, directly and detrimentally affects the myocardium: it decreases the specific activity of the SR Ca ATPase and the efficiency of the calcium pump, causes cholesterol accumulation in the SR membranes where it is usually absent, with a simultaneous fivefold to tenfold increase in the LPO products; all this can impair the intracellular calcium transport which is important for contraction and relaxation.[147] Thus, the stress-induced atherogenic dyslipidemia may apparently not only contribute to coronary atherosclerosis, but directly harm the myocardial metabolism.

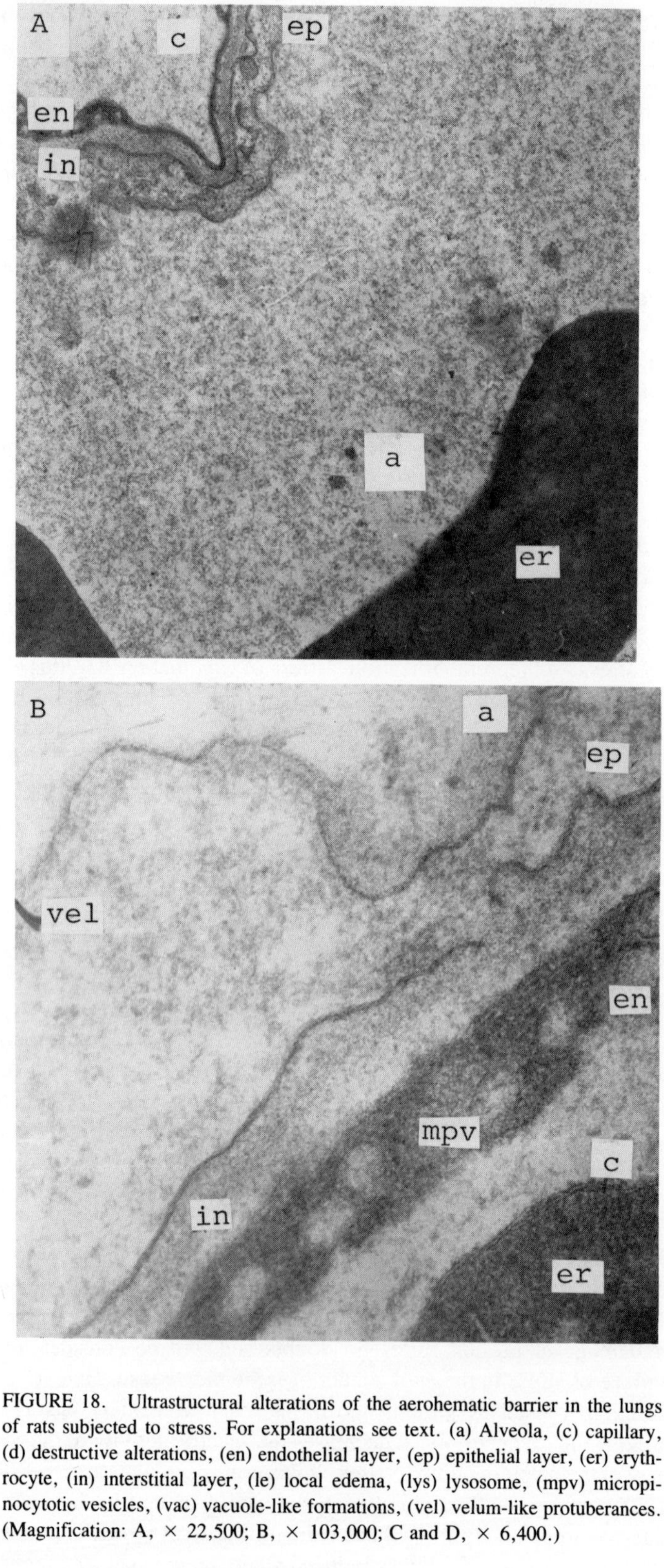

FIGURE 18. Ultrastructural alterations of the aerohematic barrier in the lungs of rats subjected to stress. For explanations see text. (a) Alveola, (c) capillary, (d) destructive alterations, (en) endothelial layer, (ep) epithelial layer, (er) erythrocyte, (in) interstitial layer, (le) local edema, (lys) lysosome, (mpv) micropinocytotic vesicles, (vac) vacuole-like formations, (vel) velum-like protuberances. (Magnification: A, × 22,500; B, × 103,000; C and D, × 6,400.)

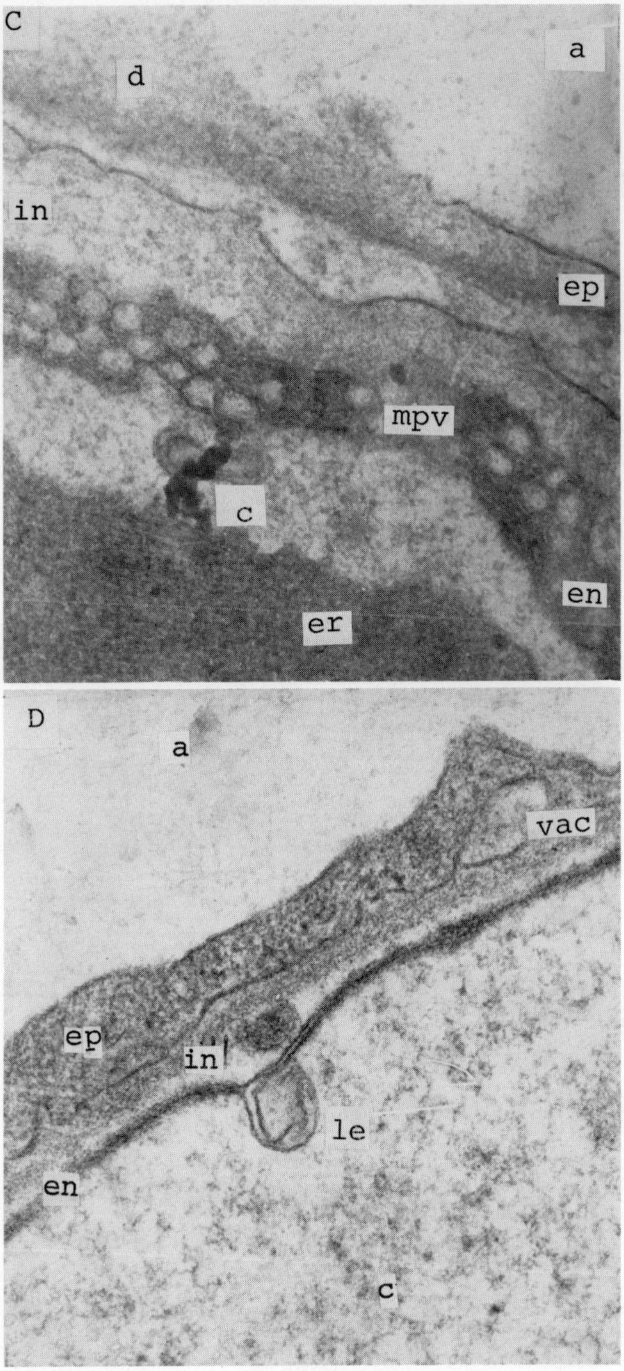

FIGURE 18C and D.

Another example of extracardiac effects of stress mediating heart damage is the stress injury to the pancreas. Initially, together with Saulya and Gudumak we found [148] that with increasing duration of immobilization stress the activity of the main proteolytic enzyme, trypsin, increases in the plasma. In this connection a special study was undertaken to correlate the plasma activities of trypsin and α_1-antitrypsin with the myocardial content of sialic acid.

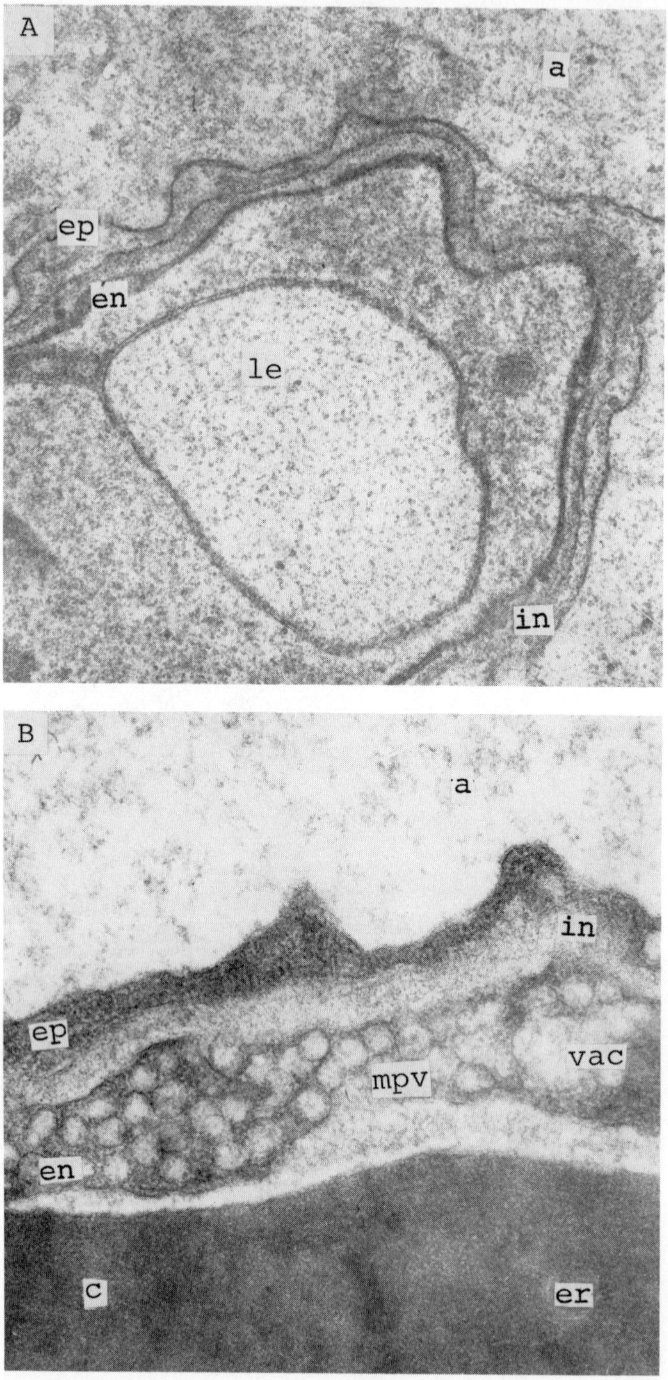

FIGURE 19. Ultrastructural alterations in the pulmonary aerohematic barrier. For explanations see text. Designations are as in Figure 18. (Magnification × 22,500.)

The rationale stemmed from the concept of Langer [149] that the sarcolemmal lipid bilayer and the glycocalyx covering it carry a large number of fixed negative charges which are the binding sites for calcium ions. The ionized calcium binds predominantly to the anionic regions of the molecules of sialic acid entering into the composition of cell membrane

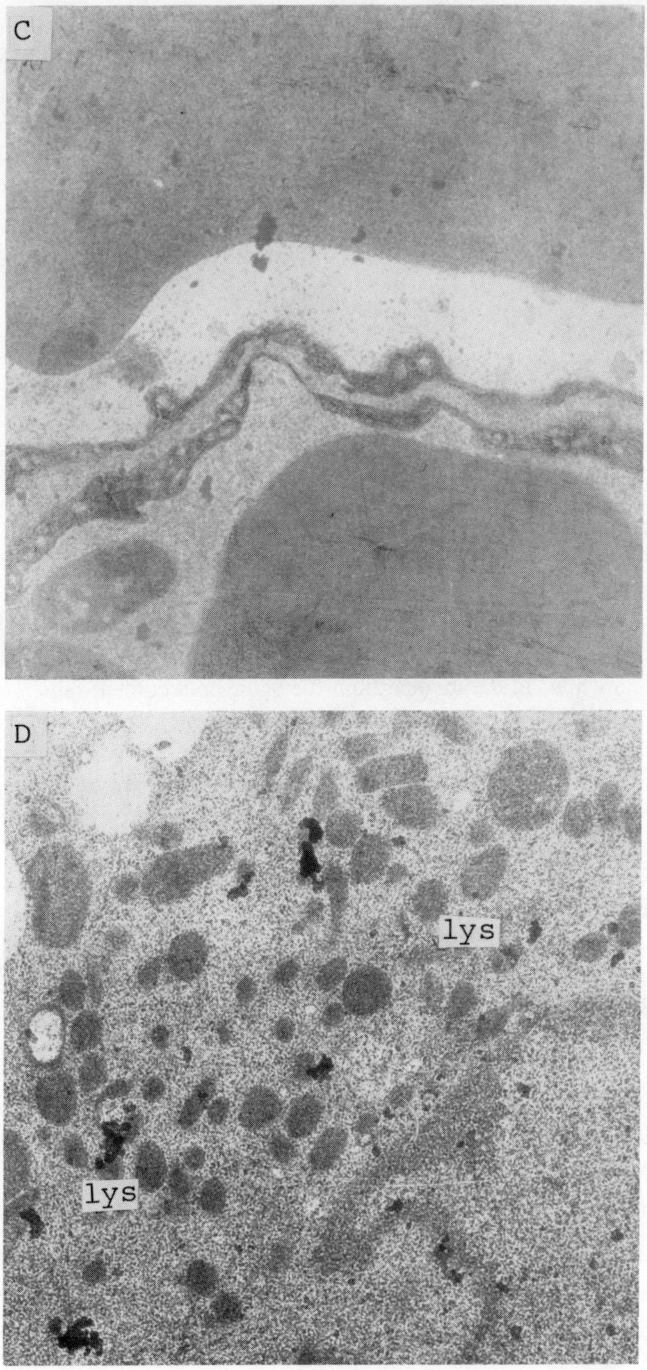

FIGURE 19C and D.

glycoproteins and glycolipids.[150] It seemed probable that glycoprotein hydrolysis by excess trypsin in stress could decrease the myocardial content of sialic acid and thereby diminish calcium binding in the zone immediately adjacent to the sarcolemma.

The biochemical indices were assayed 2 h after the end of stress exposure. *N*-Acetyl neuraminic (sialic) acid was determined in plasma and myocardial homogenates from control

TABLE 14
Effect of Prolonged Immobilization Stress on Sialic Acid, Trypsin, and Antitrypsin Levels in Myocardium and Serum

		Immobilization		
Indices	**Control (n = 12)**	**3 h (n = 10)**	**6 h (n = 11)**	**9 h (n = 12)**
Sialic acid				
Myocardial (nmol/mg wet wt)	1.27 ± 0.05	1.06 ± 0.05[a]	0.96 ± 0.05[a]	0.77 ± 0.06[a]
Serum, total (mmol/l)	3.72 ± 0.17	3.82 ± 0.17	3.77 ± 0.16	5.12 ± 0.26[a]
Serum, free (mmol/l)	0.05 ± 0.002	0.05 ± 0.001	0.05 ± 0.001	0.10 ± 0.007[a]
Trypsin activity				
Serum (μmol/l·s)	52.09 ± 5.73	75.28 ± 6.01[a]	94.78 ± 6.73[a]	141.85 ± 12.7[a]
α_1-Antitrypsin				
Serum (g/l)	1.74 ± 0.05	1.56 ± 0.05[a]	1.48 ± 0.05[a]	1.20 ± 0.06[a]

[a] $p < 0.05$.

and stress animals by a modified thiobarbituric method of Horgan.[151] Trypsin, α_1-antitrypsin, and α_2-macroglobulin were measured by agarose gel electrophoresis according to German et al.[150]

Table 14 shows that sialic acids in plasma are elevated only after a 9-h immobilization stress with the total content and the free fraction exceeding the control by 37 and 80%, respectively. Meanwhile, in the myocardium the sialic acid content falls proportionately to stress duration, declining by 39% after 9 h of immobilization.

The trypsin activity in plasma exceeds the control level by 44, 82, and 173% after 3, 6, and 9 h of stress, respectively. It is noteworthy that the increased proteolytic activity is accompanied by a decline in the major trypsin inhibitor α_1-antitrypsin responsible for 90% of the total antitryptic activity in serum.

On the whole, the data in this Section serve to emphasize that the pathogenesis of cardiac stress damage is not reducible to direct cardiomyocyte injury by various stress hormones and secondary ischemic injury resulting from stress shifts and coronary thrombosis. Disorders caused by stress in other organs through a variety of pathways also lead to heart damage.

However, the multiplicity of the pathogenetic mechanisms of cardiac stress damage does not change the basic fact that the ultimate target of all these mechanisms is the cardiomyocyte. It is essential in this context that many of the phenomena described above (myocardial stress rigidity, enhanced cardiac sensitivity to external Ca^{2+}, enzyme leakage from isolated stress heart, destruction of glycocalix, and finally the focal contractural injury to cardiomyocytes) provide unequivocal evidence to the impairment of cardiomyocyte membranes and systems of ionic, first of all calcium transport.

VII. ACTIVATED LIPID PEROXIDATION AND CARDIOMYOCYTE MEMBRANE INJURY IN STRESS

Cardiomyocyte membrane injury by the excessive lipotropic effect of stress, as already pointed out, is determined by the lipid triad, namely overactivation of phospholipases and lipases, direct damage by lysophosphatides and acyl carnitine, and overactivation of free-radical lipid peroxidation. The first two factors have already been the subject of comprehensive reviews.[153,154] Studies of the disturbances to the free-radical homeostasis in cardiac damage, and in stress in particular, have only recently been initiated.[155]

In 1979 we demonstrated that EPS is accompanied by enhanced chemoluminescence of lipids isolated from the cardiac muscle.[156] This fact per se indicated that stress may activate free-radical oxidation in the myocardium. Then we determined the primary (hydroperoxides of polyenic lipids) and final LPO products (fluorescing Schiff bases) in the heart, skeletal muscle, and brain of rats that had undergone EPS,[157] and found that they are all reliably increased already in 2 h after stress and for the next 2 to 3 d.

Thus, exposure to stress entails activation of lipid peroxidation, which is most pronounced in the heart and maintained for a long period.

A medically important question is to what extent this issue, proved experimentally in animals, is applicable to man. It is known that LPO activation in animals, through decomposition of lipid hydroperoxides and β-cleavage of the alkoxyl radicals, yields lower hydrocarbons. These gases are released with the exhaled air and their content is a specific and sensitive criterion of the intensity of LPO processes. Basing on this, Prilipko et al.[158] measured the gaseous LPO products in the exhaled air to elucidate whether or not LPO is activated in humans under stress caused by intense intellectual work under time shortage.

The stress exposure consisted in operator work requiring consecutive solution of seven complicated enough mental tasks in certainly too little time; the overall duration of such load was 2 h. The amounts of gaseous LPO products in the exhaled air and of catecholamines in the blood were assayed 24 h and 15 min before stress, during stress, and up to 5 d after. In the quantitative analysis of hydrocarbons in the exhaled air we reasoned from the fact that the preferred LPO substrate are the ω-6-unsaturated fatty acid residues and correspondingly the predominant gaseous LPO product would be pentane. Therefore, pentane was measured to ensure maximal sensitivity. Of the 20 healthy persons studied, 13 were subjected to stress.

Figure 20 depicts the typical chromatograms of exhaled air before (1) and after (2) stress. The first peak on the left of each chromatogram corresponds to pentane: one can see that the pentane content is appreciably higher after stress. Before stress the pentane content in the exhaled air was 1.71 ± 0.34 nmol/l and the epinephrine and norepinephrine contents in the blood were 0.70 ± 0.05 and 0.8 ± 0.05 μg/l, respectively. Upon stress there was an immediate but relatively short elevation of blood catecholamines and a slower but prolonged elevation of exhaled pentane (Figure 21); this reflects the excitation of the adrenergic system typical of stress that precedes maximal LPO activation.

The results obtained show that in humans, as well as in animals, an emotiogenic stress influence (not associated with direct damage to the organism from exogenous physical or chemical factors) elicits substantial activation of peroxidation as manifest by increased amounts of exhaled gaseous LPO products.

It is essential that in the cell membranes LPO activation is not isolated, but inseparably linked with activation of lipases and phospholipases, detergent action of lysophosphatides and acyl carnitine, and excessive entry of Ca^{2+} into the cell. One of the manifestations of cell membrane damage in this case is the "stress enzymemia", i.e., release of both cytoplasmic and lysosomal enzymes into the blood.

Indeed, the activities of aspartate transaminase, alanine transaminase, lactate dehydrogenase, and malate dehydrogenase have been shown to increase twofold in 2 h after EPS.[1] Acid cathepsins decrease by 25% in the myocardial lysosomal-mitochondrial fraction and increase by 45% in the supernatant. Their activity in plasma is elevated more than twice. This leakage of cytosolic and lysosomal enzymes is completely abolished by the β-blocker propranolol as well as by the antioxidant ionol (butylated hydroxytoluene), i.e., results in great measure from catecholamine-induced LPO activation.[159] The mechanism of LPO activation in stress will be considered in Chapter 5, which also presents data on LPO activation in ischemia and on antioxidant protection of the heart. Here it is important that, first, the β-adrenergic membrane stress damage linked with LPO activation can be documented for the heart, and second, that it can be blocked with propranolol. *A priori,* one can envisage that LPO activation, lysosomal labilization, and membrane injury in any case affect such membrane-bound enzymic systems central to cardiac function as the Na,K and Ca pumps.

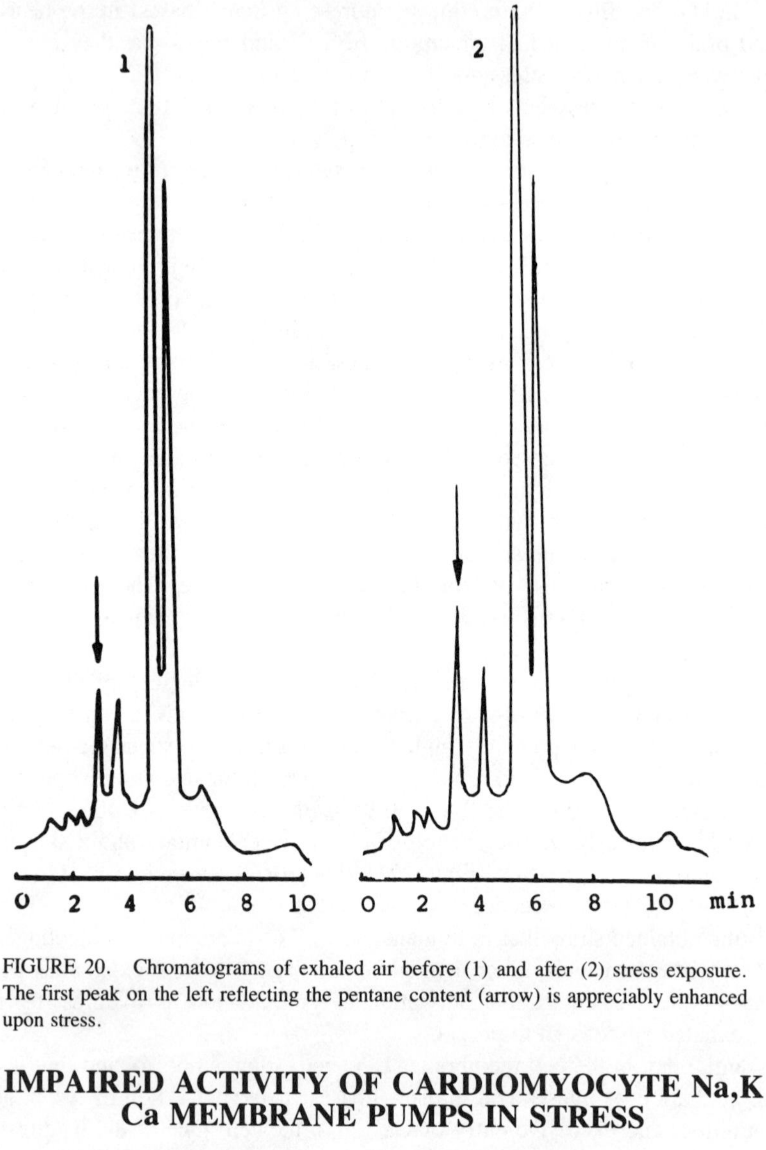

FIGURE 20. Chromatograms of exhaled air before (1) and after (2) stress exposure. The first peak on the left reflecting the pentane content (arrow) is appreciably enhanced upon stress.

VIII. IMPAIRED ACTIVITY OF CARDIOMYOCYTE Na,K AND Ca MEMBRANE PUMPS IN STRESS

The sarcolemmal Na,K pump is known to play a decisive part in maintaining the transmembrane cation gradient, the Na^+/Ca^{2+} exchange on the sarcolemma, normal cell calcium concentration, and thereby the physiological values of rest potentials, generation and conduction of action potentials, and the electric stability of the heart as a whole.

We have studied the effect of EPS on the Na,K ATPase activity in cardiac muscle and the action of a β-blocker in this system.[160] The Na,K ATPase activity in the myocardium of rats subjected to EPS proved to decrease by 25%, and this could be prevented by prior administration of propranolol.

Further, this study was reproduced in greater detail. ATPase activity was assayed in the sarcolemmal fraction by P_i accumulation with and without ouabain.[161] Protein was determined according to Lowry. Heat denaturation was carried out at 50 to 60°C. The thermodenaturation kinetics was detrmined and the thermodynamic parameters calculated as described.[162]

The diagram in Figure 22 shows that upon stress, the sarcolemmal Na,K ATPase activity decreased by 28%, and this could be prevented with the β-blocker propranolol or the antioxidant ionol, i.e., the decrease resulted from β-induced LPO activation. Interestingly,

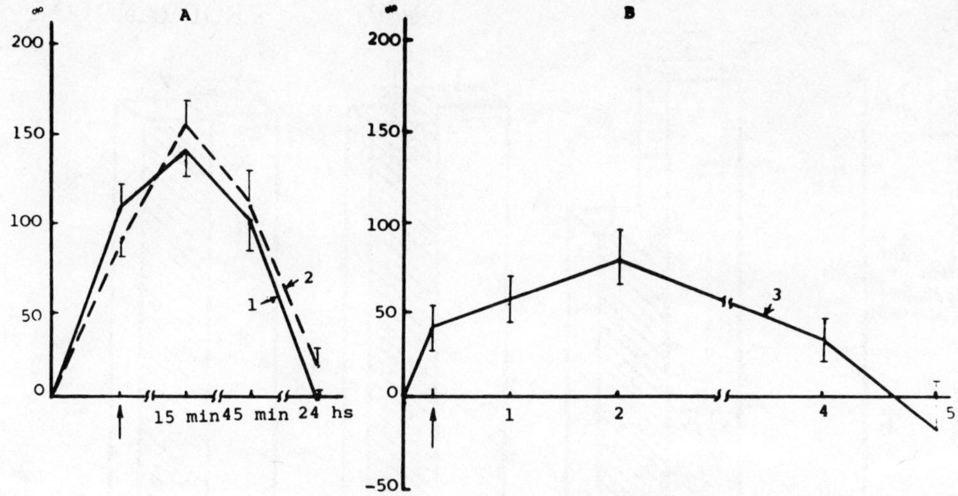

FIGURE 21. Dynamics of (A) catecholamines in blood and (B) pentane in exhaled air of subjects in and after stress. 1, Epinephrine; 2, norepinephrine; 3, pentane. The abscissa is time after the end of stress (arrows denote the values obtained during stress exposure); the ordinate is the percent excess over initial levels.

the ATPase inactivation could be reproduced *in vitro* by inducing LPO with the Fe-ascorbate system, and also prevented with ionol.

Taken together, these data furnish evidence that the mechanism "β-adrenergic LPO activation → Na,K ATPase inactivation" is actually operative in stress. The nature of damage to the sarcolemmal Na,K ATPase system was elucidated by studying the effects of stress and antioxidant on the dynamics of ATPase inactivation during heat denaturation.

Figure 23 presents the results of studies with rat myocardial sarcolemmal membrane preparations. One can see that upon EPS the enzyme loses activity much more rapidly, so that the half-inactivation time decreases by half (Figure 23A). Stress increases the denaturation rate constant for the Na,K ATPase, as shown in Figure 23B where the shaded zone quantitatively reflects this effect. It is essential that administration of ionol to animals (50 mg/kg body weight) prior to stress completely prevents such stress alterations.

The thermodynamic parameters of Na,K ATPase heat inactivation in Table 15 reveal two basic facts: the lower activation energy and a smaller change in entropy during denaturation of the enzyme from stress animals. In essence they both mean that *the stress itself brings the Na,K ATPase protein-lipid complex closer to the denatured state; these changes are prevented by prior suppression of free-radical lipid oxidation.*

Considering the decisive role of the Na,K ATPase in maintaining the rest potential (RP), one could suppose that impaired activity of this enzymic system in stress would in some way affect the ability of cardiomyocytes to preserve this principal parameter of electric stability.

In our experiments the RP was measured in isolated hearts perfused with a Krebs-Henseleit solution (pH 7.4, oxygenated with 98% 0_2/2% CO_2) at a constant hydrostatic head of 100 mm to sustain the electric and contractile activity. The heart was perfused at 36°C and the RP was recorded within ±1 mV with a glass electrode from the left ventricular surface. Then the heart was chilled to 4°C by perfusing it with a cold solution, and the RP dropped. Then the temperature of the perfusing solution was returned to 36°C and the dynamics of RP restoration was monitored.

Figure 24 shows that in the control group (curve 1) the cooling decreases the RP from −80 to −45 mV; a subsequent rise from 4 to 36°C entails restoration and overshoot of the RP to a maximum of −100 ± 5 mV in 2 to 2.5 min. The restoration rate at the half-

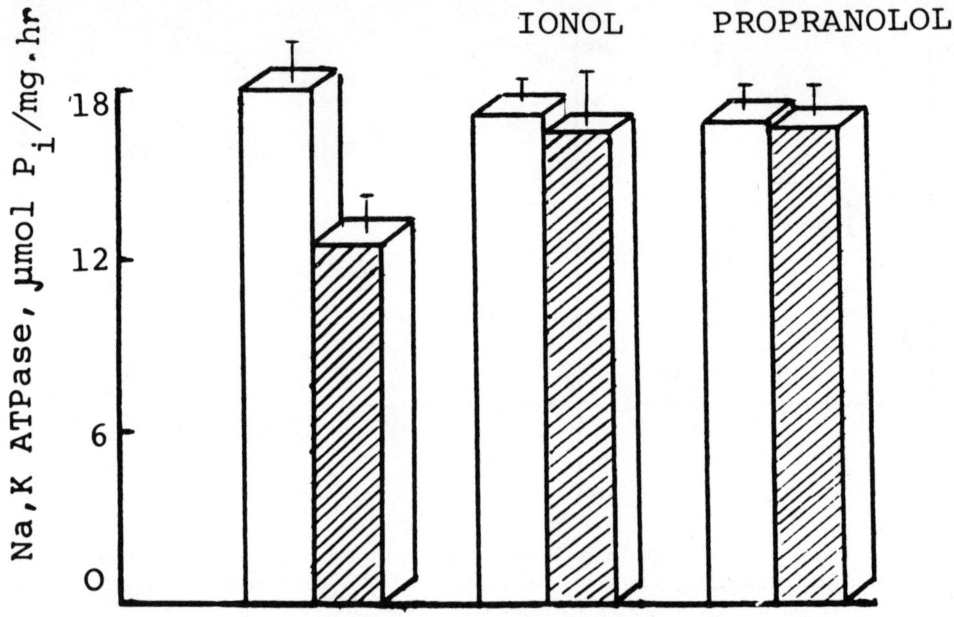

FIGURE 22. Prevention of the stress-induced inhibition of the myocardial sarcolemmal Na,K ATPase with the antioxidant ionol (butylated hydroxytoluene) and the β-blocker propranolol. Empty blocks, control; shaded blocks, stress.

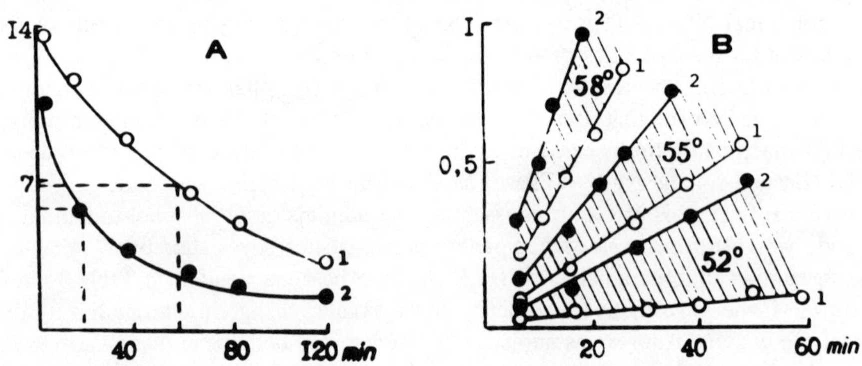

FIGURE 23. Heat inactivation of rat cardiac sarcolemmal Na,K ATPase. (A), Enzyme activity at 52°C in the control (1) and after EPS (2). The abscissa is time in min; the ordinate is activity in μmol/h per mg protein. (B), Changes in the denaturation rate constant (K = 2.303 tgα) with temperature (52°C, 55°C, 58°C). The abscissa is time in min; the ordinate is lg A_o/A_t where A_o is the initial and A_t the current activity.

maximal point was about 0.7 mV/s. In animals subjected to EPS (curve 2) the RP was initially diminished by 10 mV; upon cooling it fell to −35 ± 2 mV; in the course of restoration there was no hyperpolarization and the restoration rate did not exceed 0.2 mV/s, i.e., less than one third of the control. Prior administration of ionol to animals (50 mg/kg daily for 3 d before the experiment) prevented the stress-induced impairment of RP restoration. Curve 3 in Figure 24 is close to the control one, showing that the restoration rate and hyperpolarization are retained despite the experienced stress. Thus, *under certain conditions the β-induced LPO activation can be involved in the damage to the Na,K ATPase system and electric stability of cardiomyocytes.*

TABLE 15
Parameters of Heat Denaturation of Rat Myocardial Sarcolemmal Na,K ATPase, Effect of Stress and Antioxidant

Indices	Control (n = 26)	Stress (n = 26)	Ionol (n = 20)	Ionol + stress (n = 20)
E_a	75.6 ± 2.3	60.7 ± 2.0[a]	72.5 ± 2.8	72.1 ± 3.3
ΔH*	75.0 ± 2.3	60.1 ± 2.0[a]	71.9 ± 2.8	71.5 ± 3.3
ΔS*	156.8 ± 0.6	111.3 ± 3.6[a]	149.3 ± 2.4	146.7 ± 2.6
ΔF*	24.4 ± 1.5	23.7 ± 1.9	24.3 ± 1.6	23.9 ± 1.6

Note: E_a, Activation energy (kcal/mol); ΔH*, enthalpy change (kcal/mol); ΔS*, entropy change (kcal/mol. degree); ΔF*, free energy change.

[a] Difference from control significant at $p < 0.001$.

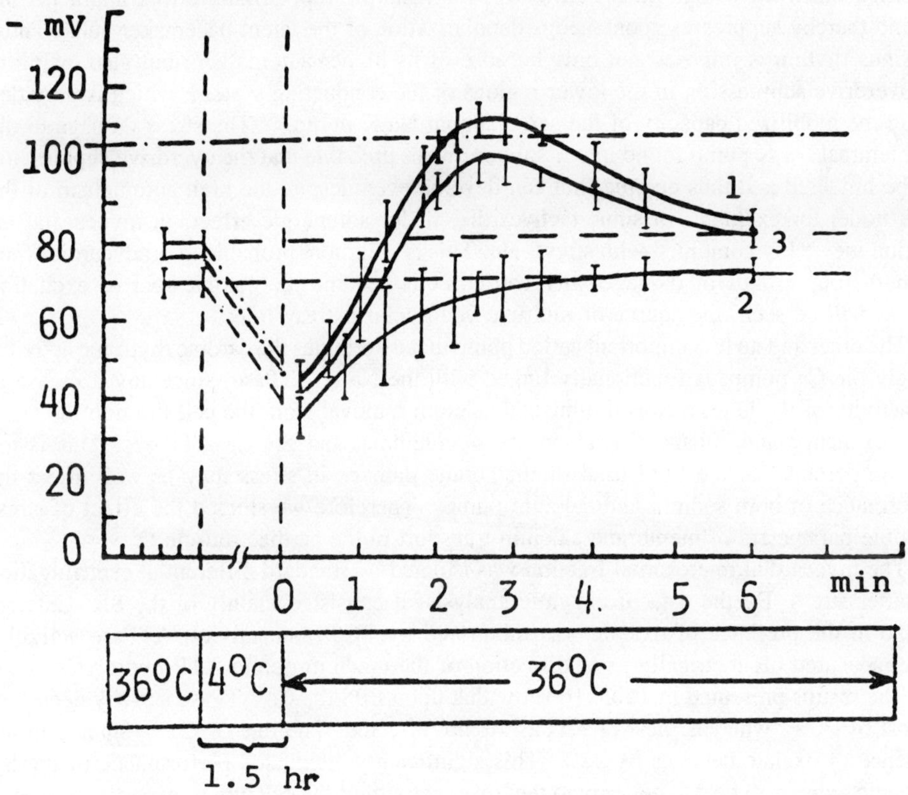

FIGURE 24. Effect of cooling and subsequent warming of isolated rat heart on the rest potential of left ventricular cardiomyocytes. The abscissa is time before and after cooling in min; the ordinate is the RP in mV. 1, Control; 2, stress; 3, ionol plus stress.

It should be borne in mind that the role of such disturbances is quite well known in modern arrhythmology. In the healthy heart the impulse from the sinus node having the highest automatism depolarizes any latent pacemakers before they can depolarize themselves. However, higher automatism and timely depolarization are not the sole mechanism by which the sinus node suppresses latent pacemakers. An important part is played by the phenomenon known as overdrive suppression. Stimulation of the cells of the conducting system and working myocardium at a frequency exceeding their own results in enhanced Na^+ entry into the cells, with ensuing marked activation of the Na,K pump; since sodium extrusion is

TABLE 16
Effect of EPS on the Enzymic System of Ca^{2+} Transport in the SR Vesicles

Indices	Control	Stress
Ca ATPase (nmol P_i/min per mg protein)	502 ± 68 (n = 12)	359 ± 127[a] (n = 10)
Mg ATPase (nmol P_i/min per mg protein)	694 ± 113 (n = 12)	642 ± 153 (n = 10)
Calcium uptake rate (nmol Ca^{2+}/min per mg protein)	37.2 ± 4.0 (n = 10)	23.1 ± 4.2[b] (n = 8)

[a] $p < 0.01$.
[b] $p < 0.001$.

increased much more than potassium entry, the resulting repolarizing efflux augments the RP and thereby suppresses spontaneous depolarization of the latent pacemaker cells. Thus, the sinus rhythm is imposed not only because of its higher automatism, but also owing to the overdrive suppression in the lower regions of the conducting system, which is provided for by the mobilized capacity of the sarcolemmal Na,K pump.[163] The stress damage to the sarcolemmal Na,K pump found in our studies makes probable that the overdrive suppression can be hindered and thus ectopic foci can develop even despite the high automatism of the sinus node; for example, in sinus tachycardia, under adrenergic effect, in myocardial infarction inevitably combined with stress, etc. This is still more probable in bradycardia when the numerous groups of damaged myocardial cells become the ectopic foci of excitation and, as will be seen, the source of multiple ventricular extrasystoles.

The other and no less important cation pump that determines the cardiac rhythmic activity, namely the Ca pump, is functionally linked with the Na,K ATPase, since any decrease in the activity of the latter means diminished calcium removal from the cell through the Na^+/Ca^{2+} exchange and enhanced load on the sarcolemmal and SR Ca ATPases. This is the more important that the lipid triad of membrane damage in stress may as well affect the performance of both sodium and calcium pumps. Therefore we studied the effect of stress on some parameters of membrane calcium transport in the cardiac muscle.[164]

The myocardial microsomal fraction was isolated by standard differential centrifugation 2 h after stress. By the data of enzymic analysis, it consisted mainly of the SR. Calcium uptake in the presence of oxalate was monitored by ^{45}Ca radioactivity. ATPase activities were measured pH-metrically as acidification of the medium due to ATP hydrolysis.

The results presented in Table 16 show that upon EPS the Ca ATPase activity decreases almost by 30%, whereas the Mg ATPase is not affected. The rate of Ca^2+ uptake in the presence of oxalate declines by 38%. This significantly attenuated performance of the SR Ca pump appears to be due not only to the lower activity of the calcium transporting enzyme, but also to a greater calcium permeability of damaged SR membranes.

For a more precise evaluation of the role that depressed calcium pumping activity may play in the damage to cardiac function and electric stability in stress, together with Sazontova and Vovk we undertook a study of calcium uptake by SR vesicles from control animals and those subjected to 1- to 2-h and 6-h immobilization stress of capitulation. Since it has been shown earlier that a 2-h stress of this type diminishes cardiac resistance to the contractural and arrhythmogenic action of calcium, these experiments allowed a quantitative comparison of the stress damage to cardiac calcium resistance and to the SR calcium pump function.

The rate of calcium uptake by the SR vesicles in the presence of oxalate was determined with a Ca-selective electrode and an Orion® EA 940 ion meter. Mitochondrial uptake was prevented with NaN_3. The uptake was monitored for 5 min with 50 to 200 μl homogenate

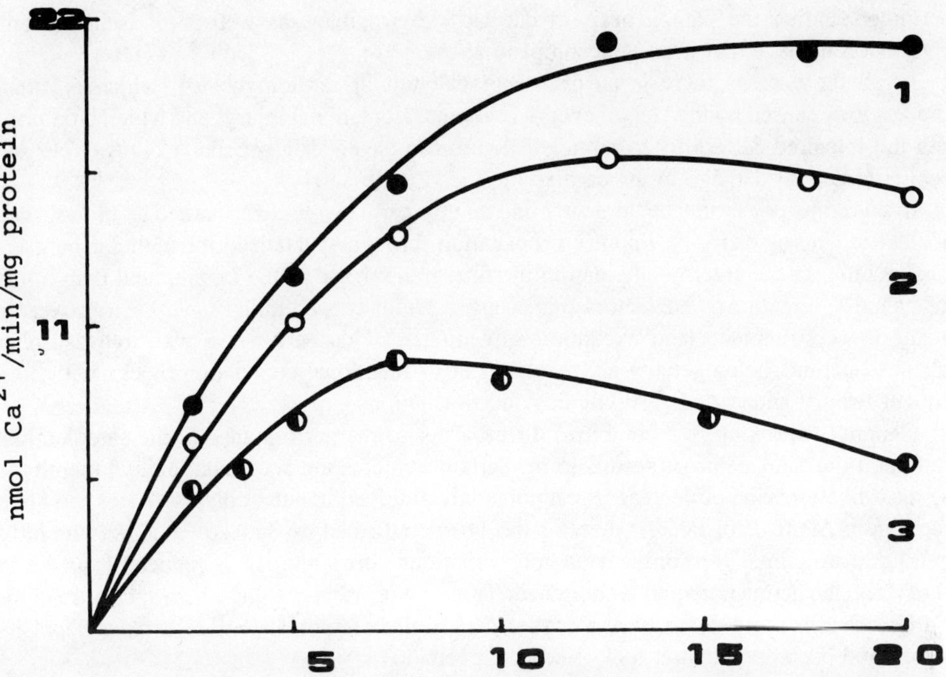

FIGURE 25. Effect of immobilization stress on the Ca^{2+} transport by rat myocardial SR vesicles. The abscissa is μM Ca^{2+}; the ordinate is nmol Ca^{2+}/min per mg protein. 1, Control; 2, 6-h stress; 3, 1-h stress.

added to 5 ml of 100 m*M* KCl, 15 m*M* potassium oxalate, 20 m*M* Hepes pH 7.0, 4 m*M* $MgCl_2$, 5 m*M* NaN_3, 4 m*M* ATP, and 1 to 20 μM $CaCl_2$. The rates were then determined by drawing tangents to the reaction curves 1.5 min after the onset and quantitated using calibration curves.

Figure 25 demonstrates the dependence of the calcium uptake rate on its concentration in the medium. It can be seen that in control SR the uptake rate increases with the ion concentration, reaching a plateau in the region 10 to $20 \cdot 10^{-6}$ *M*.

After a 1-h stress, the maximal rate is attained already at $7.5 \cdot 10^{-6}$ *M* and is only 9.4 nmol/min·mg protein as compared to 16.2 in the control. Further rise in the external concentration of Ca^{2+} inhibits its transport; at 20 μM it decreases by more than one third of the maximum and proves to be 3.5 times lower than the corresponding control value.

Curve 2 in Figure 25 shows that a 6-h stress causes qualitatively similar, but much less pronounced alterations; thus, instead of the depression of uptake at high concentrations, here one can only see a tendency to this. At the highest calcium concentration tested (20 μM) the uptake rate after 6 h of stress is 25% lower.

Thus *there is no doubt that the immobilization stress of capitulation impairs the calcium-uptake ability of the SR. It is also obvious that this is not just a test-tube artifact, since (see the end of Section II) it is the immobilization stress that markedly aggravates the propensity of the isolated heart to respond by contracture to elevated calcium in the perfusing fluid. Furthermore, the physiological and the biochemical results concur in one quite important feature: a short capitulation stress is much more effective than a long one both in impairing the calcium uptake by the SR and in aggravating the calcium-induced contracture*. Such an unexpected and ostensibly paradoxical dependence of the extent of damage on the duration of the capitulation stress is probably due to the appearance of some stabilizing factor already in the course of the stress reaction, and deserves becoming the subject of special study. Here we must emphasize that the stress damage to calcium transport proved above is essential for understanding the pathogenesis of cardiac stress damage as well as of ischemic and reperfusion damage that usually accompany stress.

In all these cases there is an excess of calcium in cardiomyocytes, which is either adrenergic or caused by the lack of energy or direct sarcolemmal injury, and which combined with the impaired SR ability to remove calcium can engender a peculiar vicious circle and focal contractural damage to the cardiac muscle.

In this context it should be borne in mind that the cardiac muscle is marked by pronounced bioelectric heterogeneity.[165] Impulse propagation through specialized intercellular contacts is more rapid in the anterograde than in the retrograde[166] and in the longitudinal than in the transverse[167] directions. All factors increasing calcium concentration have been proved to impair the cell contacts and excitation spreading.[168] This becomes a plausible cause of enhanced cardiac heterogeneity and evolvement of functional conduction blocks with consequent reentry and various arrhythmias and fibrillation.

Generally speaking, the combined disturbances to the performance of the sarcolemmal Na,K and the SR Ca pumps results in the sarcoplasmic cation accumulation and thereby is the most likely reason of decreased rest potentials observed in our studies with isolated heart (see Figure 24). It is of interest that this has been confirmed by Sudakov et al.[169] who have found that in animal cardiomyocytes upon emotional stress the RP is reduced from 83 to 69 mV and the action potential is shortened. Those myocardial regions where such alterations of bioelectric activity occur have a higher probability of spontaneous or evoked depolarization, and become potential foci of ectopic excitation.

It is noteworthy that the stress-induced decrease in the RP is in line with the observations of Wit and Cranefield[170] that *in vitro* norepinephrine can not only lower the RP by diastolic depolarization, but also trigger the automatism of a quiescent myocardial cell. It is not hard to envisage that in damaged cells with reduced RP the appearance of such adrenergically originating foci of automatism is rather probable, and they may be actuated by additional adrenergic influences, owing to the weaker inhibitory control from the sinus node, or by impulses arriving in the relative-refractory period.

On the whole, the above testifies that the lipid triad and in particular enhanced lipid peroxidation naturally found in stress damages the sarcolemmal membrane and its Na,K pump as well as the Ca pump of the SR. These defects are the key link in the pathogenetic chain of cardiac stress damage and may play a weighty part in the impairment of cardiac electric stability and evolvement of arrhythmias.

IX. STRESS DAMAGES TO CARDIAC STRUCTURES

Stress damages to cardiac function, electric stability, cation pumps, energy metabolism, and even DNA, all had a distinguishing feature which we maybe failed to clearly outline, namely their pronounced reversibility in the overwhelming majority of the myocardial cells. This is in conformity with our starting concept that the stress reaction evolved as a link of organismic adaptation to the environment, and causes damage only when excessively enhanced. Nevertheless, at the climax of the stress reaction and in certain groups of cells the stress damage finds its morphological equivalent which we made a point of study.

Our electron-microscopic investigations together with Frolov have shown that stress mainly affects the cell and intracellular membranes. The sarcolemma loses its distinct outline, becomes blurred, and in some places completely disintegrates. Normal myocardial nuclei possess a clear double-bordered nucleolemma, whereas in EPS the nucleolemma loses its integrity, and chromatin can be seen to escape from the nucleus through the ruptures. The myocardium of intact rats has few lysosomes, all of them with clearly defined membranes. In stress their number increases and their membranes become less distinct or altogether destroyed. A typical feature of the stress myocardium is the alterations in its capillaries: severe edema of endothelial cells, pronounced pinocytosis in the capillary walls in EPS.

In whole, these data correlate well with the biochemical evidence to the stress damage to membranes, nuclear DNA, and lysosomes, emphasizing thus the importance of studying further the vascular component of the stress damage.

The second step of this research was prompted by the biochemical data on the stress depression of the SR calcium pump and the physiological data on the attenuated resistance of the stress heart to excess calcium. This work[66] was an attempt to assess the amount and distribution of calcium in the cardiomyocytes in stress by combining electron-microscopic and histochemical techniques.

Left ventricular posterior papillary muscle was obtained from animals 2 and 48 h after exposure to stress and fixed with 4% paraformaldehyde in 0.6 *M* phosphate (pH 7.2). To locate calcium, the material was incubated with 2% potassium pyroantimonate,[171] 1% Os O_4, pH 7.0 to 7.1 for 1 h at 4°C, and then embedded in Araldite-Epon. Sections were poststained with lead hydroxide and uranyl acetate. Preparations incubated with 5 m*M* EGTA for 1 h prior to fixation served as control for the specificity of histochemical staining.

In control papillary muscle pretreated with EGTA (Figure 26A) there are no deposits of calcium pyroantimonate, and the cells have normal ultrastructure. Figure 26B demonstrates the localization of calcium in control myocardial cells: the deposits are seen in the SR terminal cisternae, the N strips of myofibrillar I discs, and are lacking or negligible in the subsarcolemmal space and mitochondria. (Occasional granular deposits in mitochondria appear to be nonspecific and not calcium pyroantimonate. A similar result was obtained in mitochondrial studies[171] and is in line with the biochemical data that indicates the calcium concentration in papillary muscle mitochondria of normal rats is relatively low.[172]

The micrographs in Figure 26C and 26D depict the myocardial ultrastructure 2 h after stress. One can see (Figure 26C: calcium-depleted material, no deposits) that shortly after stress there are moderate ultrastructural changes such as swelling of T-system elements and sarcomere contraction manifest as strips of contraction in place of the Z lines. Simultaneously the localization of intracellular calcium is somewhat altered: deposits are enhanced in the subsarcolemmal space, in the sarcoplasm among the myofibrils, and around mitochondria (Figure 26D). Increased amounts of disperse deposits are also observable in the myofibrils proper, especially in the strips of contraction.

The most demonstrative results were obtained 48 h after stress. Figure 26E (no calcium deposits) shows a significantly greater number of dilated elements of the T system and SR in most cardiomyocytes; there is also peculiar shrinkage of mitochondria with condensed matrix and enhanced osmophilicity of mitochondrial membranes. Simultaneously the calcium pyroantimonate deposits are markedly increased in the subsarcolemmal space, sarcoplasm, myofibrils, and especially around mitochondria (Figure 26F).

Such enhanced sarcoplasmic calcium content as we have observed in stress constitutes, according to the modern data, a common pathogenetic link of the most various forms of myocardial damage — from hereditary cardiopathies to the failure of hypertrophied heart — and becomes the cause of calcium cardiotoxicity and, in particular, of the myocardial stress rigidity described above.[87]

The next step of our research[173] combining light transmission and polarization microscopy, yielded the most essential morphological result that the membrane injury and ensuing calcium triad of cell damage are not at all uniform through the stress myocardium, but, on the contrary, reach their maximum in certain spatially separated groups of cardiomyocytes, i.e., become the basis of profound but focal damage and subsequent noncoronarogenic cardiosclerosis.

These morphological studies have determined that soon after stress the myocardium develops focal alterations which gradually lead to complete muscle cell contracture in 39 to 45 h. In some cases the contracture is attended with cell death followed by their resorption and formation of fibroplastic granuloma; in other cases the contracture regresses and the cell structures are restored.

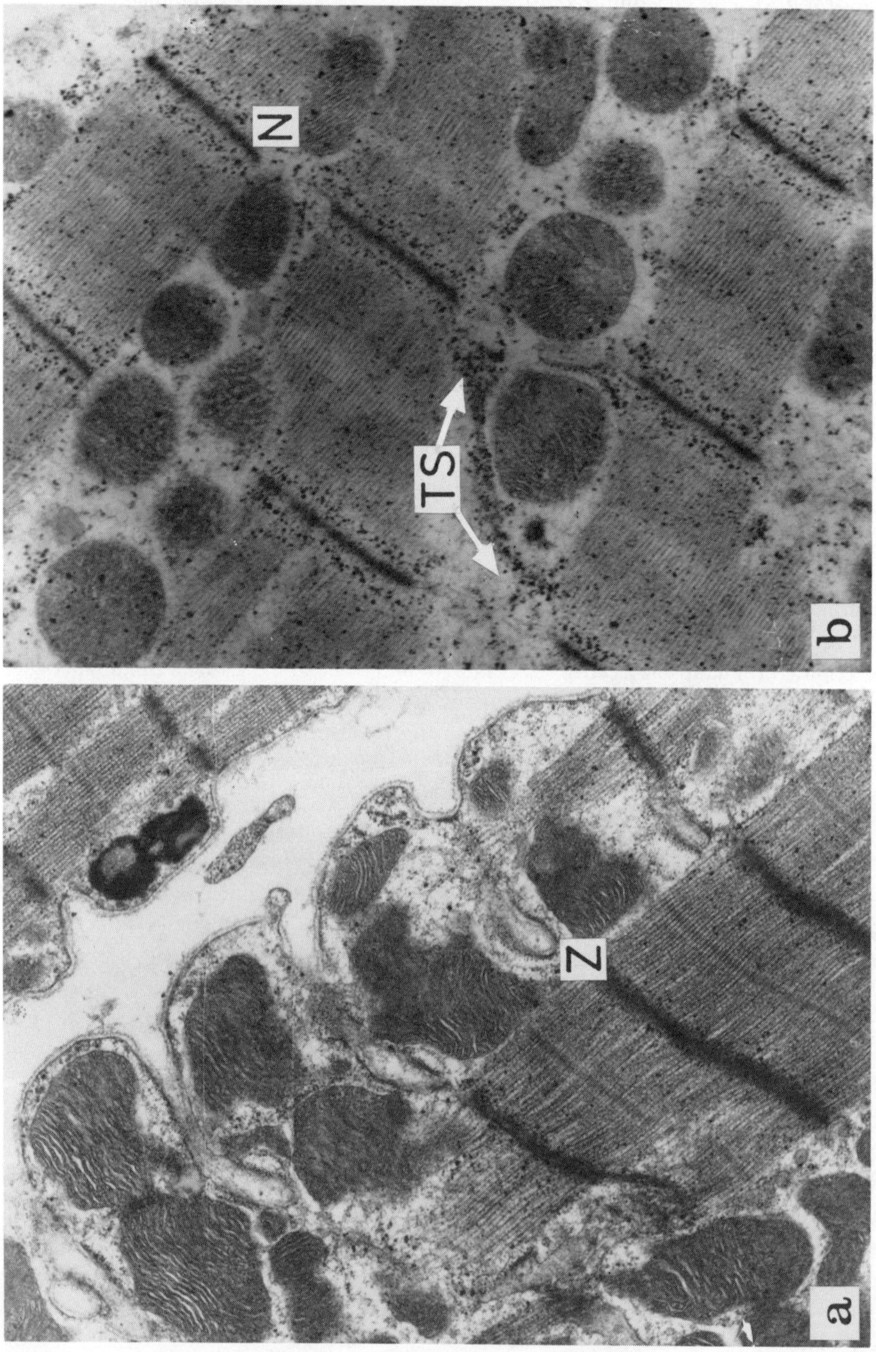
N
TS
b
Z
a

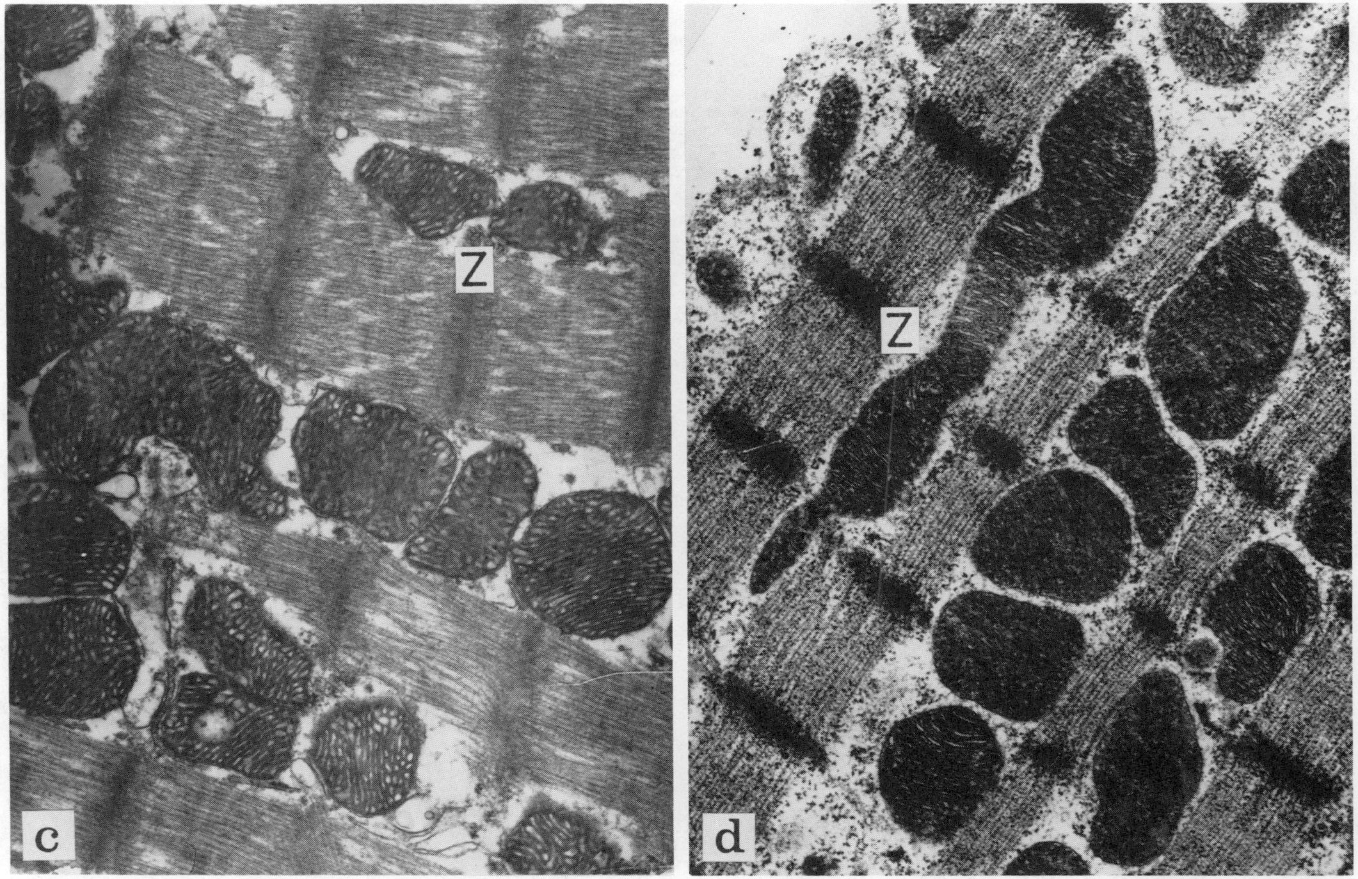

FIGURE 26. Influence of EPS on cardiomyocyte ultrastructure and calcium localization. (a) and (b), Intact myocardium; (c) and (d), 2 h after EPS; (e) and (f), 48 h after EPS. (M), Mitochondria; (N), the N strips of the I discs; (TC), terminal cisternae of the SR; (Z), the Z lines; arrows indicate dilated elements of the T system. Calcium localization is revealed in deposition of calcium pyroantimonate. (a), (c), and (e), Controls for the reaction specificity, pretreated with EGTA to remove calcium.

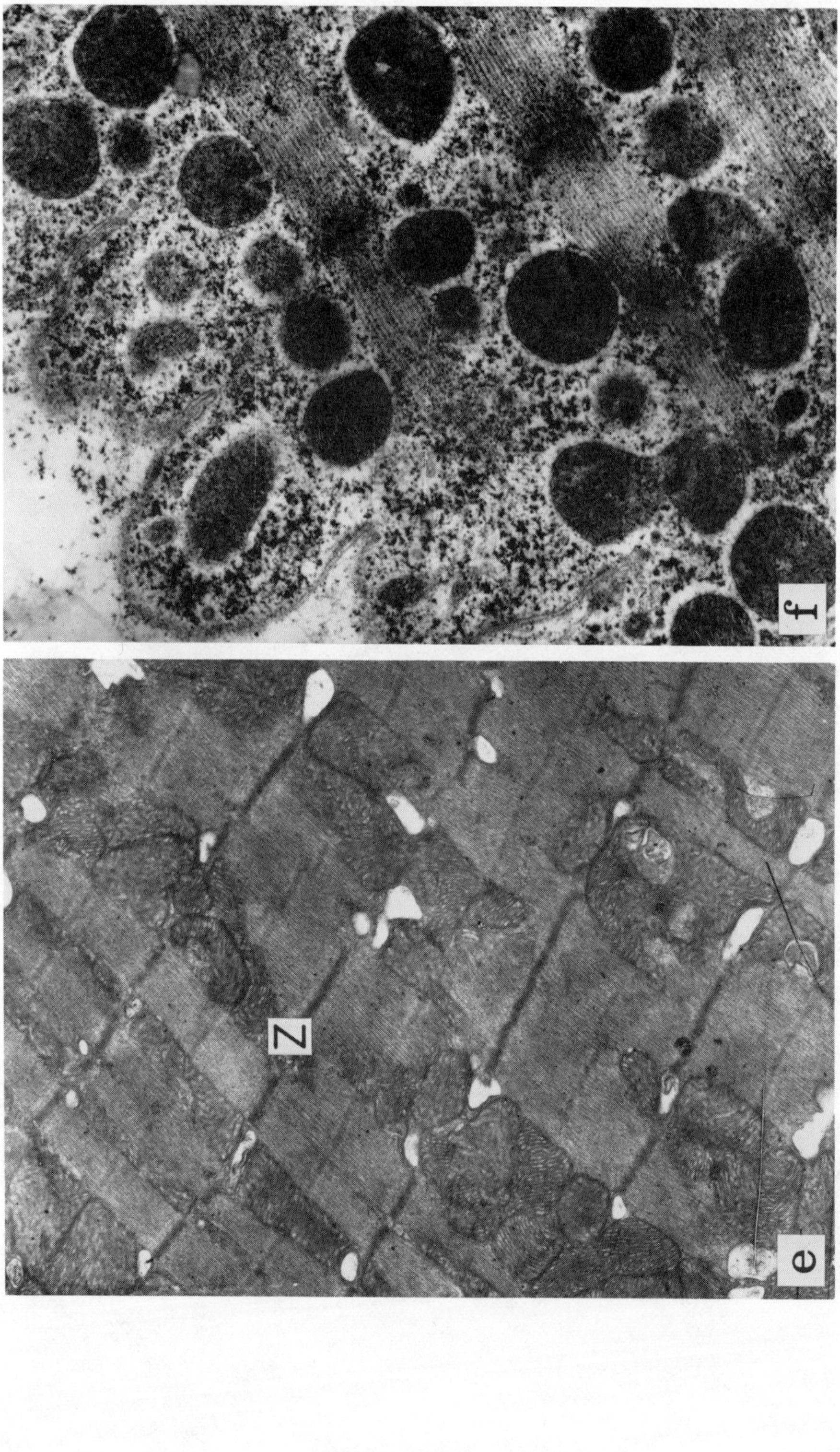

FIGURE 26E and F.

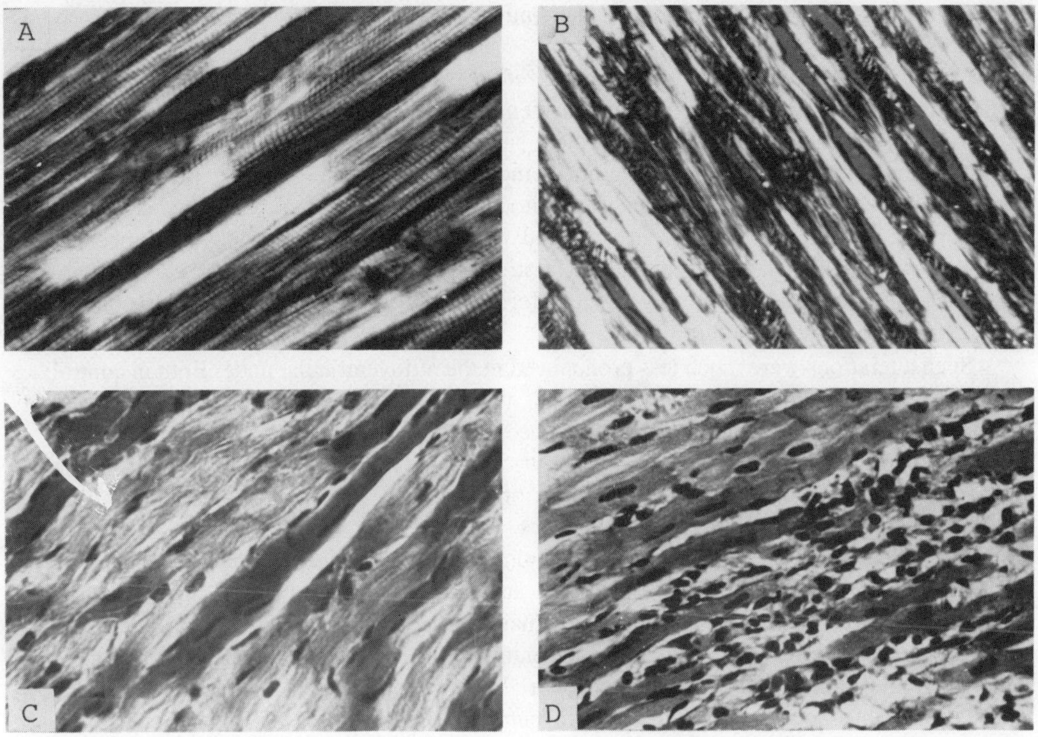

FIGURE 27. Rat myocardial damage 45 h after stress termination. (a) and (b), polarized light microscopy; (c), Pearls' reaction for iron; (d), staining with hematoxylin-eosin. (Magnification: a, × 197; b, × 49; c, × 126; d, × 49.) For explanations see text.

Figure 27 shows that 45 h after stress (i.e., in the phase of maximal morphological alterations) there is deep myocardial contracture with the merging of the A discs of the myofibrils, here and there forming anisotropic conglomerates (Figure 27A); a large number of such contracturally altered muscle fibers with pronounced anisotropy are shown at lower magnification (Figure 27B). Figure 27C shows the staining for iron and Figure 27D demonstrates formation of cell infiltrate around necrotic muscle fibers, with pyknotically altered nuclei and fiber homogenization in the necrotic locus.

Again it should be emphasized that these irreversible changes are microfocal, affect only a minority of cardiomyocytes, and just for this reason, on the one hand, may not tell on the myocardial function some time after a single stress, but, on the other, have at least two unfavorable consequences. First, they aggravate myocardial heterogeneity which, combined with impaired ionic transport, may to a large extent precondition arrhythmogenesis. Second, such damages accumulating in inevitable repeated stress exposures may underlie gradually progessive noncoronary cardiosclerosis.

Finally, our electron-microscopic study of the sinus node and downstream regions of the conducting nervous system was prompted by the widely observed and typical feature of the stress heart in the whole organism: disparity between normal parameters of contractility and markedly upset electric stability. In animals subjected to stress or receiving β-agonists, such disorders as ectopic arrhythmias or AV block occur only on the background of pronounced vagal bradycardy, which in its turn results from diminished resistance of sinus automatism to the negatively chronotropic action of the vagus nerve.

In accordance with this we[174] aimed our work at elucidating the ultrastructural changes elicited by a 6-h immobilization stress in the conducting system and contractile myocardium, and correlating the stress alterations in the sinus node with its resistance to the negatively chronotropic vagal effect.

In controls, the sinus node was characterized by exclusive location of colloid lanthanum (added during specimen fixation to assess membrane permeability),[175] in the intercellular space along the sarcolemma, and by typical small mitochondria with few cristae (Figure 28A). In the sinus nodes from stress animals the lanthanum particles clearly penetrated not only into the sarcoplasm, but also into the mitochondrial matrix of specific node cells, and the number of cristae was markedly reduced in mitochondria, some of which appeared "empty" (Figure 28B). The sinus nodes in stress specimens were also marked by disappearance of the normally present glycogen, formation of lipid droplets in the sarcoplasm, foci of myofibrillar contracture.

Such alterations were much less pronounced in the atrioventricular node. Both in control (Figure 28C) and stress (Figure 28D) animals the colloid lanthanum is mainly distributed along the sarcolemma in the intercellular space, and only occasionally penetrates into the sarcoplasm in stress. However, in the atrioventricular node region as well as in the contractile myocardium stress gave rise to a large number of contractural cells with distinct myofibrillar overcontracture (Figures 28E and 28F).

We failed to reveal any stress-induced ultrastructural changes in the subendocardial Purkinje fibers. On the whole, a qualitative analysis of electron micrographs suggests a decreasing downstream gradient of stress damage to the cardiac conducting system, alterations being maximal in the sinus node and minimal in the Purkinje fibers. A quantitative analysis shows that the number of mitochondrial cristae per unit area decreases in stress by 35% in the sinus node, by 19% in the atrioventricular node, and by 15% in the contractile myocardium of the interventricular septum.

Taken together, these data point to the preferential damage to the conducting system and first of all to the sinus node as compared to the contractile myocardium. All this is in line with the concept that stress is a weighty arrhythmogenic factor, and various damages to the sinus node upset the resistance of its automatism to the impeding action of the vagus nerve and may cause the known sinus node dysfunction syndrome[176-178] and diverse arrhythmias. Similarly, preferential or selective injury to the upstream regions of the conducting system, exemplified in Figure 28, may contribute to the evolvement of various functional and stable blocks, reentry, and grave arrhythmias. In particular, we have observed auricular and AV blocks, atrioventricular dissociation in conditions of pronounced vagal bradycardy in animals with adrenergically injured heart; these disorders were apparently determined by (1) sinus node dysfunction and profound depression of its automatism and (2) impairment of the atrioventricular node and other parts of the conducting system.

By and large, the body of morphological evidence fits into the hypothesis of selective or preferential stress damage to the cardiac conducting system, and makes expedient further morphological studies that would allow a comparison of the state of the contractile myocardium and of the different regions of the conducting system in stress.

X. THE PATHOGENETIC CHAIN OF CARDIAC STRESS DAMAGE

The scheme in Figure 29 is an attempt at summarizing the data on cardiomyocyte stress damage. It shows that in stress situations the excitation of the higher vegetative centers determining the stress reaction constitutes the first link of the process, exposing the heart to greatly increased concentrations of catecholamines, parathyroid hormones, probably vasopressin, histamine, and other agonists of the Ca-mobilizing receptors. This results in activation of two regulatory systems — adenylate cyclase and IP_3-DAG (the second link). The ensuing third link comprises the lipid triad (activation of LPO; lipases and phospholi-

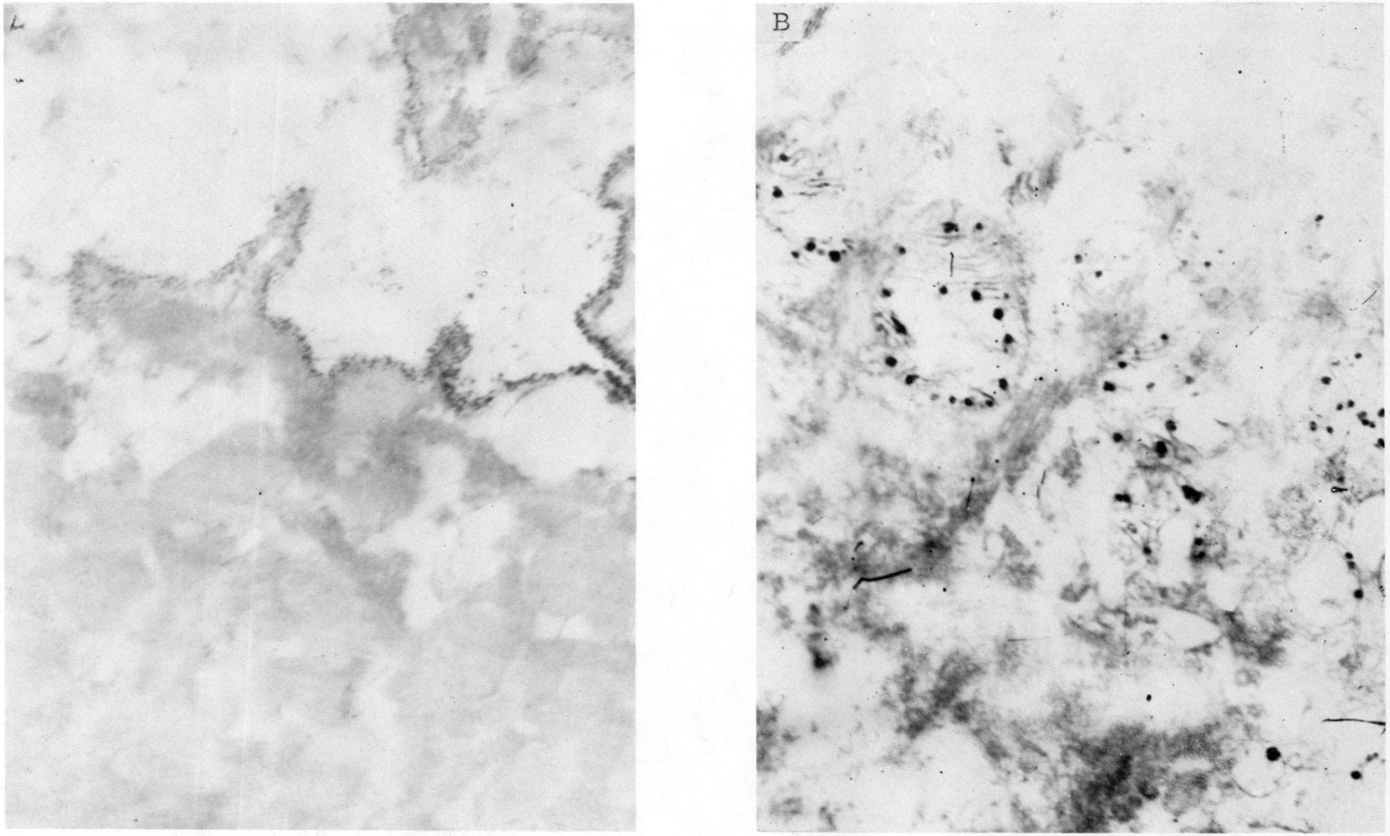

FIGURE 28. Ultrastructure of the conducting system and myocardium in stress. (A), Control, sinus node. Small mitochondria with few cristae are distributed in the sarcoplasm. Colloid lanthanum particles are seen in the intercellular space and do not penetrate through the sarcolemma. (Magnification × 5700.) (B), Stress, sinus node. Colloid lanthanum particles are found in the sarcoplasm of specific cells, on mitochondrial membranes, and in the mitochondrial matrix. (Magnification × 5700.)

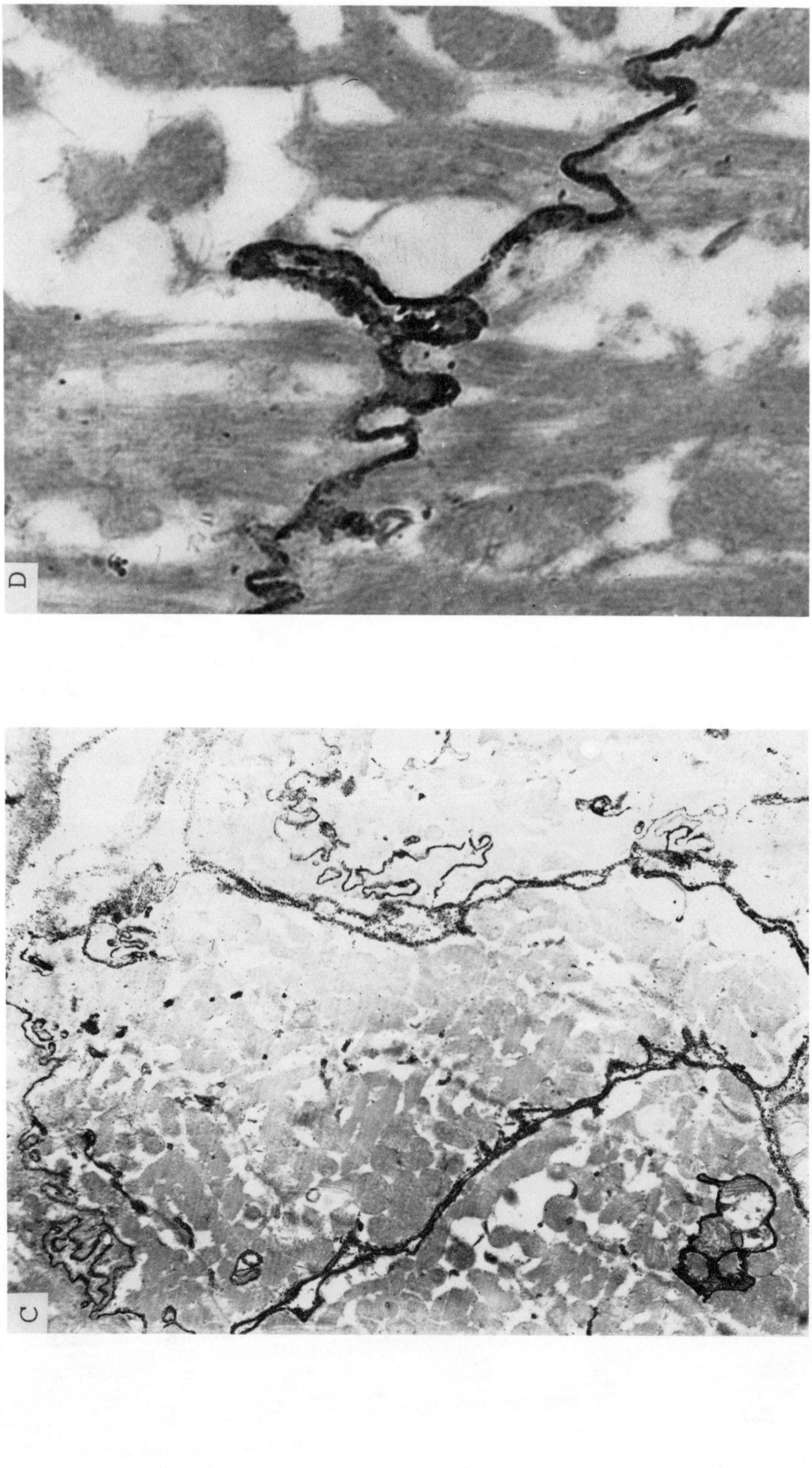

FIGURE 28. (C,D). (C), Control, atrioventricular node. Colloid lanthanum stains the intercalated discs. (Magnification × 5700.) (D), Stress, atrioventricular node. Colloid lanthanum particles are distributed in the intercellular space and on the outer surface of the sarcolemma, staining the intercalated discs of two specific conducting cells (center and top), penetrate into the cell (bottom right), and line the mitochondrial membranes without entering the matrix. (Magnification × 3200.)

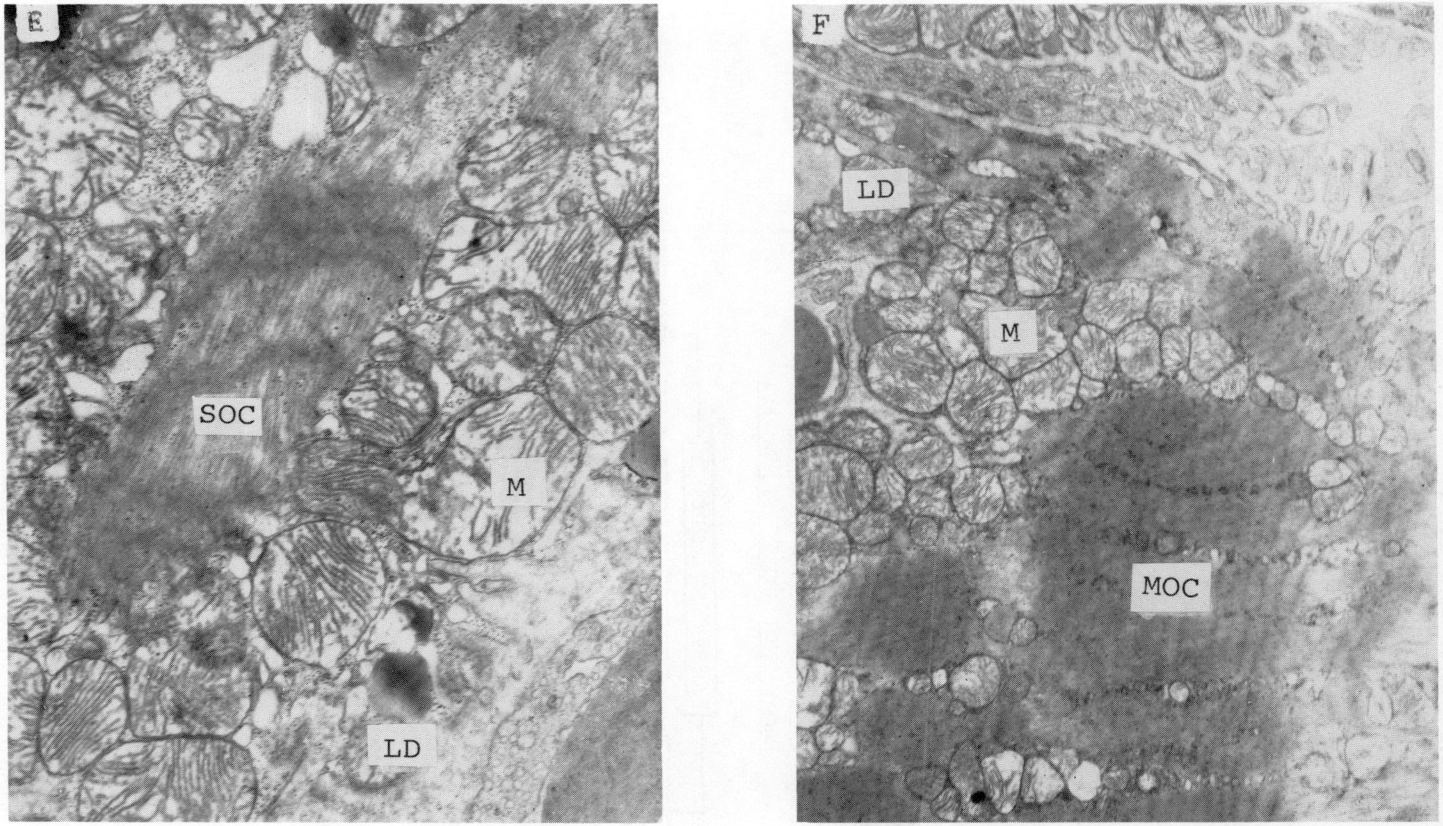

FIGURE 28. (E,F). (E), Stress, atrioventricular node. (LD), Lipid droplet; (M), mitochondria; (SOC), strips of overcontraction. (Magnification × 7200.) (F), Stress, interventricular septal myocardium. (LD), Lipid droplet; (M), mitochondria; (MOC), myofibrillar overcontraction encompassing more than 20 sarcomeres. (Magnification × 5700.).

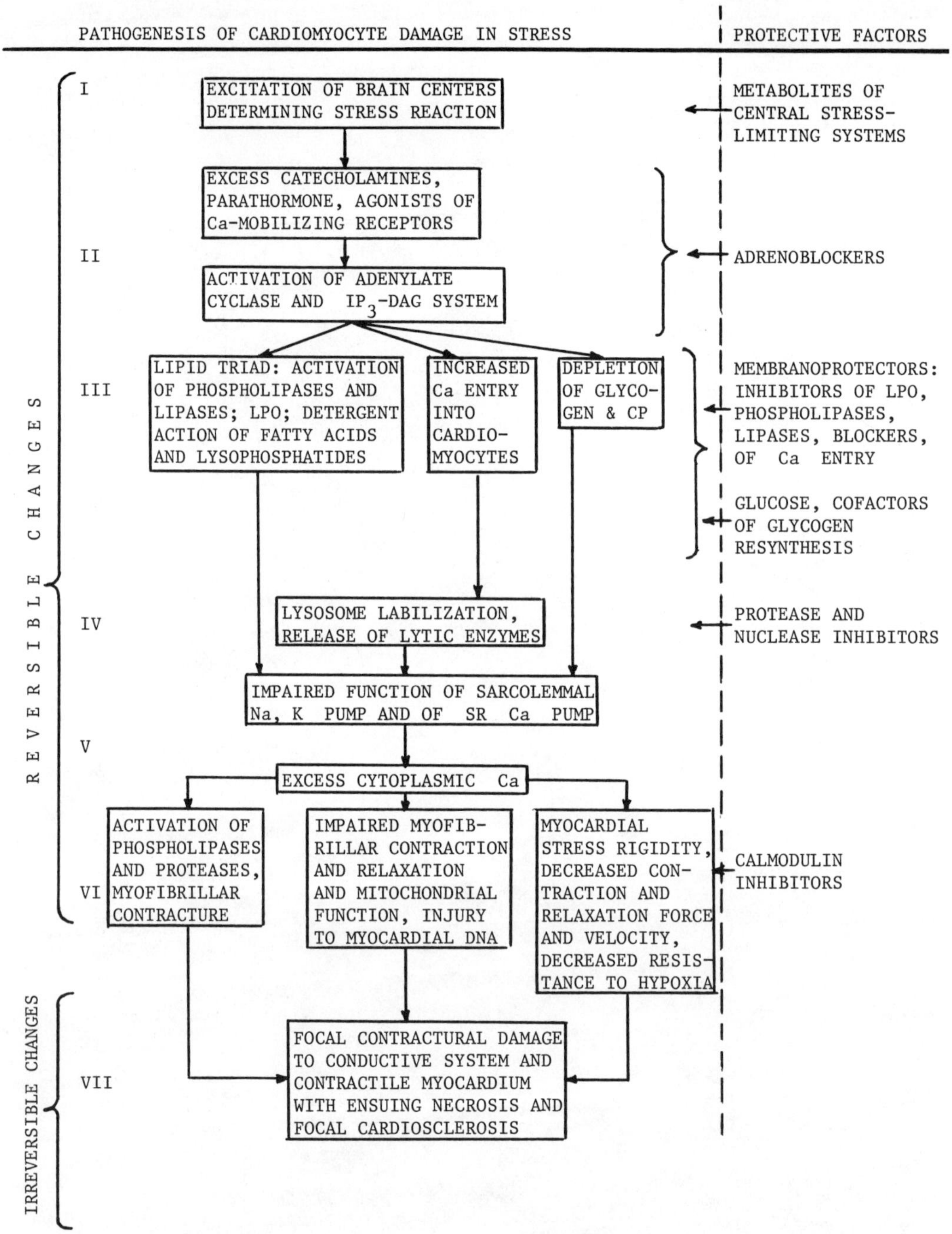

FIGURE 29. Pathogenetic scheme of stress damage to the cardiomyocyte. For explanations see text.

pases; and detergent action of lysophosphatides, acyl carnitine, and long-chain fatty acids), enhanced calcium entry, and mobilization of glycogen and creatine phosphate stores. Subsequent injury to lysosomal membranes releases lytic enzymes (the fourth link), which, together with the lipid triad and glycolytic defects, cause damage to the sarcolemmal and SR membranes responsible for calcium transport, and impair the performance of the sarcolemmal Na,K pump and the SR Ca pump (the fifth link). It is important that, among other consequences, there is a common outcome of the impairment of these two cation pumps. Depressed function of the Na,K pump increases the intracellular Na^+ content, thereby hindering Ca^{2+} removal from the cells and thus contributing to its increasing level, similar to the action of cardiac glycosides. Depressed function of the SR Ca pump diminishes calcium uptake into the SR and also contributes to its increasing cytoplasmic content. Combined with the enhanced calcium entry, all this gives rise to a real excess of intracellular calcium. This serious alteration has at least two sequelae. First, it can activate the set of processes constituting the lipid triad and thereby close the vicious circle aggravating myocardial membrane damage. Second, it is itself directly detrimental to the cells, causing the calcium triad composed of myofibrillar contracture, impaired function of calcium-overloaded mitochondria, and activation of myofibrillar proteases and mitochondrial phospholipases; this makes the damage still worse (the sixth link).

In most cardiomyocytes this chain is stopped at some point owing to an ''automatic blocking'' system inherent in the mechanism of the stress reaction and to the specialized stress-limiting systems (see Chapters 4 and 5); the alterations undergo regression, and at the level of the whole heart it goes no further than transient disturbances of its contractile function and electric stability, which will be dealt with in Chapter 2. Yet, in some cardiomyocytes, irreversible myofibrillar contracture always develops with ensuing necrobiosis and microfocal noncoronarogenic cardiosclerosis (the seventh link).

Of course, the scheme covers only the direct stress damage to the cardiomyocyte, leaving out such pathogenetic mechanisms as stress coronary spasm, thrombosis, stress-imposed load on the heart, or liver-mediated coronary sclerosis. In all these cases the stress may provoke absolute or relative ischemia, which becomes the immediate detrimental factor. Accordingly, they will be considered in the section devoted to the place of stress in the ischemic disease (Chapter 2). Here, in considering the primary stress (i.e., mainly adrenergic) damage to the cardiomyocyte, let us deal with some issues of substantial clinical import.

First, the above discussed disturbances of metabolism, structure, and function were observed after the cessation of stress; hence they are not just a reaction to stress, but relatively stable sequelae of a damage inflicted during stress. This fact, together with the vast clinical data, give grounds for believing that it is such metabolic and functional disturbances, persisting after the stress reaction has passed, that accumulate from stress episode to episode and may be involved in primary noncoronarogenic cardiosclerosis and chronic heart failure, which not infrequently develop in persons who previously had no circulatory disorders.

Second, adrenergic and parasympathetic regulation are known to be most widely represented in the cardiac conducting system,[179] which is also the most dependent for its energy provision on glycolysis profoundly upset in stress.[180] This may apparently be the cause of preferential stress damage to the conducting system, for example, the right-branch block of the bundle of His occurring early in practically healthy persons, or more grave blocks and arrhythmias in the advanced age.

Third, the right part of the scheme in Figure 29 presents some possible means of protection against the stress damage stemming from the concept of its pathogenesis. Further on, the reader will have an opportunity to see that most of these possibilities have been realized in our experiments either through preliminary adaptation which mobilizes the protective stress-limiting systems of the organism, or administering the metabolites of these systems and other chemical factors.

Fourth and finally, the data presented on the disturbances to the energy metabolism and membrane ionic transport have been obtained upon a single stress not very rich in emotiogenic moments. The observed injury to the conducting system (sinus node) and the working myocardium (focal damage) drastically increase the heterogeneity of the heart and, as we shall see, upset its electric stability. However, repeated, diverse, and — most importantly — emotionally tense stress situations abounding in the real life of animals and people would cause greater stress reactions and accordingly much greater damage. This is in our opinion the angle from which to analyse not only the electric disorders and fatal arrhythmias in animals, but also the idiopathic, often neurogenous, arrhythmias and sudden death in man, which is now known to occur without any alterations in the coronary bed (see Chapter 2). These extremely important stress pathologies of the heart will be the subject of further consideration.

REFERENCES

1. **Meerson, F. Z.,** *Adaptation, Stress and Prophylaxis,* Springer-Verlag, Berlin, 1984.
2. **Archakov, A. I.,** *Microsomal Oxidation* (in Russian), Nauka, Moscow, 1975.
3. **Salganik, R. I., Manankova, N. M., and Semenova, L. A.,** The hypocholesterolemic effect of rat liver microsomal enzyme induction (in Russian), *Vopr. Med. Khim.* 4, 468, 1977.
4. **Simonov, P. V.,** Physiology of emotions and conditional reflex activity (in Russian), in *Physiology of Higher Nervous Activity,* Nauka, Moscow, 1970, 4.
5. **Viru, A. A. and Kyrge, P. K.,** *Hormones and Sports Efficiency* (in Russian), Fizkultura i Sport, Moscow, 1983.
6. **Filaretov, A. A.,** *Regulatory Principles and Mechanisms of the Hypophysial-Adrenocortical System* (in Russian), Nauka, Leningrad, 1987.
7. **Golikov, P. P.,** *Receptor Mechanisms of the Glucocorticoid Effect* (in Russian), Meditsina, Moscow, 1988.
8. **Munck, A., Guyre, P. M., and Holbrook, N.J.,** Physiological functions of glucocorticoids in stress and their relation to pharmacological actions, *Endocrin. Rev.,* 5, 25, 1984.
9. **Meerson, F. Z., Malyshev, V. V., Ekimov, E. N., Petrova, V. A., and Lifant'ev, V. I.,** Effect of adaptation of the organism to short stress exposures on the realization of stress reaction, impairment of the cardiac metabolism and contractile function caused by prolonged emotional-pain stress (in Russian), *Vop. Med. Khim.* 1, 76, 1986.
10. **Mikulaj, L., Kvetnansky, R., Murgas, K., Parizkova, J., and Vencel, P.,** Catecholamines and corticosteroid in acute and repeated stress, in *Catecholamines and Stress,* Usdin, E., Ed., Pergamon Press, Oxford, 1976, 445.
11. **Kvetnansky, R., Sun, C. L., Lake, C. R., Thoa, N., Torda, T., and Kopin, I. Y.,** Effect of handling and forced immobilization on rat plasma levels of epinephrine, norepinephrine and dopamine-beta-hydroxylase, *Endocrinology,* 103, 1868, 1978.
12. **Galbo, H., Holst, J. J., and Christensen, N. J.,** Glucagon and plasma catecholamine responses to graded and prolonged exercise in man, *J. Appl. Physiol.,* 38, 70, 1975.
13. **Kellner, K., Hecht, K., Marck, H., and Aquino, A. M.,** Das Verhalten von Schilddrüsenhormonen, Kortikosteron, Adrenokortikotropen Hormon und Insulin in Rattenplasma unter Stressbedingungen, *Z. Gesamte inn. Med. Ihre Grenzgeb.,* 35, 418, 1980.
14. **Slepushkin, V. D., Lishmanov, Yu. B., Zoloev, G. K., and Prum, I. A.,** Modern concepts of some unorthodox neuroendocrine mechanisms of stress (in Russian), *Usp. Fiziol. Nauk,* 16, 106, 1985.
15. **Shephard, R. J. and Sidney, K. H.,** Effect of physical exercise on plasma hormone and cortical level in human subjects, *Exercise Sport Sci. Rev.,* 3, 1, 1975.
16. **Geyssant, A., Geelen, G., Denis, Ch., Allevard, A. M., Vincent, M., Jarsaillon, E., Bizollon, C. A., Lacour, J. R., and Gharib, Cl.,** Plasma vasopressin, renin activity, and aldosterone: effect of exercise and training, *Eur. J. Appl. Physiol.,* 46, 21, 1981.
17. **James, D., Burleigh, K. M., Kraegen, E. W., and Chisholm, D. J.,** Effect of acute exercise and prolonged training on insulin response to intravenous glucose *in vivo* in the rat, *J. Appl. Physiol.,* 55, 1660, 1983.
18. **Chirkov, A. M., Chirkova, C. K., and Startsev, V. G.,** *Emotional Stress in Apes* (in Russian), Nauka, Leningrad, 1987.
19. **Pierce, G. N., Rich, T. L., and Langer, G. A.,** Trans-sarcolemmal Ca^{2+} movements associated with contraction of the rabbit right ventricular wall, *Circ. Res..* 61, 805, 1987.
20. **Berridge, M. J.,** Calcium: a universal second messenger, *Triangle,* 24, 79, 1985.
21. **Berridge, M. J.,** Inositol triphosphate and calcium mobilization, *J. Cardiovasc. Pharmacol.,* 8 (Suppl 8), S85, 1986.
22. **Berridge, M. J.,** Inositol triphosphate and diacyl glycerol as second messengers, *Biochem. J.,* 220, 345, 1984.

23. **Abdel-Latif, A. A.,** Calcium-mobilizing receptors, polyphosphoinositides, and the generation of second messengers, *Pharmacol. Rev.*, 38, 227, 1986.
24. **Combettes, L., Berton, B., and Claret, M.,** Phospholipid second messengers and calcium, *Biochimie,* 69, 281, 1987.
25. **Meerson, F. Z., Samosudova, I. V., Glagoleva, E. V., Shimkovich, M. V., and Belkina, L. M.,** Impairment of myocardial contractile function and ultrastructure upon emotional-pain stress (in Russian), *Arkh. Anat. Gistol. Embriol.*, 2, 43, 1983.
26. **Csapo, Z., Dusek, J., and Rona, G.,** Early alterations of the cardiac muscle cells in isoproterenol-induced necrosis, *Arch. Pathol.* 93, 356, 1972.
27. **Takasu, N., Hashimoto, H., Miyazaki, Y., Ito, T., Ogawa, K., and Satake, T.,** Effects of phospholipase inhibitors and calcium antagonists on the changes in myocardial phospholipids induced by isoproterenol, *Basic Res. Cardiol.*, 83, 567, 1988.
28. **Fleckenstein, A., Frey, M., and Fleckenstein-Grün, G.,** Myocardial and vascular damage by intracellular calcium overload. Preventive action of calcium antagonists, in *Calcium Entry Blockers and Tissue Protection,* Godfrain, Th., Ed., Raven Press, New York, 1985, 91.
29. **Emilsson, A. and Gudbjarnason, S.,** Changes in fatty acyl chain composition of rat heart phospholipids induced by noradrenaline, *Biochim. Biophys. Acta,* 664, 82, 1984.
30. **Franson, R. C., Pang, D. C., and Weglicki, W. B.,** Modulation of lipolytic activity in isolated canine cardiac sarcolemma by isoproterenol and propranolol, *Biochem. Biophys. Res. Commun.* 90, 956, 1979.
31. **Takasu, N., Miyazaki, Y., Ogawa, K., and Satake, T.,** Activation of phospholipases play a role in the development of isoproterenol-induced myocardial damage, *J. Mol. Cell. Cardiol.*, 18 (Suppl. 1), 227, 1986.
32. **Häggendal, J., Jönsson, L., Johansson, G., Bjurström, S., Carlsten, J., and Thoren-Tolling, K.,** Catecholamine-induced free radicals in myocardial cell necrosis on experimental stress in pigs, *Acta Physiol. Scand.*, 131, 447, 1987.
33. **Kogan, A. Kh., Kudrin, A. N., and Nikolaev, S. M.,** On the question of the role of free-radical lipid peroxidation in the pathogenesis of epinephrine cardionecroses (in Russian), *Patol. Fiziol. Eksp. Ter.* 1, 66, 1979.
34. **Hirata, F. and Axelrod, J.,** Phospholipid methylation and biological signal transmission, *Science,* 209, 1082, 1980.
35. **Vladimirov, Yu. A.,** Free-radical lipid oxidation and physical properties of the biological membrane lipid bilayer (in Russian), *Biofizika,* 32, 830, 1987.
36. **Katz, A. M. and Messineo, F. C.,** Lipid-membrane interactions and the pathogenesis of ischemic disease in the myocardium, *Circ. Res.*, 48, 1, 1981.
37. **Shud, A. L. and Subramanian, R.,** Modification of adenine nucleotide translocase activity during myocardial ischemia, *Z. Kardiol.*, 76 (Suppl. 5), 26, 1987.
38. **Cao, Y.-Z., Choy, K. O. P. C., and Chan, A. C.,** Regulation by vitamin E of phosphatidylcholine metabolism in rat heart, *Biochem. J.*, 247, 135, 1987.
39. **Fiehn, W. and Hasselbach, W.,** The effect of phospholipase A on the calcium transport and the role of unsaturated fatty acids in ATPase activity of sarcoplasmic vesicles, *Eur. J. Biochem.*, 13, 510, 1970.
40. **Torda, T., Yamaguchi, I., Hirata, F., Kopin, I. J., and Axelrod, J.,** Quinacrine-blocked desensitization of adrenoreceptors after immobilization stress or repeated injection of isoproterenol in rats, *J. Pharmacol. Exp. Ther.*, 216, 334, 1981.
41. **Clark, M. G., Patten, G. S., Filsell, O. H., and Rattigan, S.,** Co-ordinated regulation of muscle glycolysis and hepatic glucose output in exercise by catecholamines acting via α-receptors, *FEBS Lett.*, 158, 1, 1983.
42. **Winder, W., Beattie, M. A., and Holman, R. T.,** Endurance training attenuates stress hormone responses to exercise in fasted rats, *Am. J. Physiol.*, 243, R179, 1982.
43. **Galbo, H., Holst, J. J., Christensen, N. J., and Hilsted, J.,** Glucagon and plasma catecholamines during beta-receptor blockade in exercising man, *J. Appl. Physiol.*, 40, 855, 1976.
44. **Tkachuk, V. A.,** Molecular regulation mechanisms of the cardiac adenylate cyclase system, in *Regulation of Myocardial Contractile Function and Metabolism* (in Russian), Chazov, E. I. and Smirnov, V. N., Eds., Nauka, Moscow, 1987, 259.
45. **Kepple, J. D., Cdacearuso, B., and Massry, S. G.,** Does parathyroid hormone cause protein wasting?, *Contribs. Nephrol.*, 20, 138, 1980.
46. **Viru, A. A. and Eller, A. K.,** Adrenocortical regulation of protein turnover in prolonged physical loads (in Russian), *Byull. Eksp. Biol. Med.*, 82, 1436, 1976.
47. **Luyckx, A. S., Dresse, A., Cession-Fossion, A., and Lefebre, P. J.,** Catecholamines and exercise-induced glucagon and fatty acid mobilization in the rat, *Am. J. Physiol.*, 229, 376, 1975.
48. **Oscai, L.,** Type L hormone-sensitive lipase hydrolyzes endogenous triacylglycerols in muscle in exercised rats, *Med. Sci. Sports Exercise* 15, 336, 1983.

49. **Filaretov, A. A., Filaretova, L. P., Podvigina, T. G., and Balashov, Yu. G.,** Relation of activities of the vasopressin-ergic and hypophysial-adrenocortical systems (in Russian), *Dokl. Akad. Nauk SSSR,* 301, 500, 1988.
50. **Frol'kis, V. V., Golovchenko, S. R., Medvedev, V. I., and Frol'kis, R. A.,** Vasopressin and the cardiovascular system (in Russian), *Usp. Fiziol. Nauk,* 44, 56, 1983.
51. **Rona, G., Chappel, C. J., and Kahn, D. D.,** The significance of factors modifying the development of isoproterenol-induced myocardial necrosis, *Am. Heart J.,* 66, 389, 1963.
52. **Simkhovich, B. Z., Meirena, D. B., Briede, Ya. L., Shutenko, Zh. V., Hagi, H. V., Kalvinsh, I. Ya., and Lukevits, E. Ya.,** Pathophysiological aspects of the disturbances in lipid metabolism in the heart under adrenergic influences, and means of their correction (in Russian), in *Physiology and Pathophysiology of the Heart and Coronary Circulation.* Stepanov, K. V., Ed., Meditsina, Moscow, 1987, 149.
53. **Verrier, R. L. and Haegeston, E. L.,** Neural mechanisms of cardiac arrhythmias, in *Mechanisms and Treatment of Cardiac Arrhythmias,* Reiser, H. J. and Horowitz, L. N., Eds., Urban and Schwarzenberg, Baltimore-Munich, 1985, 76.
54. **Pshennikova, M. G.,** Adaptation to physical loads (in Russian), in *Physiology of Adaptive Processes,* Gazenko, O. G. and Meerson, F. Z., Eds., Nauka, Moscow, 1986, 124.
55. **Vatner, S. F. and Hintze, T. H.,** Mechanism of constriction of large coronary arteries by β-adrenergic receptor blockade, *Circ. Res.,* 53, 389, 1983.
56. **Meerson, F. Z.,** *Adaptation of the Heart to Great Load and Heart Failure* (in Russian), Nauka, Moscow, 1975.
57. **Meerson, F. Z.,** Main patterns of individual adaptation (in Russian), in *Physiology of Adaptive Processes,* Gazenko, O. G. and Meerson, F. Z., Eds., Nauka, Moscow, 1986, 10.
58. **Sheehan, G. A.,** An overview of overuse syndromes in distance runners, *Ann. N.Y. Acad. Sci.,* 301, 77, 1977.
59. **Young, M. A. and Vatner, S. F.,** Regulation of large coronary arteries, *Circ. Res.,* 59, 579, 1986.
60. **Yasue, H., Takizawa, A., Nagao, M., Nishida, S., Horie, M., and Kubota, J.,** Role of coronary spasm in different anginal syndromes, *Acta Med. Scand.,* 694 (Suppl.), 83, 1984.
61. **Meerson, F. Z., Saulya, A. I., and Guduman, V. S.,** Role of the loss of sialic acid by the myocardium in the depression of the cardiac muscle contractile function (in Russian), *Vopr. Med. Khim.,* 2, 118, 1985.
62. **Meerson, F. Z., Tverdokhlib, V. P., and Nikonorov, A. A.,** Prevention of atherogenic dyslipoproteinemias and complex metabolic disturbances in liver in emotional-pain stress (in Russian), *Vopr. Med. Khim.,* 6, 104, 1988.
63. **Meerson, F. Z. and Yavich, M. P.,** The role of cytoplasmic factors in the poststress changes in RNA synthesis in heart and liver (in Russian), *Vopr. Med. Khim.* 2, 90, 1987.
64. **Drzhevetskaya, I. A., Belyaev, N. G., Karaulova, L. K., and Limanskii, N. N.,** On the expediency of blood calcium and calcitonin determination in the complex evaluation of the response of athletes to physical loads (in Russian), in *Humoral-Hormonal Regulation of Energy Metabolism in Sports,* Kravtsov, E. D., Ed., Fizkultura i Sport, Moscow, 1983, 41.
65. **Pouysségur, J.,** The growth factor-activatable Na^+/H^+ exchange system: a genetic approach, *Trends Biochem. Sci.,* 10, 453, 1985.
66. **Samosudova, N. V., Glagoleva, E. V., Shimkovich, M. V., Belkina, L. M., and Meerson, F. Z.,** Impairment of myocardial contractile function and cardiomyocyte ultrastructure upon emotional stress (in Russian), *Arkh. Anat. Gistol. Embriol.,* 2, 43, 1983.
67. **Kristt, D. A. and Freimark, S. J.,** Histopathology and pathogenesis of behaviorally induced gastric lesions in rats, *Am. J. Pathol.,* 73, 411, 1973.
68. **Pare, W. P. and Livingston, A.,** Brain norepinephrine and stomach ulcers in rats exposed to chronic conflict, *Physiol, Behav.,* 5, 215, 1970.
69. **Weiss, J. M.,** Effects of punishing the coping response (conflict) on stress pathology in rats, *J. Comp. Physiol. Psychol.,* 77, 14, 1971.
70. **Vald'man, A. V.,** Psychopharmacological aspects of emotional stress (in Russian), *Vestnik Akad. Med. Nauk SSSR,* 8, 26, 1975.
71. **Vedyaev, F. P.,** The brain limbic system, emotional stress and its endocrine and vegetative manifestations (in Russian), *Vestnik Akad. Med. Nauk SSSR,* 8, 57, 1975.
72. **Samokhvalov, V. G.,** Dynamics of the vegetative and bioelectric shifts in emotional-stress conditions in rats (in Russian), *Fiziol. Zh. SSSR,* 62, 831, 1976.
73. **Randall, D. C., Kaye, M. P., Randall, W. C., Brady, J. V., and Martin, K. H.,** Response of primate heart to emotional stress before and after cardiac denervation, *Am. J. Physiol.,* 230, 988, 1978.
74. **Miller, D. G. and Malov, S.,** Quantitative determination of stress-induced myocardial damage in rats, *Pharmacol. Biochem. Behav.,* 7, 139, 1977.
75. **Desiderato, O., MacKinnon, J. R., and Hissom, H. J.,** Development of gastric ulcers in rats following stress termination, *J. Comp. Physiol. Psychol.,* 87, 208, 1974.

76. **Manukhin, B. N., Pavlova, V. I., Putintseva, T. G., Volina, E. V., Berdysheva, L. V., Kurbanova, G. D., Selivanova, G. P., and Meerson, F. Z.**, Functional state of the rat sympathoadrenal system in emotional-pain stress (in Russian), *Fiziol. Zh. SSSR,* 68, 1182, 1981.
77. **Fallen, E. T., Elliot, W., and Gordin, R.**, Apparatus for study of ventricular function and metabolism in isolated perfused rat heart, *J. Appl. Physiol.*, 22, 836, 1967.
78. **Spieckermann, P. G.**, Role of energy metabolism in enzyme retention. A study on isolated perfused canine hearts, *Experientia,* 31, 1046, 1975.
79. **Meerson, F. Z. and Kapel'ko, V. I.**, Modern notions of the mechanism of cardiac muscle contraction and relaxation (in Russian), *Usp. Fiziol. Nauk,* 9, 21, 1978.
80. **Jacobus, W. E. and Lehninger, A. L.**, Creatine kinase of rat heart mitochohondria, Coupling of creatine phosphorylation to electron transport, *J. Biol. Chem.*, 248, 4803, 1973.
81. **Neely, J. R., Libermeister, H., Battersby, E. J., and Morgan, H. E.**, Effect of pressure development on oxygen consumption by isolated rat heart, *Am. J. Physiol.*, 212, 804, 1967.
82. **Morad, M. and Goldman, J.**, Excitation-contraction coupling in heart muscle; membrane control of development of tension, *Prog. Biophys. Mol. Biol.*, 27, 259, 1973.
83. **Saulya, A. I., Golubeva, L. Yu., and Meerson, F. Z.**, Effect of emotional-pain stress on the contractile function of hypertrophied cardiac muscle (in Russian), *Byull. Eksp. Biol. Med.*, 2, 145, 1985.
84. **Tillisch, J. and Langer, G.**, Myocardial mechanical responses and ionic exchange in high-sodium perfusate, *Circ. Res.*, 24, 40, 1974.
85. **Poole-Witson, P.**, Effects of acidosis and weak acids on the normal, hypoxic, and ischaemic myocardium, in *Symposium on Anaerobic Metabolism and Lactic Acid,* Berlin, 1980, 197.
86. **Adams, K. and Welch, H.**, Oxygen uptake, acid-base status, and performance with varied inspired oxygen fractions, *J. Appl. Physiol.*, 49, 863, 1980.
87. **Meerson, F. Z. and Ugolev, A. A.**, Impairment of membrane calcium transport as the common pathogenetic link of various forms of cardiac insufficiency (in Russian), *Kardiologiya,* 20, 68, 1980.
88. **Kapel'ko, V. I.**, Effect of hypoxia and ischemia on ionic transport and contractile function of the cardiac muscle (in Russian), *Byull. Vses. Kardiol. Nauch. Tsentra,* 103, 1981.
89. **Malyshev, V. V., Lifant'ev, V. I., and Meerson, F. Z.**, Functional state of cardiac mitochondria in the dynamics of emotional pain stress (in Russian), *Kardiologiya,* 6, 118, 1982.
90. **Jacobus, W. E.**, Respiratory control and integration of heart high-energy phosphate metabolism by mitochondrial creatine kinase, *Annu. Rev. Physiol.*, 47, 707, 1985.
91. **Saks, V. A., Rosenshtraukh, L. V., Chazov, E. I., and Smirnov, V. N.**, Role of creatine phosphokinase in cellular function and metabolism, *Can. J. Physiol. Pharmacol.*, 56, 691, 1978.
92. **Saks, V. A. and Kupriyanov, V. V.**, Intracellular energy transport and control of cardiac contraction, in *Advances in Myocardiology,* 3, Chazov, E. I., Smirnov, V. N., and Dhalla, N. S., Eds., Plenum Press, New York, 1982, 475.
93. **Sharov, V. G., Saks, V. A., Smirnov, V. N., and Chazov, E. I.**, The electron microscopic histochemical investigation of the localization of creatine phosphokinase in heart cells, *Biochim. Biophys. Acta,* 468, 495, 1977.
94. **Kupriyanov, V. V., Lakomkin, V. L., Kapelko, V. I., Steinschneider, A. Ya., Ruuge, E. K., and Saks, V. A.**, Dissociation of adenosine triphosphate levels and contractile function in isovolumic hearts perfused with 2-deoxyglucose, *J. Mol. Cell. Cardiol.*, 19, 729, 1987.
95. **Kapel'ko, V. I., Kupriyanov, V. V., Novikova, N. A., Lakomkin, V. L., Steinschneider, A. Ya., Zueva, M. Yu., and Saks, V. A.**, Mechanisms of adaptation of the contractile function and energy metabolism of the heart to chronic deficiency of phosphocreatine (in Russian), *Fiziol. Zh.* 34, 3, 1988.
96. **Nikitovich, S. N.**, Effect of stress on glycogen content in rat liver cells, in *Physiological-Biochemical Studies on Nervous and Endocrine Systems* (in Russian), Yaroshenko, M. F., Ed., Shtiintsa, Kishinev, 1973, 86.
97. **Skinner, J. E., Beder, S. D., and Ehtman, M.**, Psychological stress activates phosphorylase in the heart of the conscious pig without increasing heart rate and blood pressure, *Proc. Natl. Acad. Sci. U.S.A.* 80, 4513, 1983.
98. **Raiskina, M. E., Shargorodskii, B. M. Dolgov, V. V., Dolgova, N. P., Pavlovich, L. A., Wollenberger, A., Krause, E., and Bartel, C.**, On the dependence of the physiological and pathological effects of epinephrine on the changes in cardiac metabolism (in Russian), *Kardiologiya,* 2, 83, 1978.
99. **Seraydarian, M., Sato E., and Harary, I.**, In vitro studies of beating heart cells in culture, *Arch. Biochem. Biophys.*, 138, 233, 1970.
100. **Kruta, V. Z.**, Über die Bienflussung der Tätigkeit des isolierten Sängerherrzens durch Glycolisehemmung mittels der Monojodessigsäure, *Z. Gesamte Exp. Med.*, 92, 612, 1934.
101. **Baum, H., Murer, E., Slauterback, D., and McConnell, D.**, Association of integrated metabolic pathways with membranes. II. Electron micrographic studies on glycolytically active preparations from erythrocytes, *Arch. Biochem. Biophys.*, 113, 487, 1966.

102. **Weisser, A., Kruger, F., Baba, N., Scarpelli, D., Leighbon, R., and Gallimore, J.,** Role of anaerobic metabolism in preservation of functional capacity and structure of anoxic myocardium, *J. Clin. Invest.*, 47, 403, 1968.
103. **Meerson, F. Z. and Larionov, N. P.,** Role of glycolysis in the energy provision for the heart contractile function (in Russian), *Kardiologiya,* 1, 17, 1969.
104. **Meerson, F. Z., Arkhipenko, Yu. V., Rozhitskaya, I. I., and Kagan, V. E.,** Damage to the Ca^{2+}-transporting system of the cardiac sarcoplasmic reticulum in emotional pain stress (in Russian), *Byull. Eksp. Biol. Med.*, 4, 405, 1981.
105. **Bricknell, O. L., Daries, P. S., and Opie, L. H.,** A relationship between adenosine triphosphate, glycolysis and ischaemic contracture in the isolated rat heart, *J. Mol. Cell. Cardiol.*, 13, 941, 1981.
106. **Jamarkani, J. M., Nagatomo, T., and Langer, G. A.,** The effect of calcium and high energy phosphate compounds on myocardial contracture in the newborn and adult rabbit, *J. Mol. Cell. Cardiol.*, 10, 1017, 1978.
107. **Humphrey, S. M., Gavin, J. B., and Herdson, P. B.,** The relationship of ischemic contracture to vascular reperfusion in the isolated rat heart, *J. Mol. Cell. Cardiol.*, 12, 1397, 1980.
108. **Opie, L. H. and Owen, P.,** Effect of glucose-insulin-potassium infusion on arteriovenous differences of glucose and free fatty acids and on tissue metabolic changes in dogs with developing myocardial infarction, *Am. J. Cardiol.*, 38, 310, 1976.
109. **Burke, W., Asokan, S., Moschos, C., Oldewurtel, H., and Regan, T.,** Effect of glucose and non-glucose infusion on myocardial potassium ion transfers and arrhythmias during ischemia, *Am. J. Cardiol.*, 24, 713, 1969.
110. **Kypson, J., Hait, G., and Mathew, R.,** Effects of uridine on the performance and the metabolism of oxygenated and hypoxic rabbit hearts, *J. Mol. Cell. Cardiol.*, 10, 545, 1978.
111. **Meerson, F. Z., Pavlova, V. I., Sukhikh, T. T., Pshennikova, M. G., Efimenko, T. P., Solomatin, V. B., Frolov, B. A., and Vorontsova, E. Ya.,** Poststress activation of nucleic acid and protein synthesis and its role in the organismic adaptive reactions (in Russian), *Patol. Fiziol. Eksp. Ter.*, 5, 3, 1982.
112. **Meerson, F. Z. and Vasil'ev, V. K.,** Cardiac muscle DNA injury and reparation in emotional pain stress (in Russian), *Byull. Eksp. Biol. Med.*, 1, 297, 1981.
113. **Meerson, F. Z. and Vasil'ev, V. K.,** Prevention of damage to cardiac muscle DNA structure caused by emotional pain stress with the use of agents blocking the beta-adrenoreceptors and lipid peroxidation (in Russian), *Vopr. Med. Khim.*, 2, 115, 1982.
114. **Meerson, F. Z., Yavich, M. P., and Rozhitskaya, I. I.,** Effect of emotional pain stress on the rate of DNA synthesis in heart and liver cells (in Russian), *Vopr. Med. Khim.*, 5, 59, 1988.
115. **Cleaver, J. E.,** Repair replication of mammalian cell DNA, *Radiat. Res.*, 37, 334, 1969.
116. **Cohn, S. M., Krawicz, B. R., Dresler, S. L., and Liberman, M. V.,** Induction of replicative DNA synthesis in quiescent human fibroblasts by DNA-damaging agents, *Proc. Natl. Acad. Sci. U.S.A.*, 81, 4828, 1984.
117. **Castellot, J. J., Miller, M. R., Lehtanahi, D. M., and Pardee, A. B.,** Comparison of DNA replication and repair enzymology using permeabilized baby hamster kidney cells, *J. Biol. Chem.*, 254, 6904, 1979.
118. **Chin, M. L. and Irvin, J. L.,** Effect of inhibition of DNA synthesis on histone synthesis, turnover and deposition in the rat, *Arch. Biochem.*, 236, 260, 1985.
119. **Khanson, K. P. and Ivanova, D. V.,** Animal mitochondrial deoxyribonucleic acid (in Russian), *Usp. Sovrem. Biol.*, 72, 56, 1971.
120. **Meerson, F. Z. and Alekhina, G.,** Action of intensity of contractile function of muscle cells of the heart on the DNA synthesis in intermediate connective tissue of the myocardium, *Acta Anat.*, 70, 559, 1968.
121. **Meerson, F. Z., Yavich, M. P., Rozhitskaya, I. I., and Golubeva, L. Yu.,** Abolishment of the stress activation of reparative DNA synthesis in the myocardium in cardiac hyperfunction (in Russian), *Byull. Eksp. Biol. Med.*, in press.
122. **Meerson, F. Z.,** *The Failing Heart: Adaptation and Deadaptation,* Raven Press, New York, 1983.
123. **Morkin, E. and Ashford, T.,** Myocardial DNA synthesis in experimental cardiac hypertrophy, *Am. J. Physiol.*, 215, 1409, 1968.
124. **Florini, J. R. and Dankberg, F. L.,** Changes in ribonucleic acid and protein synthesis during induced cardiac hypertrophy, *Biochemistry,* 10, 530, 1971.
125. **Friedberg, E. C.,** *DNA Repair,* W. H. Freeman, New York, 1985.
126. **Posner, B. I. and Fanburg, B. L.,** Ribonucleic acid synthesis in experimental cardiac hypertrophy in rats, *Circ. Res.*, 23, 137, 1968.
127. **Javitch, M. P. and Meerson, F. Z.,** The role of cytoplasmic factors in RNA synthesis activation during hyperfunction of heart and liver, *Basic Res. Cardiol.*, 78, 83, 1983.
128. **Pelham, H. R. B. and Brown, D. D. B.,** A specific transcription factor that can bind either the 5S RNA gene or 5S RNA, *Proc. Natl. Acad. Sci. U.S.A.*, 77, 4170, 1980.
129. **Hammond, G. L., Weiben, E., and Markert, C. L.,** Molecular signals for initiating protein synthesis in organ hypertrophy, *Proc. Natl. Acad. Sci. U.S.A.*, 76, 2455, 1979.

130. **Breslav, I. S.,** *Respiration Patterns; Physiology, Extreme States, Pathology* (in Russian), Shik, L. L., Ed., Nauka, Leningrad, 1984.
131. **Vagin, Yu. E., Koplik, E. V., and Vedyaev, D. F.,** A study of the respiration rhythm in rats under acute emotional stress (in Russian), *Byull. Eksp. Biol. Med.,* 5, 524, 1984.
132. **Kondrashova, M. N., Grigorenko, E. V., Guzar, I. B., and Okon, E. B.,** Removal by negative aeroions of the changes in mitochondrial respiration in stress (in Russian), *Biofizika,* 26, 687, 1981.
133. **Helmholz, H. F.,** The abbreviated alveolar air equation, *Chest,* 75, 748, 1979.
134. **Seredenko, M. M., Minyailenko, T. D., and Pozharov, V. P.,** Peculiarities of the development and compensation of secondary tissue hypoxia during muscular activity (in Russian), *Fiziol. Cheloveka,* 13, 831, 1987.
135. **Stroev, E. A.,** *Biological Chemistry* (in Russian), Vysshaya Shkola, Moscow, 1986.
136. **Dukov, L. G.,** Pulmonary shunt and its regulation (in Russian), *Usp. Fiziol. Nauk,* 12, 112, 1981.
137. **Piiper, J., Huch, A., Kötter, D., and Herbst, R.,** Pulmonary diffusing capacity at basal and increased O_2 uptake levels in anesthetized dogs, *Respir. Physiol.,* 6, 219, 1969.
138. **Seredenko, M. M., Pozharov, V. P., and Rozova, E. V.,** On the adequacy of the pulmonary blood oxygenation and mass transfer of O_2 across the aerohematic barrier to the organismic oxygen demand (in Russian), in *Actual Problems of Modern Physiology,* Kostyuk, P. G., Ed., Naukova Dumka, Kiev, 1986, 224.
139. **Shakhlamov, V. N.,** *The Capillaries* (in Russian), Meditsina, Moscow, 1971.
140. **Kovalenko, T. N., Pozharov, V. P., and Seredenko, M. M.,** Effect of acute hypoxic hypoxia on the thickness of the lung aerohematic barrier (in Russian), *Byull. Eksp. Biol. Med.,* 58, 51, 1980.
141. **Drinker, C. K.,** *The Clinical Physiology of the Lungs,* Springfield, 1954.
142. **Walters, D. V.,** The role of beta-adrenergic agents in the control of surfactant secretion, *Biochem. Soc. Trans.,* 13, 1089, 1985.
143. **Torda, T. and Kopin, I. J.,** Lack of preventive effect of 6-hydroxy dopamine on a decrease of beta-adrenergic receptors induced by repeated stress in heart of rats, *Endocrinol. Exp.,* 19, 47, 1985.
144. **Oyarzum, M. J. and Clements, J. A.,** Control of lung surfactant by ventilation, adrenergic mediators, and prostaglandins in the rabbit, *Am. Rev. Respir. Dis.,* 117, 879, 1978.
145. **Meerson, F. Z., Tverdokhlib, V. P., Nikonorov, A. A., Fillipov, V. K., and Frolov, B. A.,** Role of suppressed cholesterol 7-alpha-hydroxylase activity in the liver in evolvement of atherogenic stress dyslipidemia (in Russian), *Kardiologiya,* 9, 85, 1987.
146. **Meerson, F. Z., Tverdokhlib, V. P., and Nikonorov, A. A.,** Prevention of atherogenic dyslipoproteinemias and complex metabolic disturbances in liver in emotional pain stress (in Russian), *Byull. Eksp. Biol. Med.,* 6, 104, 1988.
147. **Tverdislova, I. L. and Rigov, V. B.,** Lipid peroxidation as the main cause of modification of the catalytic function of the sarcoplasmic reticular Ca ATPase in hypercholesterolemia (in Russian), *Byull. Eksp. Biol. Med.,* 4, 415, 1987.
148. **Kuz'mina, I. L. and Rigov, V. B.,** Modification of the functional properties of the sarcoplasmic reticular Ca ATPase in hypercholesterolemia (in Russian), *Byull. Eksp. Biol. Med.,* 4, 419, 1986.
149. **Langer, G. A.,** The structure and function of the myocardial cell surface, *Am. J. Physiol.,* 235, H461, 1978.
150. **German, N. G., Guduman, V. S., and Madan, N. I.,** Electrophoretic resolution of lactate dehydrogenase isoenzymes in agarose gel (in Russian), *Lab. Delo,* 9, 545, 1982.
151. **Horgan, L. E.,** A modified spectrophotometric method for determination of nanogram quantity of sialic acid, *Clin. Chem. Acta,* 116, 409, 1981.
152. **Jacoes, L. W., Brown, E. B., and Barrnett, J. M.,** Sialic acid, a calcium-binding carbohydrate, *J. Biol. Chem.,* 252, 4533, 1977.
153. **Sobel, B., Corr., P., Robinson, A., Goldstein, R., Witkowski, F., and Klein, M.,** Accumulation of lysophosphoglycerides with arrhythmogenic properties in ischemic myocardium, *J. Clin. Invest.,* 65, 546, 1978.
154. **Katz, A. and Messineo, F.,** Lipid-membrane interactions and the pathogenesis of ischemic damage in the myocardium, *Circ. Res.,* 48, 1, 1981.
155. **Meerson, F. Z., Golubeva, L. Yu., Kagan, V. E., Shimkovich, M. V., and Ugolev, A. A.,** Activation of lipid peroxidation as the decisive link in the pathogenesis of stress damage to the heart, and prevention of stress and hypoxic injuries with the antioxidant ionol (in Russian), in *Proc. Soviet-Am. Symp. Myocardial Metabolism,* Smirnov, V. I., Ed., Meditsina, Moscow, 1981, 59.
156. **Meerson, F. Z., Kagan, V. E., Prilipko, L. L., Rozhitskaya, I. I., Giber, L. M., and Kozlov, Yu. P.,** Activation of lipid peroxidation in emotional pain stress (in Russian), *Byull. Eksp. Biol. Med.,* 10, 404, 1979.
157. **Meerson, F. Z., Didenko, V. V., Belkina, L. M., and Manukhina, E. B.,** Lipid peroxidation and antioxidant protection of the heart in stress, ischemia, and arrhythmias, in *Cellular Antioxidant Defense Mechanisms,* Chow, Ch. K., Ed., CRC Press, Boca Raton, FL, 1988, 215.

158. **Prilipko, L. L., Orlov, O. M., Ivanova, S. M., Kagan, V. E., Meerson, F. Z., Ushakov, L. S., and Gazenko, O. G.,** Activation of lipid peroxidation in stress in man assayed by the pentane content in the exhaled air (in Russian), *Dokl. Akad. Nauk SSSR,* 265, 1010, 1982.
159. **Meerson, F. Z.,** The role of lipid peroxidation in the myocardium in stress and antioxidant protection of the heart, in *Oxygen Radicals in the Pathophysiology of Heart Disease,* Singal, P. K., Ed., Kluwer Academic Boston, 1988, 285.
160. **Meerson, F. Z., Medvedev, L. N., Golubeva, L. Yu., and Ustinova, E. E.,** Effect of emotional pain stress on the Na,K ATPase activity in the cardiac muscle (in Russian), *Byull. Eksp. Biol. Med.,* 8, 61, 1982.
161. **Rathbun, W. B. and Betlach, M. V.,** Estimation of enzymatically produced orthophosphate in the presence of cystein and adenosine triphosphate, *Anal. Biochem.,* 28, 436, 1969.
162. **Johnson, F. H., Eyring, H., and Stover, B. J.,** *The Theory of Rate Processes in Biology and Medicine,* John Wiley & Sons, New York, 1974.
163. **Vassalle, M.,** The relationship among cardiac pacemakers: overdrive suppression, *Circ. Res.,* 41, 269, 1977.
164. **Meerson, F. Z., Arkhipenko, Yu. V., Rozhitskaya, I. I., and Kagan, V. E.,** Damage to the sarcoplasmic reticular Ca-transporting system in emotional pain stress (in Russian), *Kardiologiya,* 4, 60, 1981.
165. **Kuo, C. S., Amlie, J. P., Munakata, K., Reddy, C. P., and Surawicz, B.,** Dispersion of monophasic action potential durations and activation times during atrial pacing, ventricular pacing and ventricular premature stimulation in canine ventricle, *Cardiovasc. Res.,* 17, 152, 1983.
166. **Abildskov, J. A.,** Ventricular repolarization and arrhythmia, in *Diagnosis and Treatment of Cardiac Arrhythmias,* Bayes, A. and Cosin, J., Eds., Pergamon Press, New York, 1980, 71.
167. **Barr, L., Dewey, M., and Berger, W.,** Propagation of action potentials and the structure of the nexus in cardiac muscle, *J. Gen. Physiol.,* 48, 797, 1965.
168. **Weingart, R.,** Cell-to-cell coupling in cardiac tissue, in *Cardiovasc. Physiol. Heart, Peripheral Circ. and Methodol,* Proc. 28th Int. Congr. Physiol. Sci., Budapest, 1980, Academic Press, Oxford, 1981, 59.
169. **Sudakov, K. V., Yumatov, E. A., and Ul'yaninskii, L. S.,** Systemic mechanisms of emotional stress (in Russian), in *Stress Development Mechanisms,* Furdui, F. I., Khaidarliu, S. Kh., Shtirtu, E. I., Nadvodnyuk, A. I., and Mamalyga, L. M., Eds., Shtiintsa, Kishinev, 1987, 52.
170. **Wit, A. L. and Cranefield, P. E.,** Triggered and automatic activity in the canine coronary sinus, *Circ. Res.,* 41, 435, 1977.
171. **Legato, M. J. and Langer, G. A.,** The subcellular localization of calcium ion in mammalian myocardium, *J. Cell Biol.,* 41, 401, 1969.
172. **Samosudova, N. V., Skrebnitskaya, L. K., and Klimov, A. A.,** Localization of Ca^{2+} in muscle with dual calcium regulation (in Russian), *Biofizika,* 26, 319, 1981.
173. **Meerson, F. Z., Malyshev, V. V., Kagan, V. E., Treschuk, L. I., and Rozhitskaya, I. I.,** Activation of lipid peroxidation and focal contractural damage in cardiac muscle in emotional pain stress (in Russian), *Arkh. Patol.,* 42, 9, 1980.
174. **Meerson, F. Z. and Usynin, A. F.,** Electron-microscopic alterations in the conducting system of the heart and disturbances in its electric stability in immobilization stress (in Russian), *Arkh. Patol.,* 1989 in press.
175. **Chervova, I. A. and Pavlovich, E. R.,** Morphology of the main regions of the rat heart conducting system (in Russian), *Arkh. Anat. Gistol. Embriol.,* 8, 67, 1979.
176. **Doschitsin, V. L., Grudtsyn, G. V., and Gendlin, G. E.,** The sinus node dysfunction syndrome (in Russian), *Kardiologiya,* 3, 56, 1976.
177. **Strauss, H. C., Bigger, J. Th., and Saroff, A. L.,** Electrophysiologic evaluation of sinus node function in patients with sinus node dysfunction, *Circulation,* 53, 763, 1976.
178. **Smetnev, A. S., Shevchenko, N. M., and Grosu, A. A.,** Dysfunction and sinus node weakness syndrome (in Russian), *Kardiologiya.* 2, 5, 1988.
179. **Levy, M. W. and Martin, P. J.,** Neural control of the heart, in *Handbook of Physiological Circulation, Section 2, The Cardiovascular System,* Berne, R. M. and Sperelakis, N., Eds., American Physiological Society, Bethesda, 1979, 581.
180. **Meerson F. Z., Pavlova, V. I., Kamilov, F. Kh., and Yakushev, V. S.,** Impairment of energy metabolism in the liver in emotional pain stress and their prevention with sodium gamma-hydroxybutyrate (in Russian), *Vopr. Med. Khim.,* 24, 744, 1978.

Chapter 2

THE PLACE OF PRIMARY CARDIAC STRESS DAMAGE IN THE PATHOGENESIS OF ARRHYTHMIAS, ISCHEMIC DISEASE, AND SUDDEN CARDIAC DEATH

I. INTRODUCTION

The conventional idea of the place of stress in the pathogenesis of arrhythmias and sudden death is that man, as compared to other species, is most open to the influence of mainly biosocial stressful situations which he either enters himself or is put in by social circumstances. In our opinion, however, the problem is not so straightforward since intelligence, which is an exclusive property of *Homo sapiens,* allows the person to clearly understand many of the ambient events and thereby obviates groundless fear and stress reaction. Indeed, Laughlin[1] has shown that in subjects aware of the particulars of the centrifugal test there was no or minor increase in the blood catecholamines. Accordingly, the most thorough clinical examination, and in some cases post-mortem studies upon incidental death, failed to reveal any damage to the cardiac muscle. On the contrary, for animals the centrifugation proved to be a drastic stress factor: the blood catecholamine concentration rose up to fiftyfold with ensuing grave cardiac damage manifest in subendocardial hemorrhages, myofibrillar contractures evolving into micronecroses, etc. In other words, the mental mechanisms often certainly avert the stress reaction hazardous to the organism and, in particular, detrimental to the heart. With all this it should be borne in mind that just the same mechanisms and linked associative activity may cause reiteration of stress situations that either have really occurred or are quite probable. That is to say, a person going through multiple brief or prolonged stress episodes may not only ignore them by virtue of the mental mechanisms, but, vice versa, amplify and aggravate them through the same mechanisms.

Taking into account these important peculiarities of the psychics and cardiac neural regulation, in this chapter we shall first consider the experimental data on the role of cardiac stress damage in the pathogenesis of arrhythmias and sudden death, and then the materials directly pertaining to man.

II. ROLE OF STRESS DAMAGE TO THE HEART IN IMPAIRMENT OF ITS ELECTRIC STABILITY AND DEVELOPMENT OF ARRHYTHMIAS IN THE EXPERIMENT

Researchers concerned with the place of stress in arrhythmias, fibrillation, and cardiac arrest never fail to mention that the literary heritage provides us with numerous examples of sudden cardiac death of apparently healthy people brought about by acute stressful situations.

Abiding by the tradition, I can cite A. K. Tolstoi's famous drama, *Ivan the Terrible,* where the Tsar receives a prophecy that he will die on one particular day, namely St. Philip's Day; one of his officers, having thoroughly consulted the physician, and assured that emotions are all important in the Tsar's illness, kills his sovereign with a single, perfectly timed remark, "St. Philip's Day is not yet over, Sire."

Getting on to the gist of the matter, it must be recalled that as far back as early in this century it has been found that direct introduction into the brain of drugs or chemicals such as nicotine, barium chloride, caffeine, epinephrine, acetylcholine, or strophanthin causes ventricular arrhythmias and fibrillation. Further studies using more precise techniques of stereotaxic electrode introduction have shown that ventricular arrhythmias are elicited upon stimulation of the frontal, orbital, motor, and premotor cortical zones, anterior temporal zone, island, and convolution of the cingula. Arrhythmias are relatively easy to evoke by stimulation of subcortical regions such as posterior hypothalamus and lamina quadrigemina (for review see Korteweg et al.).[2] Similarly, the probability of arrhythmias and susceptibility to ventricular fibrillation increase upon electric stimulation of peripheral neural structures such as cardial sympathetic nerves and stellate nodes. These artificial pathological phenomena are of interest as indications of the possible central genesis of arrhythmias, but of course do not themselves prove their stress origin. Important in this context are the experiments of Lown et al.,[3-5] who reproduced the emotional pain stress (EPS) by placing dogs in a stanchion according to Pavlov and delivering moderate electric pain stimulation. This procedure was repeated for 3 d, after which the stress reaction as manifest by blood catecholamine elevation developed without electric pain stimulation, as a conditioned response to the experimental setting. In the process, the heart was stimulated by electric current through an electrode implanted in the apex cordis. It turned out that the stress situation substantially lowered the threshold current, causing extrasystoles and cardiac fibrillation, i.e., substantially increased their probability.[3-5]

Further studies of Lown's group[6] showed that the decisive part in the arrhythmogenic action of stress on the heart is played by inordinately intense and protracted excitation of adrenergic regulation.

In our experiments we used two main approaches to assessing the effect of stress on cardiac electric stability: determining the cardiac fibrillation threshold and evaluating the resistance of cardiac automatism and its ectopic activity upon stimulation of the distal end of the dissected vagus nerve.

Figure 1 illustrates the technique used to determine the fibrillation threshold. A premature single impulse delivered to the apex cordis from a stimulator triggered by the ECG R wave is seen to evoke transitory fibrillation attended by a drop in arterial pressure. The fibrillation threshold is defined as the current sufficient to cause fibrillation; it is an index of the probability of cardiac fibrillation and death of fibrillation.

Figure 2 presents another approach to evaluating the electric stability of the heart: the normal automatism of the sinus node is hindered by stimulating the vagus nerve. On the background of the resulting vagal bradycardia, extrasystoles are very rare in control animals, but quite common in experimental infarction and postinfarction cardiosclerosis.

Before considering the data obtained with the use of these approaches, it must be noted that the results of all experiments on the effects of stress on cardiac electric stability differed basically from what had been found for the contractile function. Indeed, the contractile function had to be studied with isolated heart preparations, since in the whole organism it was only little or not at all altered even upon appreciable exposure to stress. On the contrary, the electric stability parameters, and first of all the cardiac fibrillation threshold, changed markedly in the intact organism. A similar dissociation between the preserved contractile function and the impaired electric stability was observed by us in cardiac damage with the selective β-agonist isoproterenol. Moreover, such dissociation is now demonstrable with 24-h monitoring in both diseased and practically healthy persons; many of them develop more or less pronounced arrhythmias with quite intact pump and contractile functions of the heart.[7,8] This essential dissociation is one of the causes of often sudden cardiac death; its mechanism is of great interest, and we shall return to it again.

At the first stage we studied the effect of stress on the cardiac fibrillation threshold and reactivity to the inhibitory action of the vagus nerve.[9] Immobilization stress was created in male Wistar rats by fixing them in the supine position for 10 h. It turned out that 2 h after the end of the stress exposure the fibrillation threshold fell more than twofold and remained decreased for the next 2 d, with a minor tendency to restitution by the end of this period.

Simultaneously, the stress substantially enhanced the sensitivity of the sinus pacemaker to vagal inhibition. This was only pronounced enough 12 and 24 h after stress, but regressed by the end of the second day (Figure 3).

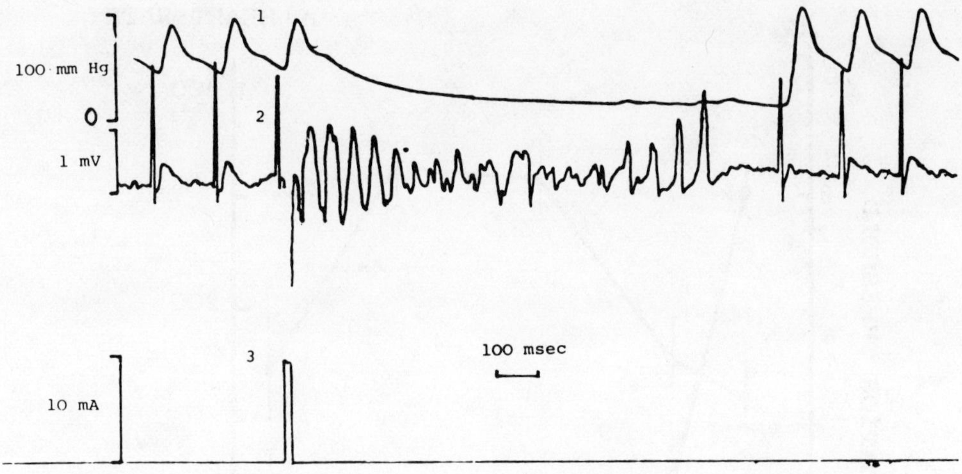

FIGURE 1. Determination of the electric threshold of cardiac fibrillation. (1) Pressure in the carotid artery, (2) ECG, (3) recording of the stimulating impulse.

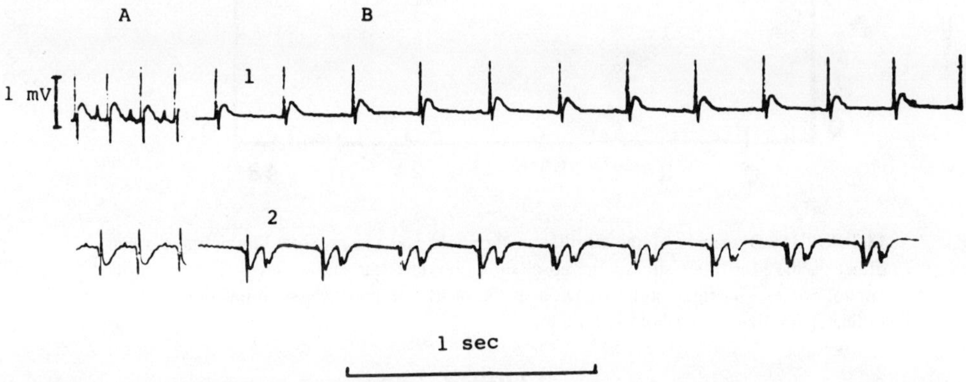

FIGURE 2. Ectopic activity of the heart in vagal stimulation. (A) ECG before stimulation, (B) ECG during stimulation. (1) Control: bradycardia caused by stimulation of the vagal periphery; (2) postinfarction cardiosclerosis: bradycardia attended with bigeminy.

Obviously, in the whole organism the lower cardiac fibrillation threshold, together with the lesser ability of the sinus node to withstand vagal inhibition, significantly increase the probability of appearance of heterogenous foci of excitation and consequently of arrhythmias and fibrillation.

It is quite important that all these electric stability disorders, as in other studies, could be completely prevented with prior administration of a β-blocker. The data in Table 1 show that the β-blocker itself raises the fibrillation threshold in control animals, while the α-blocker has no such effect.

When administered before a 6-h immobilization stress, the β-blocker totally prevented the stress-induced decline in the electric fibrillation threshold, while the α-blocker exhibited no effect. It thus seems likely that the observed stress impairment of contractile function and electric stability is in essence a β-injury. The studies of recent years with whole organisms in behavioral stress situations fit in with this idea.

Thus, Verrier and Lown[10] studied the changes in cardiac susceptibility to fibrillation, and in so doing tried to assess the mechanism through which the adrenergic action on the heart affects its electric stability. It turned out that various stress conditions evoked by pain,

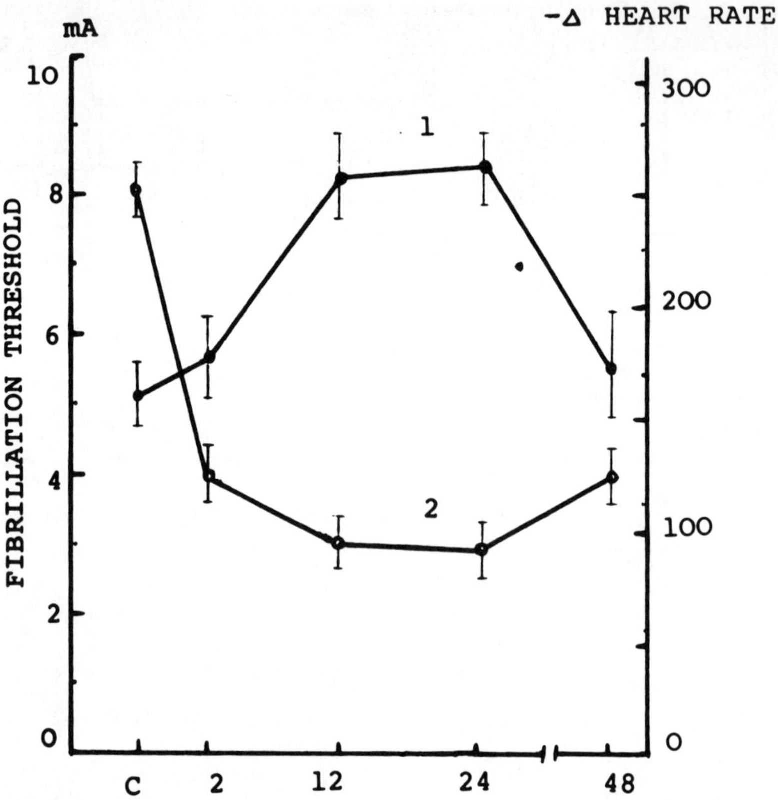

FIGURE 3. Dynamics of the fibrillation threshold and the negative chronotropic vagal effect on the heart after stress. The abscissa is time after the end of stress; C denotes the control values. (1, right ordinate) Drop in the heart rate upon vagal stimulation; (2, left ordinate) fibrillation threshold in milliamperes.

TABLE 1
Effect of α- and β-Adrenoblockers on the Cardiac Fibrillation Threshold in Control Animals and in Animals Subjected to Stress

Conditions	Fibrillation threshold (mA)[a]
Control (n = 12)	6.5 ± 0.63
Propranolol (β-blocker) (n = 10)	11.0 ± 1.50[b]
Prazosin (α-blocker) (n = 10)	6.1 ± 0.54
Stress (n = 19)	2.9 ± 0.26[b]
Propranolol + stress (n = 17)[c]	6.6 ± 0.44
Prazosin + stress (n = 17)[c]	3.1 ± 0.40[b]

[a] The threshold was determined 1 h after the end of a 6-h immobilization stress.
[b] $p < 0.05$ as compared to the control.
[c] The adrenoblockers were administered at 1 mg/kg body wt 30 min before stress.

fear, or rage caused by taking away food significantly enhance the myocardial blood flow, i.e., in the healthy animal behavioral stress elicits not ischemia, but hyperemia of the myocardium. However, the myocardial oxygen consumption greatly increases therewith;[11] therefore in stress hyperemia there still can be inadequate supply of oxygen to the myocardium, i.e., relative hypoxia. In this connection the authors made use of the calcium antagonist nifedipine, which causes coronary vasodilation and at the same time prevents the stress-induced increase in myocardial oxygen consumption. With nifedipine, stress can evoke neither ischemia nor hypoxia of the myocardium, and yet nifedipine does not affect the drop in fibrillation threshold in stress. On the other hand, the β-blocker methoprolol does not change the myocardial oxygen consumption, but averts the stress decline in the fibrillation threshold.

We can see that the propensity of the normal heart to ventricular fibrillation in behavioral stress (decline in the fibrillation threshold) is due to direct catecholamine action on the myocardial β-adrenoreceptors, and takes place at the background of enhanced coronary blood flow. Essentially similar data have been obtained by Vatner and Hintze[12] in continuous measurement of coronary blood flow in primates. The diurnal variations can be fivefold, with minimal flow during the night sleep and maximal in the behavioral emotional stress, when the blood supply to the heart proves quite adequate to its metabolic demands. In other words, we can conclude that acute stress situations engender not myocardial ischemia, but, on the contrary, hyperemia, which is nevertheless attended by a strong β-adrenergic effect on the heart and ensuing upset of its electric stability.

This can be stated to conform to the present day concepts of the differential reaction of the cross-striated cardiac muscle and of the smooth muscle of coronary arteries to catecholamines. While the β-adrenergic effect in the cross-striated cardiac muscle via enhanced cAMP formation and calcium entry into the sarcoplasm (see the scheme in Figure 29, Chapter 1) results in enhanced contraction force typical of stress, the β-adrenergic stimulation of the coronary vessels conversely leads to hyperpolarization of the smooth-muscle cell membranes, greater cAMP formation promotes calcium removal by the ion pumps, and the smooth muscle relaxes providing for enhanced coronary blood flow, i.e., myocardial hyperemia.[13] Catecholamines acting on the α-receptors of the vascular wall set in motion another chain of events including depolarization of the vascular smooth-muscle cells and increased calcium permeability of the cell membranes; elevated cytoplasmic calcium activates the contractile proteins with ensuing smooth-muscle cell contraction.

The above data on the cardiac effects of stress give grounds for believing that when an initially healthy organism encounters a heavy enough stress situation, the β-adrenergic effect of stress on the heart certainly dominates over the α-adrenergic one and, accordingly, the discovered complex of rather stable alterations in the function and electric stability retained after the end of the stress is the result of the stress β-adrenergic damage to the heart. This complex, completely preventable with β-blockers, has been shown to comprise myocardial stress rigidity; depressed force and velocity of contraction and velocity of relaxation; greatly increased myocardial response to calcium, sodium, and hydrogen ion shifts; and, finally, lower cardiac fibrillation threshold and lower resistance of the sinus node automatism to the negatively chronotropic vagal action.

The question arising in this connection is how a healthy human or animal heart in the absence of ischemia, only under adrenergic influence, develops not just arrhythmia, but pronounced fibrillation. To answer this question it is essential to recall the already mentioned concept of the electric heterogeneity of the healthy heart as well as the fact that it may be increased by the marked hypercalcium effect of stress. With this in mind it can be envisaged that upon stimulation of the apex cordis in the works of Lown et al.[3] and Verrier and Lown,[10] or in our experiments, an impulse evoked in the vulnerable period and slowly propagating in the retrograde direction may even in a healthy myocardium encounter zones of increased resistance. Circumventing them and spreading further to the base, it can concurrently propagate anterograde, returning to the recently blocked zone which now becomes patent. This results in cyclic excitation which becomes the basis of cardiac fibrillation.[14]

It is essential that *the probability of reentry caused by retrograde and anterograde impulse propagation is much higher in the stress than in the healthy heart, since excessive stress damages the cell membranes and nexuses and markedly increases the number of zones with decreased RP and conductivity which can give rise to reentry.* As a result, for the first fixed reentry to appear in stress animals the excitation should spread over a comparatively small region of the myocardium and the stimulation need be much weaker than in the norm, as the electric threshold of extrasystole is lowered. Accordingly, much weaker current is required for multiple nonfixed reentries which trigger and replace each other to encompass the heart, i.e., become the basis of ventricular fibrillation. The decreased cardiac resistance to arrhythmias and fibrillation is due not only to the presence of one-way conduction blocks and potential pacemakers, but also to the impulse getting through a zone of partial blockade (where the rapid response linked with sodium entry is mostly inhibited) which turns out to be deformed. It has a flat excitation front and diminished amplitude, i.e., it is transformed into the slow response provided mainly by the calcium influx. Hence there is a significantly higher probability that this impulse would be subsequently blocked and would participate in formation of reentry.

These considerations are important not only for explaining the drop in the electric threshold of fibrillation in stress, but also for understanding some weighty realities of the cardiological clinics. The matter is that at the background of microfocal cardiac stress damage and markedly enhanced bioelectric heterogeneity, an ectopic impulse arising in the zone of a long-existing organic injury (e.g., in the subendocardial cells of the postinfarct scar zone) or in the region of partial or complete ischemia is much more likely to entail arrhythmias and cardiac fibrillation than in the absence of stress damage.

It should be emphasized that the essentially β-adrenergic damage to the heart not associated with ischemia was discovered and described in detail 30 years ago in excellent studies of Rona, et al.,[15] who were the first to find that large doses of the synthetic norepinephrine analog, β-agonist isoproterenol, act through the adenylate cyclase of the heart, adipose tissue, and other organs to cause enhanced calcium entry into myocardial cells; this, together with excess fatty acids, uncouples oxidative phosphorylation in mitochondria and decreases the cell contents of ATP and CP; simultaneously, excess calcium induces myofibrillar contracture. These mostly microfocal lesions develop at the background of cardiac hypertrophy, and at moderate doses of the agonist may not impair the contractile function, whereas at large doses they depress it. The outcome, if not lethal, is focal necrobiotic damage with ensuing focal cardiosclerosis.

Later, Waldenström et al.,[16] basically following up the works of Rona et al., replaced isoproterenol with norepinephrine and ran experiments with the isolated heart excluding the changes in coronary flow. In this case, certainly ruling out coronary spasm and ischemia, increasing dosage of norepinephrine consistently caused myocardial damage as manifest by declining ATP level and leakage of creatine kinase and transaminases into the perfusate. These alterations were proportionate to the acting catecholamine concentration in the perfusing solution and duration of the exposure, and were attended with depression of the cardiac contractile function. Pathological changes such as myofibrillar contracture developed in the myocardial cells. These alterations could in great measure be prevented with β-blockers or verapamil, which is known to block calcium entry into the cells.

Thus, *β-adrenergic nonischemic damage to the myocardium, caused not by a synthetic, but by the natural catecholamine, taking place both in the whole organism and in the isolated heart and attended with marked impairment of the contractile function and — most importantly — electric stability of the heart, is an undebatable reality and is very probably involved in arrhythmias and sudden death.*

The data available on the molecular bases of β-adrenergic damage in stress have been considered in Chapter 1. Here it must be pointed out that the direct β-adrenergic injury to the contractile myocardium and to the conducting system of the heart is not the sole pathway through which the stress damage can be realized.

The contractile myocardium, the conducting system, and, what is most important, the coronary arteries, are rich in α_1-adrenoreceptors which, under the action of catecholamines, activate Ca^{2+} entry into muscle cells through slow channels[17] and probably its release from the sarcoplasmic reticulum (SR) mediated by inositol triphosphate.[18,19] Unlike the β-adrenergic effect, this is not accompanied by cAMP formation or increase in contraction and relaxation velocities and, notably, is not blocked by endogenous adenosine.[20] Accordingly, the α-adrenergic effect, if inordinately amplified, may be directly arrhythmogenic as well as cause coronary spasm. The arrhythmogenic action of α_1-adrenoreceptors has been demonstrated by Thandroyen et al.[21] administration of the α-agonist methoxamine results in a pronounced inotropic effect and a 2.5-fold decrease in the fibrillation threshold.

Both these shifts could be prevented with the α-blocker prazosin, the slow-channel blocker nizoldipine, or rianodine blocking Ca^{2+} release from the SR. The authors arrive at a conclusion that both the positive inotropic and the arrhythmogenic effects of overactivation of α-adrenoreceptors are actualized through excess calcium coming both from the extracellular space and from the SR.

The vasoconstrictive effect of α-receptor activation has been demonstrated in experiments with intact animals as well as in clinicophysiological studies on human subjects. Thus Murray and Vatner[22] used a flowmeter to measure the animal coronary blood flow under physical load. The flow increased according to the metabolic demands of the myocardium; however, the α-blocker phentolamine caused additional increase in the blood flow, indicating the existence of a constant tonic vasoconstrictive α-adrenergic influence on the coronary vessels.

The clinicophysiological studies of Mudge et al.[23] show that in coronary disease this tonic α-adrenergic influence may increase and result in coronary spasm. Thus, immersion of the hand into cold water proved to elevate the ST segment and cause pectoral pains in patients with coronary disease; this was preventable with the α-blocker phentolamine.

Of principal importance in this context is the fact that all effects of α-adrenoreceptor stimulation are consistently enhanced upon blocking the β-receptors with propranolol[12,24] or their desensitization by sustained high catecholamine levels in the blood.[25]

The latter is most essential for us as it suggests that desensitization of the β-adrenoreceptors in prolonged or chronic stress may result in coronary spasms. Indeed, Verrier and Haegeston[11] justly recall that a primary decrease in the coronary flow independent of shifts in the systemic hemodynamics has been observed not only in variant stenocardia,[26] but also in classical and unstable angina pectoris.[27-29] Deanfield et al.[27] reported recurrent episodes of ST segment depression during ambulatory monitoring of patients with stable angina; they were not associated with changes in the cardiac pace and appeared to indicate transitory myocardial ischemia. Further, it was found that coronary spasm could be brought about by a stress situation[29] and in particular by conditioned verbal stimuli.[30] In the context of our discourse it is important that in all these cases the coronary spasm is apparently realized on the basis of β-receptor desensitization and is due to the fact that the α-adrenergic effect involving calcium release from the SR cannot be rectified by such a physiological factor as excess adenosine. These data also give grounds for thinking that in chronic stress situations attended with β-desensitization, coronary spasms damaging the myocardium may be elicited by other agonists of the calcium-mobilizing receptors: vasopressin, histamine, etc. Such spasms develop in impaired function of the central stress-limiting systems, one of which is the parasympathetic system restricting the stress adrenergic effects on the heart.

This stress-limiting cardioprotective action is manifest in that at a high adrenergic tonus and lowered fibrillation threshold, stimulation of the vagus nerve raises the threshold, returning it to normal; administration of atropine, conversely, decreases the threshold still further and is conducive to fibrillation.[31] In line with this, atropine has been shown to act on muscarine receptors to suppress norepinephrine release from adrenergic terminals[32] and to restrain the adrenoreceptor response to norepinephrine and the cyclic nucleotide formation.[23] However, such cardioprotective vagal influence can also become detrimental. In prolonged, heavy enough stress, when catecholamine consumption outstrips its resynthesis and the catecholamine levels decline not only in the nervous centers,[34] but also in the working organs including the heart,[35] the vagus nerve starts to predominate in cardiac regulation. This is initially expressed as bradycardia, but may accrue with more grave sequelae. Hazards of this type prove common in stress situations when escape or avoidance are precluded and reactions of capitulation and immotility prevail.

Indeed, a number of researchers who had studied susceptible animals in drastic stress situations observed not only vagal bradycardia, but asystolia and cardiac arrest. Engel[36] has systematized these works to substantiate his concept of the role of vasovagal cardiac arrest in the pathogenesis of sudden death. Of the most interesting in this respect are the studies of Corley et al.,[37-39] who put forward an idea of sudden parasympathetic activation or cessation of sympathetic influences that occur when the stress becomes excessive and the animal capitulates. Similar conclusions were arrived at by other researchers.[40,41]

In this connection we believe that *at least three factors evolving in prolonged stress may participate in the switchover of cardiac regulation from sympathetic to parasympathetic domination.*

The first factor appears to consist in profound alteration of the functioning of the higher divisions of the nervous system when, in the face of insurmountable difficulties, the stress of struggle (attack or flight) changes over to the stress of capitulation (resignation and standstill) with attending significant activation of the parasympathetic system. Engel[36] has shown that in humans this phenomenon is realized as a vasodepressive syndrome in which vagal asystolia is combined with neurogenic vasodilation and a deep drop of arterial pressure. This syndrome may result in more or less heavy syncopes as well as sudden death. Again, the capitulation stress has been shown (Chapter 1) to cause rather pronounced and rapid cardiac damage and to upset its arrhythmogenic resistance.

The second factor is the desensitization of cardiac adrenoreceptors by high catecholamine concentrations, or impairment of their function because of membrane damage by the lipid triad. Such decreased adrenoresponsiveness of the cardiac muscle has been observed in our experiments with rats subjected to a 6-h EPS.[42]

The third factor is that the preceding adrenergic action on the heart may damage the sinus node and other parts of the conduction system, with the resultant decreased resistance of the cardiac automatism to the negatively chronotropic vagal influence and loss of sinus node control over the downstream ectopic pacemakers. This is in line with the direct electron-microscopic observations of sinus node lesions and the data on the greater vagal effect on the automatism of the sinus node in stress (Chapter 1, Section IX, and above).

Notably, the β-adrenergic damage to the sinus node and other parts of the conduction system may under certain conditions cause pronounced disturbances of the cardiac rhythm. In our studies with Belkina and Kolarova this effect was achieved by administration to animals of 10 mg/kg of the selective β-agonist isoproterenol.

Rats subjected to such treatment were tested for (1) the contractile function of the heart at physiological rest and during aortic clamping and (2) electric threshold of cardiac fibrillation and the effect of increasing stimulation of the vagus nerve. The tests were run 1 d after isoproterenol administration. It turned out that isoproterenol, like EPS, had no effect on the contractile parameters in the whole organism.

At the same time, the ventricular fibrillation threshold fell on average from 7.5 ± 0.55 to 3.1 ± 0.94 mA, i.e., 2.5-fold. This upset of the electric stability was accompanied by

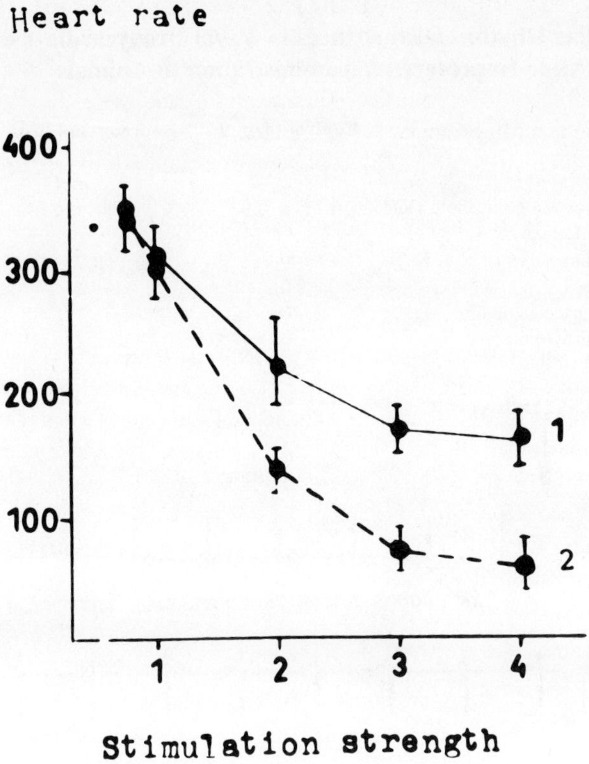

FIGURE 4. Effect of vagal stimulation on the heart rate in control animals (1) and 24 h after isoproterenol administration (10 mg/kg) (2). The abscissa is the strength of vagal stimulation, multiples of the threshold current.

a decrease in the resistance of sinus node automatism to the negatively chronotropic vagal influence. Figure 4 shows that stimulation of the vagus nerve depresses the sinus node automatism to a much greater extent in animals with isoproterenol damage than in controls: at the same strength of stimulation the heart rate decreased to 68 beats per minute vs. 168 beats per minute in the control.

The data in Table 2 demonstrate that in animals with β-adrenergic damage such vagal bradycardia was attended with rhythmic disorders not seen in controls; arrhythmias were observed in seven out of nine animals.

Figure 5 displays the main types of these ectopically originating arrhythmias: unlike the controls (1) where vagus stimulation only elicits sinus bradycardia, animals with cardiac β-adrenodamage exhibit (2) atrioventricular (AV) rhythm with ventricles being excited prior to auricles, (3) idioventricular rhythm intermittent with sinus and AV rhythms, and (4) I-degree AV block with regular atrial complexes, but every second ventricular complex omitted.

On the whole the results of this work are in accord with the concept that *cardiac β-adrenergic damage at the early stage of reaction associated with struggle is conducive to dangerous vagal arrhythmias and cardiac arrest at the late stage of reaction, in exhaustion of adrenergic regulation, and behavioral capitulation. The experimental data appear to agree with the clinical situations considered further in which stress arrhythmias, fibrillation, and sudden cardiac death may occur. For the initially healthy heart without organic alterations we can discern several situations of this kind.*

TABLE 2
Cardiac Rhythm Disturbances in Vagal Bradycardia 1 d After Isoproterenol Administration to Animals

	Control (n = 9)	Isoproterenol (n = 9)
Heart rate (min^{-1})	344 ± 42	353 ± 13
Vagal stimulation threshold (V)	0.17 ± 0.03	0.20 ± 0.04
Number of cases of:		
Arrhythmias	0	7
AV block	0	2
Idioventricular rhythm	0	4
Bradyarrhythmia	0	2

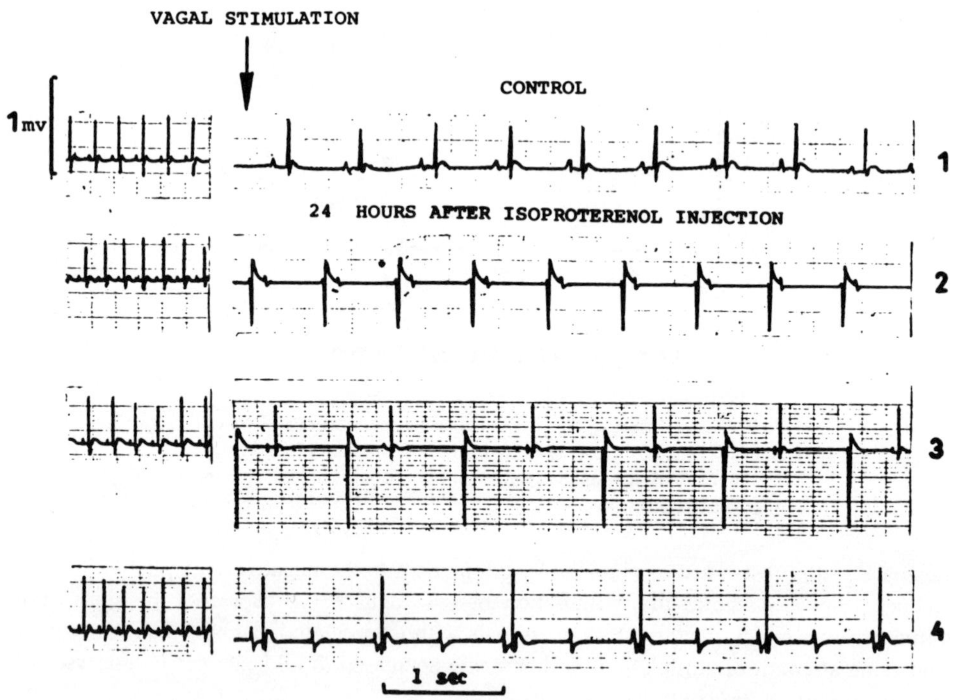

FIGURE 5. Effect of isoproterenol damage on the cardiac rhythm upon vagal stimulation. Stimulation of the vagus nerve in the control elicits sinus bradycardia (1), while after isoproterenol administration it gives rise to atrioventricular (AV) rhythm (2), idioventricular rhythm (3), and first-degree AV block (4).

1. A stress situation engendering reactions of anxiety, rage, or struggle exerts a strong β-adrenergic effect on the heart, resulting in cardiac damage that is not ischemic, but takes place in coronary dilation and manifests itself first of all as impairment of the electric stability of the heart, and also as upset contractile function. This acute β-adrenergic damage is the most plausible cause of sudden cardiac death directly in the stress episode with no observable organic lesions in the heart.
2. Prolonged action of the same stress situation also prolongs the adrenergic effect on the heart. Owing to desensitization of the β-adrenergic receptors, it may transform into a mainly α-adrenergic effect and potentiate the action of other agonists of the calcium-mobilizing receptors — vasopressin, histamine, etc. Activation of all such receptors in the coronary arteries is realized as constriction and can result in coronary spasms with more or less pronounced ischemic injury to the myocardium. This may

explain some cases of myocardial infarction in aging persons with intact or moderately atherosclerotic coronary arteries, or in patients with vague invariant angina.

3. Still further persisting stress situation, and especially stress of capitulation, engenders a fearful behavioral reaction of "freezing" reflected, in particular, in depressed circulation and respiration and in vagal bradycardia. With exhausted adrenergic regulation and preexisting β-adrenergic lesions of the heart and its conduction system, this may lead to dangerous bradycardias and vagal cardiac arrest. The latter is most probable in the Pokkuri disease and in epidemics of sudden nocturnal deaths among contingents of people finding themselves in alien and often hopeless circumstances.

In assessing these possible variants it is easy to see that *their pivot is the strong β-adrenergic effect on the heart. In the final analysis it is this factor that causes initial injury, preconditions the α-adrenergic effect, and through the damage to the conduction system and contractile myocardium makes the heart highly vulnerable to the vagally elicited ectopic arrhythmias and functional disturbances.*

Now it seems expedient to elucidate to what extent this experimentally substantiated notion of the role of stress in the pathogenesis of arrhythmias can be applied to man.

III. ROLE OF PRIMARY STRESS DAMAGE IN ARRHYTHMIAS AND SUDDEN CARDIAC DEATH IN MAN

Since any normal person goes through multiple, more or less serious, stress episodes, and we could see that stress induces disturbances of cardiac electric stability, a reasonable conclusion is that stress and adrenergic effects on the heart may rather often entail transient and therefore nonhazardous arrhythmias.

Indeed, this suggestion is favored by the now commonly known fact that with continuous monitoring various disturbances of cardiac rhythm and conduction are found no less frequently than the inevitable stress situations of everyday life. Thus cardiac arrhythmias with variation of intervals between contractions up to 8% were recorded at least once in 86% of subjects while 50% showed pronounced sinus arrhythmias with interval variation of 100% and more.[7]

The data of Bjerregaard[8] testify that a large part of those examined reveal episodes of bradycardia with pauses between contractions reaching 1500 to 1750 ms and sometimes 2000 ms.

Such episodes of transitory sinus bradycardia, caused in all probability by enhanced negative chronotropic influence of the vagus nerve, are not infrequently associated with sinoauricular block and are designated as a secondary sinus node dysfunction syndrome.[43] It can be easily envisaged that damage to the sinus node (e.g., from previous adrenergic stress attack) and decreased vagal resistance of its automatism can aggravate this phenomenon to the extent of blocked sinus rhythm and activation of the downstream ectopic foci of automatism. The data of continuous monitoring[8] demonstrate that atrial extrasystoles are found in more than half of uncomplaining subjects examined. Ventricular extrasystoles are observed with approximately the same incidence, and their daily number in practically healthy persons may exceed 1800; the proportion of people with such extrasystoles steadily increases with age, hence it is a progressing condition. It is noteworthy that multifocal and multiple extrasystoles in the form of bigeminy and trigeminy, and in 4 cases out of 260 even ventricular tachycardia, have been revealed in uncomplaining subjects.

In discussing the question of whether or not people with such extrasystoles can be considered completely healthy, it should be borne in mind that besides extrasystoles, 24-h monitoring also reveals conduction defects, albeit much more seldom. Thus in several cases, especially during sleep, unstable I- and II-degree AV blocks[44-46] as well as intermittent elongation of the Q-R interval have been reported. In a 6-h monitoring by Von Dietz and Kirchhoff,[47] three of nine uncomplaining subjects displayed a transitory block with Wenckebach's periods. Clearly the combination of ectopic impulses with transitory conduction defects is conducive to formation of reentry and heavy arrhythmias. In general, even a brief analysis of the results of continuous monitoring of the so-called healthy subjects allows one to point out at least two moments.

First, many of these transitory arrhythmias in "healthy" people verge on pathology, progress with age, and therefore make probable a gradual evolvement of a grave enough "arrhythmic heart disease" in the absence of recorded organic alterations.

Second, some of these at first glance causeless, idiopathic arrhythmias are most likely the sequelae of influenzal or other toxinfectious myocarditis, hereditary abnormalities, etc. Along with this, the transient or, more exactly, recurrent character of these arrhythmias suggests that many of them result from transitional processes in the cardiac neural regulation provoked by either exogenous or endogenous (emotional) stress.

This point of view is supported by numerous clinicophysiological studies on healthy subjects and patients.

It has been shown that among certain contingents whose occupation involves repeated stress situations, cardiac disturbances of nonischemic origin may develop that are characterized by more or less pronounced arrhythmias despite high tolerance to physical load. In other words, there is the same dissociation between impaired electric stability and intact pump function of the heart that we have described in detail in the stress damage to animal heart. Thus in our work[48] we correlated the cardiac resistance to physical and stress loads in men of such indisputably stressful occupation as international airline pilots. These people have to pass systematic examinations and are not admitted to work if showing an ischemic response to standard physical load.

As the first step, we analyzed the test results for 807 pilots that had passed the examination, and found that in the younger age group (30 to 39 years) ischemic responses were never observed, but 3% (14 cases) showed disturbances of automatism mainly in the form of atrial rhythm, and 4 cases exhibited supraventricular extrasystoles.

In the elder age group (40 to 52) rhythm disorders were found in 17% (58 cases), with equal extent of both ventricular and atrial extrasystole in 17 cases and atrial rhythm in others.

Notably, the overwhelming majority of the arrhythmic responses to physical load were observed not at peak load, but in relief, i.e., were not ischemic. *This phenomenon, not infrequently encountered in any functional diagnosis unit, is in all probability explained by the fact that when the load is relieved the rapidly increasingly vagal tonicity suppresses the sinus node automatism while the adrenergic regulation is still excited and the potential pacemakers being depolarized by excess blood catecholamines become real sources of ectopic excitation and extrasystoles.* It is essential that under conditions of such nonischemic arrhythmias there may evolve a more striking and in a sense paradoxical phenomenon when a physical load or an orthostatic test abolishes the arrhythmia steadily observed without load.

At the next stage of our work,[49] 54 pilots of the highest class aged 35 to 53 were compared in a standard test with veloergometric load (VEL) and in solving professional tasks in a flight simulator (takeoff, landing, failures, etc.). Arrhythmias turned out to occur only in 5 pilots under VEL, but in 34, i.e., more than 60%, in the simulator. In all cases extrasystoles in the simulator proved only occasional and mostly appeared during "breakdown in flight" and "flight continued after breakdown". Despite the small number of extrasystoles during flight simulation, further studies with the use of ECG monitoring showed these results to be really significant. Figure 6 displays the results of monitoring a group of pilots who either had (seven individuals) or did not have (four individuals) extrasystoles during flight simulation. It can be seen that in persons who had rhythmic disturbances in simulation the number of atrial extrasystoles is several times greater than in those who had

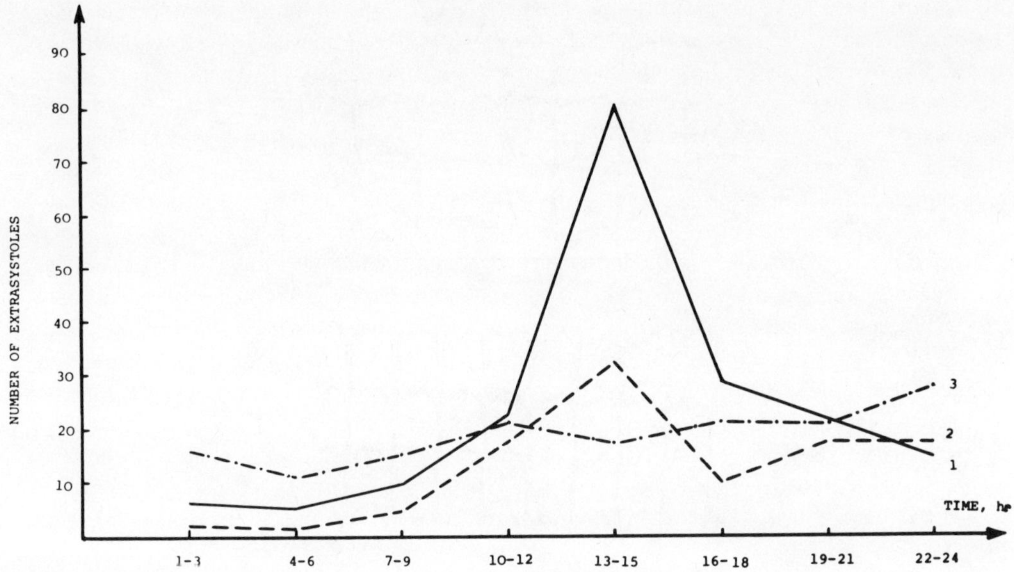

FIGURE 6. Dynamics of extrasystoles in pilots during continuous ECG monitoring. (1) Atrial extrasystoles in pilots with rhythm disturbances observed in flight simulation; (2) ventricular extrasystoles in pilots with rhythm disturbances in flight simulation; (3) atrial extrasystoles in pilots without rhythm disturbances in flight simulation.

none. Ventricular extrasystoles were completely absent from the latter group, but observable throughout the day in the former.

Much more vivid stress disturbances of cardiac rhythm and conduction in some of these people were brought on not by simulation or real flight, but by a qualitatively different stress situation — apprehension of the results of examination which could deprive them of their job.

An interesting example in this respect is pilot Z, 40, whose ECGs are presented in Figure 7. Appreciable ventricular extrasystole is seen during examination in the recuperative period after VEL and in clinical monitoring, but is totally absent at maximal physical load and during real flight including takeoff and landing. In other words, the arrhythmogenic effect is highly pronounced under stress of examination and wholly lacking in normal occupational activity, albeit involving certain risk of life. Thorough analysis revealed two more similar cases. In the aggregate these data unequivocally testify to stress-induced rhythmic disorders in apparently healthy persons (without ischemic disease). Notably, it is the more socially significant factor that proves to cause greater stress and dangerous arrhythmogenic effect.

The fact that some situations can provoke arrhythmias in practically healthy persons highly tolerant to physical load is in line with the idea that many arrhythmias may be of stress origin.

This is supported by, among other things, the very existence of a peculiar condition that had been called cardiac neurosis,[50] cardiac form of neurocirculatory dystonia,[51,52] and in recent years has been referred to in both Russian and English literature as idiopathic arrhythmias, i.e., arrhythmias the cause of which is unknown.[53,54] Of course this term can cover arrhythmias of toxinfectious origin or those resulting from congenital defects. Notwithstanding, there are several circumstances favoring the neurogenous or simply stress origin of like arrhythmias.

First, many patients with such idiopathic arrhythmias exhibit neurotization in the form of hypochondriac, anxiety depressive, cardiophobic, and less frequently hysteric syndromes

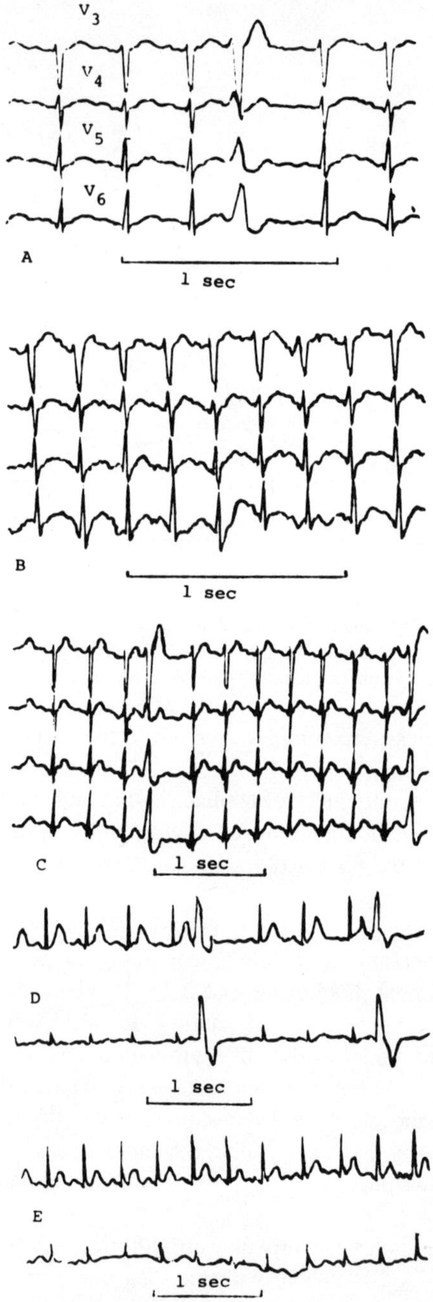

FIGURE 7. Electrocardiograms of pilot Z, age 40. (A) During examination before VEL; (B) at maximal VEL; (C) immediately upon termination of VEL; (D) continuous monitoring in the clinic during examination; (E) during real flight.

of varying degrees of severity; and arrhythmias are often proportionate to the neurotic syndrome and may disappear as the syndrome is eliminated by successful pharmacotherapy.

Second, along with the complete absence of myocardial ischemia and rather high tolerance to physical loads in such arrhythmias there often are defects in specific stress-limiting systems which will be specially considered later. Thus Skibitskii[52] has shown that in 40 patients with neurocirculatory dystonia suffering from attacks of paroxysmal supraventricular tachycardia, a GABA derivative phenibut (acting like the known GABA-receptor activator baclophen) decreased the number of attacks by a factor of 5.5 and prolonged the fitless period to 6 months. In half of 32 patients with ventricular extrasystole, this activator of the GABA-ergic system completely abolished or decreased the number of extrasystoles by 75% or more. The antiarrhythmic effect was observed not only in neurocirculatory dystonia, but also in IHD, and was accompanied by a positive psychotropic effect. It is known that the GABA-ergic system can be activated via the benzodiazepine receptors; accordingly, benzodiazepine receptor agonists have been also successfully used as antiarrhythmics.

The abolishment of arrhythmias by activation of the GABA-ergic system is in itself an indication of the important role of this central stress-limiting system (Chapter 4) in the so-called idiopathic arrhythmias.

The studies of Smetnev et al.[55] demonstrate the involvement of defects in a cellular stress-limiting system, the prostaglandin one, in arrhythmogenesis. In patients with idiopathic paroxysmal supraventricular rhythm disorders the attacks of tachycardia develop with the blood flow in both coronary arteries enhanced proportionally to the heart rate owing to decreased coronary bed resistance. In IHD patients similar attacks are not accompanied by adequately enhanced coronary flow and may in some cases lead to coronary insufficiency. Further studies have shown that persistence of idiopathic nonischemic arrhythmias and increasing frequency of spontaneous paroxysms are attended by progressive impairment of the regulatory system of prostaglandins (PG) and cyclic nucleotides: decreasing PGF/$PGF_{2\alpha}$ ratio in coronary sinus blood, and increasing thromboxane/PG and decreasing cAMP/cGMP in the blood flowing to the heart.

Thus, a *preexisting or evolving deficiency of the systems limiting the adrenergic effects on the heart may play a substantial part in development of arrhythmias having no organic basis in the heart, and this can be evidence for the stress origin of such arrhythmias.*

The third argument in favor of idiopathic arrhythmias caused by stress is that myocardial needle biopsy in such patients often reveals focal alterations and fibrosis resembling those described in experimental stress damage to animal hearts. Neglia et al.[56] studied 44 patients without ischemic disease or cardiac failure, but who complained of palpitation, heart pains and faints, and had complex ventricular arrhythmias or conduction defects. In up to 73% of these patients bidimensional ECG revealed impaired contractility of the left and/or the right ventricle. Myocardial biopsy performed on 13 of such patients demonstrated hypertrophy of muscle fibers and focal interstitial fibrosis of both ventricles in 7 and of only the left ventricle in 5 cases.

Finally, the most weighty evidence for the role of stress in evolvement of idiopathic arrhythmias has been obtained in clinical use of psychoemotional or stress loads (SL). Such techniques have been rather popular in recent years.[57-61] Of special interest are the studies where the inducibility of arrhythmias with SL has been correlated in IHD patients and those with neurocirculatory dystonia or idiopathic arrhythmias with pronounced neurasthenic syndrome. According to Rizhinashvili et al.,[62] among the whole contingent of cardiological patients with potentially possible cardiac rhythm disorders the SL test elicited arrhythmias in 18% of cases; whereas, in patients with idiopathic arrhythmias and anxiety depressive syndrome, the respective portion was 42 to 46%. These arrhythmias could be abolished with a benzodiazepine receptor agonist, seduxen, which is known to activate the brain stress-limiting GABA-ergic system. Thus, even such moderate, standard clinical tests can evoke arrhythmias in a large proportion of people with certain disturbances of cardiac neural regulation.

Together with Khalfen and Lyamina we studied the adrenergic and cardiac responses to physical and stress load in 98 healthy male subjects (mean age 35) and in 48 male patients of the same age with neurocirculatory dystonia. Since this approach was further used for patients with coronary disease, it seems expedient to consider the technique in more detail.

Stress was created by an operator type of psychoemotional load associated with time shortage for solving information tasks.[63] There were three steps of increasing complexity, each of 5-min duration.

At step 1, the subject had to respond to words heard from a tape recorder by choosing a pencil of corresponding color and striking out from a form the word denoting this color. At step 2, he had to strike out two words: one heard from the tape recorder and the other corresponding to the color of a word projected on a screen. At step 3, he had to strike out three words: one heard, one read, and one corresponding to the color of the projected word.

The performance was evaluated by a qualified observer who responsed to the subject's errors (missed word, wrong word, or wrong pencil) by actuating a sharp and unpleasant audio signal. Besides, regardless of the quality of work the testing was accompanied by standard comments, "Your work is poor", "Too many mistakes", "All men before you were better".

The subjects were tested with a stepwise-increasing VEL (initial load 25 W with 25-W increments, each step of 3-min duration), 2 d before the stress load.

The cardiovascular response was assessed by arterial pressure (AP), heart rate (HR), the index HR × APs/100, and myocardial contractility indices.

The response of the adrenergic system was assayed by catecholamine excretion in urine collected from 9 to 11 a.m. at the day of testing and the day before when there were no examinations or procedures.

As follows from Table 3, in healthy subjects the SL enhanced cardiac function by about one third as judged by the index of Katz (HR × APs/100), which characterizes myocardial O_2 consumption; the contraction and relaxation velocities increased approximately to the same extent so that the contraction and relaxation indices remained unchanged.

The VEL produced a much more pronounced mobilization of the cardiac contractile function: the Katz index increased 1.7-fold and contraction and relaxation velocities 1.3 to 1.4-fold; this resulted in a small decrease in the contraction and relaxation indices. On the whole, the heart is much more responsive to physical than to stress loads.

Another situation was found for catecholamine excretion with urine, which in response to the SL increased by more than 80% for epinephrine, 24% for norepinephrine, 87% for dopa, and 27% for dopamine. Under physical load the elevation in all catecholamines except norepinephrine was significantly smaller (only 18% for epinephrine or 12% for dopamine).

Despite the somewhat greater norepinephrine excretion under VEL, the overall adrenergic response (i.e., the sum increment in norepinephrine and epinephrine excretion) at moderate standard SL exceeds by half that at maximal VEL. Since catecholamine excretion depends on its concentration in the blood, this means that the blood catecholamine levels directly acting on the heart were higher in SL than in VEL. Accordingly, the antidiuretic effect proved to be twice as great in SL.

The same studies carried out on patients with the cardiac form of neurocirculatory dystonia (Table 4) show that at rest the excretion of epinephrine is 50% higher than in healthy subjects, and the relative response to SL is the same. *Norepinephrine excretion, unchanged at rest, drastically increases in SL (the increment is over threefold that in healthy subjects). In sum, this signifies that the adrenergic response in patients with neurocirculatory dystonia is greater than in healthy people.*

Further, it can be seen that neurocirculatory dystonia moderately decreases dopamine excretion at rest; the significance of this shift will be considered later in connection with the effect of SL in IHD.

The standard VEL revealed no ischemic or arrhythmic reactions in any of the patients examined. At the same time, upon SL arrhythmic reactions in the form of supraventricular and ventricular extrasystoles were observed in 12 patients (i.e., 25% of those examined). In other words, in dystonic patients the SL called for much lesser enhancement of cardiac

TABLE 3
Responses to Stress Load and Maximal Physical Load in Healthy Subjects

Indices	Stress load			Physical load		
	Before	After	Δ, %	Before	After	Δ, %
Heart rate (beats/min)	73	85	16	73	146	100
APs (mmHg)	123	144	17	121	160	32
APd (mmHg)	80	94	13	83	92	15
Katz index (HR × APs/100)	90	122	36	88	234	166
Diastolic relaxation velocity (cm/s)	3.56	4.76	34	3.58	8.46	136
Systolic contraction velocity (cm/s)	3.80	5.13	35	3.71	8.98	142
Relaxation index	4.22	4.20	−0.5	4.22	3.84	−9
Contraction index	4.00	3.90	−2.5	4.01	3.61	−10
Urine excretion (ml)	105	82	−22	105	96	−9
Epinephrine excretion (ng/min)	3.60	6.50	81	3.60	4.25	18
Norepinephrine excretion (ng/min)	6.25	7.73	24	6.25	9.06	45
Dopa excretion (ng/min)	5.10	9.85	87	5.10	5.46	7
Dopamine excretion (ng/min)	292	372	27	292	327	12

TABLE 4
Effect of Neurocirculatory Dystonia (NCD) on the Adrenergic Response to Stress Load (SL) (Excretion, ng/min)

Indices	Healthy subjects (n = 21)		NCD patients (n = 19)	
	Before SL	After SL	Before SL	After SL
Epinephrine (E)	3.60 ± 0.80	6.50 ± 0.81	5.40 ± 0.82[a]	10.40 ± 0.90
Norepinephrine (NE)	6.25 ± 0.81	7.77 ± 0.83	6.02 ± 0.78	11.60 ± 0.91[a]
E/NE	0.57 ± 0.06	0.84 ± 0.09	0.89 ± 0.06[a]	0.89 ± 0.06
Dopamine	292 ± 18	372 ± 22	260 ± 21	315 ± 31
Dopamine/E + NE	29.6 ± 1.81	26.0 ± 1.61	22.8 ± 1.00	18.8 ± 1.00[a]

[a] Difference with respective healthy controls significant at $p < 0.05$.

function than VEL, as in healthy subjects, but therewith caused much greater activation of the adrenergic system and in 25% of cases elicited potential arrhythmias. It is easily conceivable that in such patients with increased adrenergic reactivity the multitudinous biosocial stress episodes can cause and gradually aggravate adrenergic damage to the heart, and this process underlies the pathogenesis of the peculiar arrhythmic stress disease.

Another weighty argument in favor of the actual existence of the stress disease associated with attenuated organismic and first of all cardiac resistance to adrenergic injury is, in our opinion, the data on fibrillation and sudden cardiac death in families with marked stress intolerance. Thus Green et al.,[64] reported on sudden death in three generations, which included a 14-year-old girl who fell dead after being told that her 15-year-old brother had died immediately after a running competition. In a family studied by McRae et al.,[65] one son suddenly died at the age of 17, having been frightened by his pal, another at 12 while swimming, the third also at the age of 12 was startled by a spider and fell dead while running to tell his comrades. Their mother had about 25 syncopal episodes in the period between age 15 and 25 which had always been preceded by emotional stress causing fear and anger. Her fourth son showed no symptoms, but at 11 was found to have a shortened P-R interval and a pronounced U wave; his first syncopal episode occurred at the age of $12^1/_2$ when he got angry during a game of baseball. In the clinic no rhythm disorders were observed when the patient was left alone and quiet, but any diagnostic procedures from venipuncture to application of anesthesia and heart catheterization caused great anxiety and, as a consequence, sinus tachycardia, multifocal ventricular extrasystoles, and sometimes ventricular tachycardia developing into ventricular fibrillation.

In other words, in all these cases cardiac fibrillation and sudden cardiac death were predetermined by genetically attenuated resistance of these individuals to stress exposures. As will be shown further, such decreased resistance to the arrhythmogenic effect of stress not only can be explained by insufficiency of stress-limiting systems, but also can be rectified by adaptive activation of these systems or introduction of their metabolites.

Generally speaking, sudden cardiac death is the most grievous, but at the same time the most significant, natural phenomenon that can be used to evaluate the role of stress as a primary heart-damaging factor.

It is noteworthy that pathomorphological examination of people that have died of cardiac fibrillation reveals cases and whole groups of cases with no alterations indicative of atherosclerosis or ischemia.[66,67] A typical example is the case reported by Davies et al.[68] A 20-year-old girl suddenly fainted during her wedding ceremony and, despite intensive medical care, died of ventricular fibrillation. The autopsy revealed a nonhypertrophied, macroscopically and microscopically normal heart, without coronary atherosclerosis, focal, or other myocardial alterations. The medical history gave no indications of heart pathology; she had never complained about her heart and did not take medicinal drugs. No pathology could be found in other organs and systems. In evaluating this quite representative case, attention should be paid to the fact that fibrillation occurred during an event of great psychological significance for the young girl; this stress element was the only meaningful finding.

There are also studies covering selected groups of cases where stress appears to be the direct cause of sudden cardiac death. Thus, Cebelin and Hirsh[69] carried out a comparative pathomorphological examination of 15 persons who had died of sudden cardiac death immediately upon heavy stress, 15 who had been killed in traffic accidents, and 15 who had died of stenosing coronary atherosclerosis.

The fatal stress situations included conflicts with parents or neighbors, homicidal assaults, etc. Pathoanatomical examination of these cases revealed groups of cardiomyocytes with contractural injuries and dispersion of myofibrils, and the interstitial connective tissue had homogeneous regions alternating with zones of granulation.

Such microfocal alterations bear much resemblance to those demonstrated in the myocardium by us in EPS (Chapter 1) or by Rona et al.[15] upon administration of isoproterenol, and the authors[69] justly attributed these lesions to the action of catecholamines and calcium. As already said, these alterations substantially increase the heterogeneity of the myocardium and may give rise to ectopic foci of recurrent excitation, i.e., seriously upset the cardiac electric stability. The above data testify that in a certain proportion of cases by the moment of sudden death the heart had no irreversible organic alterations that could be regarded as the cause of death.

In accordance with this, Lown,[66] Wolf,[70] Meerson and Pshennikova,[71] and many others searched for a cause of fibrillation and sudden cardiac death beyond the heart, and pointed to biosocial stress as the most likely environmental factor. Indeed, there is a considerable body of evidence that stress may lead to fibrillation and sudden death not only through aggravation of atherosclerosis or ischemia, but directly through neurogenic or hormonal action on undamaged myocardium.

There is thus a case of a 22-year-old girl who suffered her first attack of cardiac fibrillation and clinical death in September 1983 on her first day in medical school. After resuscitation she had a defibrillator implanted; further on (in 1984 and 1985) fibrillation was sure to happen on the first day of studies, and only actuation of the defibrillator prevented sudden death.[72] Quite similar cases have been reported by Wellens et al.[73] and Lown.[66] *It is important that such "conditioned" attacks of cardiac fibrillation were not accompanied by any coronary or valvular damage or other organic alterations upon thorough clinicophysiological examinations.*

This unambiguously proves the basic possibility of primary stress fibrillation and sudden death, but gives no idea of their incidence. Of special interest therefore are descriptions of thoroughly examined patients in whom cardiac fibrillation and clinical death with subsequent resuscitation were not attended with any alterations in the coronary arteries (i.e., were primary).

The first work along this line appears to have been undertaken by Lown,[66] who, upon a complex cardiological and psychiatric examination of 117 patients revived after sudden death, discerned 25 with the least pronounced pathological alterations in the heart, but the most clear triggering of dangerous arrhythmias by external stress.

Two more groups of similar patients have recently been described in different clinics.[74,75]

Further, account should be taken of the reports of peculiar "epidemics" of sudden cardiac death among young people without coronary atherosclerosis, such as the one among Malay and Cambodian immigrants in the U.S.[76] The overwhelming majority of those who suddenly died had no or minimal coronary sclerosis, but differed from others of the same nationality in poorer prospects of social adaptation, i.e., an element of desolation. These people usually died at night, practically instantly, as apparently healthy young Japanese males die of the "Pokkuri disease" which has now been shown to result from ventricular flatter.[77]

Stress not involving direct physical action also can definitely affect people without IHD and adapted into society. Thus Helsing and Szklo[78] and Helsing et al.[79] have shown that among young adults sudden cardiac mortality is increased after bereavement.

In an interesting study by Rabkin et al.,[80] 3983 cases of sudden cardiac death in men were analyzed with respect to the day of the week. Among men with no manifestations of IHD, increased mortality fell on Monday. It is essential that such increased mortality associated with going back to work after the weekend was not observed either in cancer patients or in those with myocardial infarction; hence its mechanism differed from that in IHD.

In the aggregate, the available clinical evidence (apparently healthy persons with arrhythmias revealed with the wide use of continuous monitoring, patients with neurocirculatory dystonia, and cases of sudden cardiac death in clear absence of coronary atherosclerosis) throws doubt on the validity of the term "idiopathic arrhythmias" and at the same time seems to outline the dynamics of a certain progressive stress disease of the heart. The main role in its pathogenesis is played not at all by ischemic, coronarogenic cardiac injuries, but by direct adrenergic damage to the conduction system and contractile myocardium.

As individuals with decreased resistance to stress diseases (i.e., with defects in the stress-limiting systems considered in detail in Chapters 4 and 5), like all others, encounter numerous stress situations, the stress injuries inflicted every time may accumulate to cause considerable damage to the myocardium and especially to its conduction system, which has the most dense adrenergic and cholinergic innervation.[81,82]

Of considerable interest in this respect are the results of autopsies performed from 1963 till 1981 on 200 patients with electrocardiographically proved complete AV block. These summarized data presented in an excellent book of Davies et al.[68] testify that only in 17% of cases the pathoanatomical examination allows one to put down ischemic disease as the cause of impaired conduction. Even leaving out calcification of the node, congenital cardiomyopathy, and other causes, we still have 38% of cases where the condition is underlain by a process of unknown etiology, i.e., idiopathic bilateral His bundle-branch fibrosis. We believe that the possible part of adrenergic stress injury in the development of a chronic process leading to this rather frequent finding deserves special study.

Another morphological phenomenon often observed in autopsies for sudden cardiac death — pronounced myocardial hypertrophy — may also be caused by prolonged action of high catecholamine concentrations[83] and, combined with focal cardiosclerosis, is a plausible factor impairing the electric stability of the heart. Finally, there are reports of myocardial infarction with angiographically normal coronary arteries. The number of cases is not large, e.g., 10 out of 528 infarction patients examined by Salem et al.[84] Still, the very existence of this phenomenon justifies further studies concerned with the possbility of large adrenergic myocardial necroses under natural heavy stress. At present it can be thought that hypertrophy, fibrotic AV block, and necrobiotic foci can also be of stress origin.

By and large, it can be said that stress damage is really involved in the pathogenesis of arrhythmias, fibrillation, and sudden death, setting in through noncoronary impairment of metabolism and electric stability with only minor lesions in myocardial structures, yet under certain conditions resulting in pronounced injury to the cardiac muscle. On the other hand, it should not be forgotten that in many cases the stress acts not as a self-contained factor, but combines with ischemia brought on by stenosing coronary sclerosis. This combination stands out quite definitely in the analysis of the pathogenesis of grave arrhythmias and sudden cardiac death.

Accordingly, we shall first consider the role of stress in the pathogenesis of ischemic disease, and then the relation of stress and ischemia in arrhythmias and sudden cardiac death.

IV. ROLE OF STRESS REACTION IN ISCHEMIC DISEASE

Obviously, to assess the contribution of stress cardiac damage to the pathogenesis of ischemic heart disease it is necessary to analyze first the pathogenetic chain of the ischemic damage itself. Our analysis will be only brief, as the vast material on this problem has been comprehensively covered in the proceedings of international symposia,[85-88] fundamental reviews, and handbooks[89-91] of the last decade.

These works demonstrate that, on the one hand, the ischemic injury to the myocardium constitutes the basis of the most common disease of the century — IHD and myocardial infarction — and on the other the very concept of its pathogenesis is far from being complete and final, and in many aspects is obscure or rapidly changing. In the framework of this book a description of this pathogenetic chain is not an end in itself, and for the sake of clarity we shall use the body of evidence available to discern four basic stages of the development of ischemic damage,[92] mostly with a view to evaluating the contribution of stress usually associating with ischemia.

A general overview in Figure 8 shows that at first the two major etiological factors of IHD — excess cholesterol in food and genetically determined defects in hepatic uptake and elimination of cholesterol — combine to cause atherogenic dyslipidemia and ensuing stenosing coronary atherosclerosis. At the same time the environmental stress situations combined with defects in the stress-limiting systems cause hepatic damage (to be considered) and thereby aggravate the dyslipidemia. It can further be seen that the role of stress reactions in IHD is not restricted to this, as excessive stress entails primary cardiac stress damage, coronary spasm, and alterations in blood rheological properties conducive to coronary thrombosis. At this first stage the process is reversible and can be stopped by various factors suppressing the stress reaction, causing coronary dilation, and preventing blood clotting, either through medical intervention or by endogenous means (like metabolites of the stress-limiting systems).

However, under certain conditions when ischemia evokes endogenous stress of pain and fear that potentiates the stress reaction, the process goes into the second stage: interruption of the mitochondrial respiratory chain, despite transient activation of glycolysis, leads to an energy-deficient inhibition of the Na,K and Ca pumps of the sarcolemma and of the Ca pump of the SR. Simultaneously, excess catecholamines and other stress hormones act through cAMP and inositol triphosphate and diacyl glycerol (IP_3-DAG) to cause enhanced entry of calcium and loss of potassium in the cardiomyocytes. The resulting excess of calcium

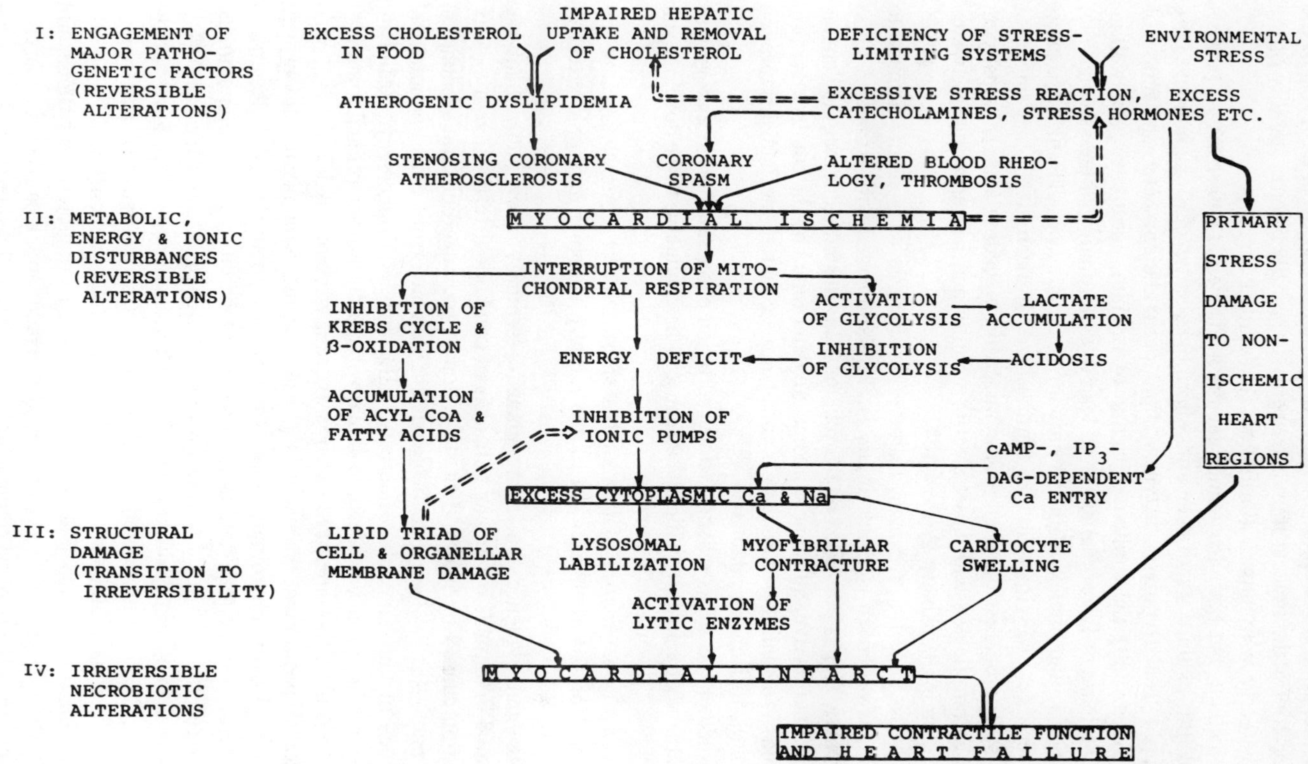

FIGURE 8. Role of stress reaction in the pathogenesis of ischemic disease. For explanations see text.

and sodium in the cells of the contractile myocardium and the conduction system, with the consequent decrease in the rest potential underlie the profound impairment of the cardiac electric stability. In principle this stage is also reversible since the endogenous mechanisms considered further can abolish ischemia by, e.g., opening the collaterals or suppressing the stress reaction through activation of the stress-limiting systems. Yet in the combination of heavy ischemia and intense stress reaction the upset of cationic transport at all levels of the conduction system or contractile myocardium can deeply impair the electric stability of the heart and cause grave early arrhythmias, fibrillation, and cardiac arrest.

If this does not happen, but both detrimental factors — ischemia and stress — persist, the process develops into its third stage when stress hormones and excess calcium and fatty acids activate the lipid triad (lypolytic enzymes, lipid peroxidation, detergent action of lysophosphatides); concurrently the cardiotoxic action of calcium, cardiomyocyte swelling from excess sodium, release of lysosomal enzymes lead to deterioration of the sarcolemma, myofibrils, mitochondria, and nuclei. With the growing deficiency of ATP all these alterations become irreversible, evolving into the fourth stage — necrobiosis that underlies myocardial infarction. The depression of cardiac contractility preceding and accompanying the infarction may be complicated with upset electric stability and late arrhythmias, which have been dealt with comprehensively.[14,93]

Here I would like to underline the main feature characteristic of ischemic damage to the heart: in a conscious organism ischemic injury is always attended with a marked stress reaction; the pathogenetic stages presented on the scheme allow a statement that the damage is not purely ischemic, but its dynamics and outcome are determined by the combined action of stress and ischemia. We shall therefore further consider the concrete mechanisms through which stress contributes to ischemic damage.

Regardless of whether the stress reaction is caused by an exogenous or an endogenous factor, there are several mechanisms by which it can cause or be conducive to the development of IHD.

The first pathogenetic mechanism of this kind is stress hypercholesterolemia and hyperlipidemia resulting from overenhancement of the initially adaptive lipotropic effect of stress.

There is experimental evidence that neurogenous, essentially stress-induced atherosclerosis can be created in animals by frequent changes of conditional-reflex stereotypes, or by emotional excitation caused by intermittent starvation or prolonged electric stimulation of the ventromedial nucleus.[94-96] These data are consistent with the results of epidemiological studies. The incidence of coronary atherosclerosis, IHD, and IHD-linked myocardial infarction is especially high in people whose occupation involves continual emotional strain.[97,98] An important development in this line of research is a recent work of Clarkson et al.[99] who correlated the biosocial position of primates in a stable group with plasma lipoprotein composition and found that in subordinate animals the ratio of total plasma cholesterol to high-density lipoproteins is more than half as great again compared to dominating animals; this was naturally accompanied by a fourfold greater percentage of coronary stenosis in subordinate females and an almost twofold increase in subordinate males than in respective dominating specimens. Thus, a protracted biosocial stress is a real cause of atherogenic shifts and progressive coronary atherosclerosis. We have further demonstrated[100] the atherogenic effect of a single emotional pain stress on rat blood lipoprotein and cholesterol levels, and were the first to prove the involvement of hepatic stress damage in this phenomenon. In this work the effects of prolonged stress according to Desiderato et al.[101] were studied in respect of serum lipoproteins on the one hand, and indices of hepatic function and metabolism on the other.

The correlation with atherosclerotic damage to coronary vessels in humans is known to be negative for high-density lipoproteins (HDLP)[102,103] and positive for low-density and very low-density lipoproteins (LDLP).[104,105] This has been confirmed in wide epidemiological and experimental studies and gave grounds for the concept of an antiatherogenic role of HDLP and the atherogenic role of LDLP as well as for the use of the atherogenicity index (AI) for prognosing the probability of coronary atherosclerosis:

$$AI = \frac{Ch_{tot} - Ch_{HDLP}}{Ch_{HDLP}}$$

where Ch_{tot} is total plasma cholesterol and Ch_{HDLP} is cholesterol in the HDLP fraction.

Table 5 shows that a 6-h EPS does not appreciably alter the total cholesterol content, but causes a substantial decrease in cholesterol contained in the fraction of antiatherogenic HDLP, which is clearly seen already 2 h after stress and reaches a maximum (over twofold) in 24 h. As a result the AI proves to be 1.5 times greater in 2 h and more than 4 times greater in 24 h after stress as compared to the control. Thus, a single long stress indeed gives rise to pronounced atherogenic dyslipidemia.

We further suggested that the decreased cholesterol content in the HDLP fraction may be due to decreased activity in the blood of the enzyme lecithin:cholesterol acyltransferase (LCAT) that catalyzes transfer of an unsaturated fatty acyl residue from position 2 in lecithin to free cholesterol, producing cholesterol esters and promoting thus formation of HDLP.[106-108]

The data in Table 6 demonstrate that upon exposure of rats to stress their overall serum esterifying capacity reliably decreased to 78% of the control value in 2 h and to 70% in 24 h after the end of a 6-h EPS. Still more marked was the decline in LCAT, which fell more than threefold in 2 h and then was restored to the initial level.

The observed alterations in lipid metabolism in EPS fit in with the suggestion that impaired esterification of cholesterol is essential to stress dyslipidemia and specifically to the decline in HDLP cholesterol. LCAT is a ''short-lived'' protein synthesized in the liver and then supplied to the blood where it participates in lipoprotein conversions.[109,110] The short half-life and high rate of biosynthesis of this enzyme is the most plausible explanation for the marked but transient drop in its activity in serum upon stress impairment of hepatic metabolism.

In further experiments we evaluated the activation of hepatic lipid peroxidation (LPO) in stress by the level of its products, and hepatic damage by the blood level of a hepatocyte-specific enzyme such as fructose 1,6-diphosphate aldolase.

Table 7 shows that stress consistently causes LPO activation as manifest by a twofold increase in the hepatic content of malonic dialdehyde, a marked decrease in the hepatic activity of the antioxidant enzyme superoxide dismutase, and a 2.5-fold rise in the plasma fructose 1,6-diphosphate aldolase. These alterations are most pronounced 2 h after stress and abate to some extent in 1 d.

This supports the idea that stress acts through LPO activation to cause damage to the key organ of cholesterol metabolism, the liver, but leaves open the main question of how the hepatic stress damage interferes with cholesterol elimination and leads to atherogenic dyslipidemia. A reasonable suggestion was that it affects cholesterol 7-α-hydroxylase; to test this we studied the effect of EPS on hepatic cholesterol oxidation.[111]

Hydroxylation of cholesterol (assayed by the amount of ^3H_2O excreted with urine after administration of labeled cholesterol to rats) proved to be appreciably diminished upon EPS (Figure 9).

Thus, hepatic stress damage is associated with impaired activity of the cytochrome P_{450} system and specifically of its important functional form cholesterol 7-α-hydroxylase that limits cholesterol conversion to bile acids and elimination from the organism.

In whole, these data prompt one to think that stabilization of the hepatic hydroxylase

TABLE 5
Effect of EPS on the Serum Lipid Content and the Atherogenicity Index

Series	Cholesterol Total	Cholesterol HDLP[a]	Triglycerides	Atherogenic index
1. Control (n = 9)	70.8 ± 3.5	52.6 ± 2.8	52.8 ± 4.2	0.35
2. 2 h after EPS (n = 10)	66.4 ± 2.0	43.6 ± 2.1	46.3 ± 2.7	0.52
3. 24 h after EPS (n = 9)	58.6 ± 4.5	22.7 ± 1.7	40.8 ± 3.2	1.60
	$p_{1\text{-}3}$ >0.05	$p_{1\text{-}3}$ <0.01	$p_{1\text{-}3}$ <0.05	

[a] HDLP = High-density lipoproteins.

TABLE 6
Cholesterol Esterification in Rat Blood Serum After EPS

Time after EPS	Total cholesterol (mg/dl)	Cholesterol-esterifying activity (nmol/ml·h)	LCAT[a] activity (nmol/ml·h)
Control	65 ± 2.1	141 ± 13	23.4 ± 2.3
2 h	65 ± 1.3	110 ± 12	8.0 ± 1.5
24 h	62 ± 1.1	99 ± 13	21.1 ± 2.3
48 h	67 ± 0.9	133 ± 12	27.4 ± 1.5

[a] LCAT = Lecithin:cholesterol acyltransferase.

TABLE 7
Effect of EPS on the Content of Malonic Dialdehyde (MDA) and Superoxide Dismutase (SOD) Activity in the Liver, and Fructose 1,6-Diphosphate Aldolase (FDA) Activity in Rat Serum

Time after EPS	MDA (nmol mg protein^{-1})	SOD (U g protein $^{-1}$)	FDA, (μmol ml^{-1} · h^{-1})
Control (n = 9)	0.30 ± 0.03	64.63 ± 7.31	0.124 ± 0.08
2 h (n = 8)	0.64 ± 0.05	30.84 ± 2.08	0.316 ± 0.02
	$p_{1\text{-}2}$<0.001	$p_{1\text{-}2}$ <0.001	$p_{1\text{-}2}$ <0.001
24 h (n = 8)	0.37 ± 0.02	50.33 ± 3.89	0.282 ± 0.02
	$p_{1\text{-}3}$ >0.05	$p_{1\text{-}3}$ >0.05	$p_{1\text{-}3}$ <0.001

activity or induction of this enzyme is a promising way of preventing atherogenic dyslipidemias of various origins and may be important in designing new means of prophylaxis of atherosclerosis. Of course this in no way contradicts the concept of Brown and Goldstein[112] about the decisive role of hepatic receptors; on the contrary, there arises a rather interesting question of the effect of stress on these receptors.

There is thus unambiguous evidence that *stress causes deep alterations in the liver and impairs cholesterol elimination from the organism. Therefore, even when there is no excess of cholesterol in food, stress can be conducive to stenosing coronary sclerosis and plays an important part in the development of IHD.*

The second pathogenetic mechanism by which stress may aggravate the dangerous consequences of myocardial ischemia is the primary cardiac damage from stress arising endogenously in response to pain and fear caused by ischemia. At least two components of this aggravating effect should be distinguished: exaggeration of arrhythmias in ischemia, and impairment of the contractile function in nonischemic cardiac regions in infarction.

The arrhythmogenic effect of the neural factor in acute ischemia is well known. Thus

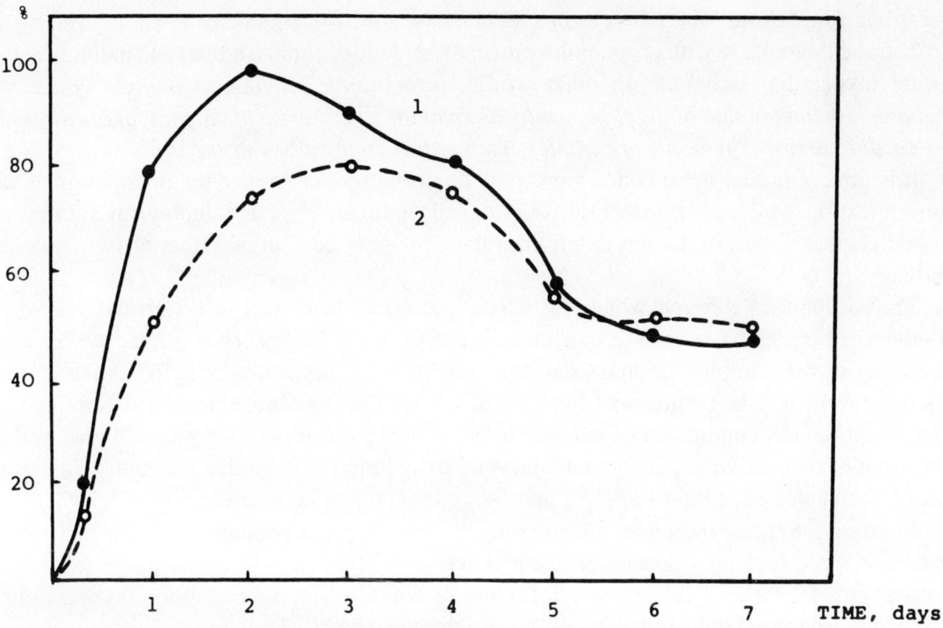

FIGURE 9. Effect of EPS on ^{3}H-cholesterol oxidation assayed by the amount of ^3H_2O in rat urine. (1) Control; (2) after EPS.

Satinsky et al.[113] found out that under deep anesthesia ligation of the descending branch of the left coronary artery causes cardiac fibrillation only in 6.3% of cases, whereas upon stimulation of posterior hypothalamic centers that control the circulatory function arrhythmias are ten times more frequent. Similarly, stress situations increase threefold the incidence of fibrillation caused by coronary occlusion.[114] Then again, the cardiac fibrillation threshold decreases in acute ischemia with the probability of fibrillation increasing twofold to threefold.[11]

It is noteworthy that these arrhythmogenic effects of stress can be restricted or prevented by removal of local sympathetic nodes or administration of adrenoblockers.[115,116]

At the same time, stimulation of cardiac sympathetic nerves and sympathetic nodes allows the arrhythmogenic effects of the midbrain to be reproduced even under conditions of stabilized blood pressure and heart rate.[117] Numerous clinical studies testify to the excitation of the sympathoadrenal section of the nervous system during attacks of arrhythmia in humans, with enhanced catecholamine excretion as well as increased cAMP and decreased cGMP production.[118]

There is thus no doubt that excitation of the sympathetic nervous centers and the adrenergic effect on the heart are essential to the pathogenesis of arrhythmias caused by neurodynamic shifts in the higher divisions of the brain.

In studying these shifts it was observed that some known antiarrhythmics such as noricisin (ethmazin) and dysopiramide (norpace) not only suppress the activity of ectopic foci and abolish cardiac arrhythmias, but also affect the bioelectric activity of the frontal lobe cortex in animals and humans, decreasing the amplitude of slow potentials, and these two effects are in good quantitative correlation.[118,119] Skinner and Jingling[120] and Skinner[121] recorded in parallel the bioelectric activity of the heart and of the frontal cortex in arrhythmias caused by stress or acute ischemia, and came to the conclusion that stress evoked by ischemia excites a certain zone in the frontal lobe cortex, and in both cases the further chain of events leading to cardiac fibrillation proves to be cortically determined.

The most essential experimental result obtained by Skinner is that in occlusion of the coronary artery and acute myocardial ischemia in pigs, excitation of this zone is accompanied by cardiac fibrillation, whereas cold blockade of the subcortical zone or tonsil as well as a corticotruncal blockade with propranolol prevent fibrillation, cardiac arrest, and animal death despite myocardial ischemia. In other words, *myocardial ischemia is a mere result of mechanically interrupted blood flow, while the reaction to ischemia in the form of fibrillation and cardiac arrest is a result of complex intercentral connections in the brain.*

It is important that these connections may be primarily determined by an environmental stress situation which gives rise to a pathological dominant[122] or a pathological system of excited centers[123] that in its turn determines the damaging adrenergic effect of ischemia on the heart.

The mechanism through which the adrenergic effect leads to cardiac arrhythmias can be envisaged on the basis of the experimental data from our laboratory presented earlier and pertaining to the complex of stress damages upon EPS. This complex is indicative of the impairment of microstructures and function of the cardiac membrane apparatus responsible for generation and conduction of excitation. Such damage can play a prominent part in the formation of two essential pathogenetic links of arrhythmias and fibrillation, namely ectopic foci of premature excitation impulses and foci of functional conduction blocks.[124,125]

In infarction, acute ischemia, and microfocal stress injury, a premature impulse generated in such ectopic foci may encounter a functional conduction block arising again from microfocal stress-induced (i.e., adrenergic) injury to nonischemic regions of the myocardium. In this case the premature impulse will not go through the blocked zone, but bypass it and return later when the conduction block will have passed, forming thus a reciprocal excitation wave and the well-known phenomenon of reentry which is the generally recognized cause of ventricular tachycardia and cardiac fibrillation.[125,126]

The second component of aggravation of ischemic damage by stress is the impairment of the contractile function of nonischemic heart regions in infarction. This was the subject of our special study in which we assessed the changes in a certainly nonischemic part of the heart — right auricle in experimental infarction of the left ventricle. The auricles were taken from animals 1 d after ligating the left coronary arterial descending branch according to Selye, and their contractile function was studied under isometric conditions as described earlier.[127]

The auricles obtained from animals that had undergone myocardial infarction did not differ from the controls in their mass and initial length, but had significantly decreased extensibility (Figure 10A) and accordingly responded to stretching with smaller increments in developed tension (Figure 10B), i.e., with a smaller Starling effect.

These data fit in with the concept that stress caused by the infarction affects the nonischemic regions of the myocardium. The resulting arrhythmias and depressed contractile function of these uninjured sections can be fatal for the myocardial infarction patient, and this justifies the wide use of β-adrenoblockers and agonists of GABA and benzodiazepine receptors in the acute infarction period.

Obviously, if stress arrhythmias and impairment of contractility were realized to the full in every infarction, then without timely drug protection most afflicted people would die a sudden death. Yet most of the myocardial infarction cases do not have such a fatal outcome, and it will be later shown that this is due to activation of the central stress-limiting systems (opioidergic, GABA-ergic, serotoninergic) that opportunely restrain the stress reaction and thereby prevent death from stress that complicates myocardial ischemia.

The third pathogenetic mechanism consists in that the strong adrenergic component of the stress reaction may cause spasm of the smooth muscle of anatomically intact coronary arteries, and this rather stable spasm results in secondary ischemic damage to the myocardium.

It has already been said (see Section II) that the vascular smooth muscle responds by contraction to α-adrenoreceptor and by relaxation to β-adrenoreceptor stimulation by catecholamines. Since the β-adrenergic effect, as we have shown, prevails in stress situations,

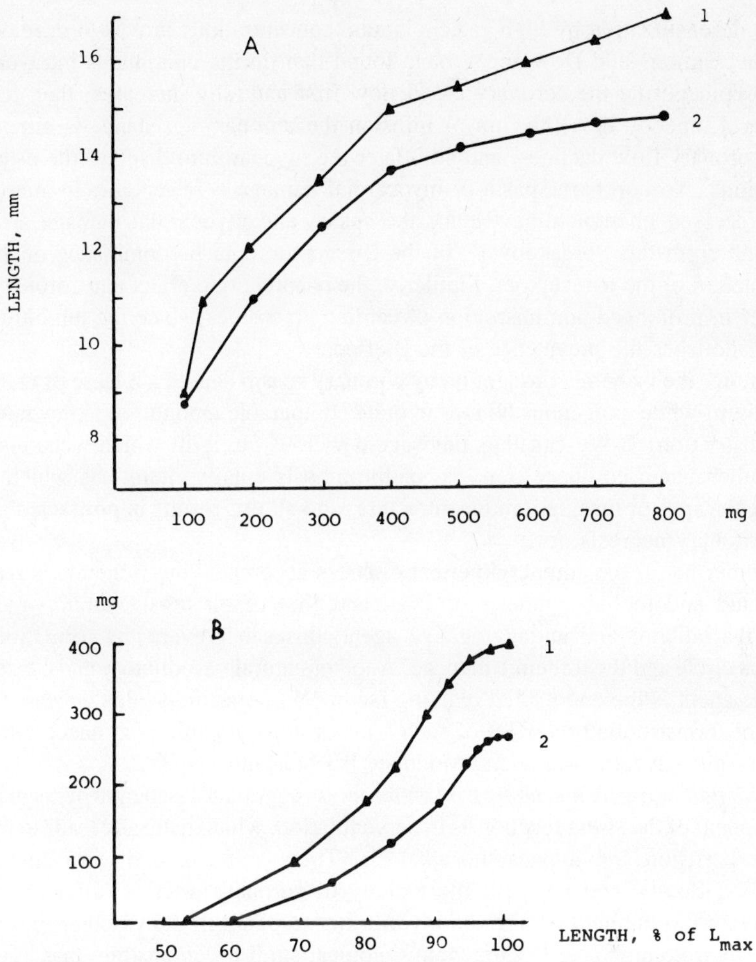

FIGURE 10. Depression of (A) extensibility and (B) developed tension of the right auricle in experimental infarction of the left ventricle. (1) Control, (2) infarction. (A) Abscissa, applied external load, mg; ordinate, atrial length, mm. (B) Abscissa, atrial length, percent of L_{max}; ordinate, developed tension, milligrams.

this design of the neural apparatus of the coronary vessels should, and really does, ensure their dilation and enhancement of coronary blood flow during stress, physical work, etc. Still, recent studies demonstrate that this does not at all exclude a stress-induced coronary spasm. The matter is that in the healthy organism, when the resistive coronary vessels are dilated owing to activation of ''β-receptor-cAMP'' system and action of local metabolites, there is still a certain tonic vasoconstrictive influence from the α-receptors. Thus the high coronary flow observed under large physical load is still further augmented upon blocking the α-adrenoreceptors with phentolamine.[22] In the healthy organism this tonic influence of sympathetic nerves on postsynaptic α-receptors of the coronary vessels serves to prevent the wasteful excessive coronary flow under physical load. On the other hand, this means that any naturally occurring or pharmacologically induced blockade of the β-adrenoreceptors may lead to coronary spasm. In particular, propranolol has been found to cause coronary constriction,[129] i.e., to demask the sympathetic vasoconstrictive action of α-receptors by blocking the β-receptors. Under natural conditions a decline in the coronarodilatory effect of β-receptors can be due to their lower (as compared to α-receptors) resistance to desensitization in protracted stress or prolonged elevation of blood catecholamines[130] in cardiac failure. This desensitization by high catecholamine concentrations proves to develop rather quickly. Thus, Simons and Downing[131] have found that during continuous intravenous infusion of norepinephrine the coronary blood flow first naturally increases, then returns to the initial level, and by the 40th min of infusion the coronary resistance is almost twice higher, the coronary flow declines, and 48 h later the myocardium displays the usual set of ischemic lesions. No coronary spasm or myocardial damage is observable in animals who beforehand received phentolamine. Hence the spasm and myocardial damage are indeed likely to result from the "breakdown" of the β-receptors and predominance of the vasoconstrictive action of the α-receptors. Similarly, the α-adrenergic effect and coronary spasm can take over in prolonged administration of cardiac glycosides, since the inhibition of the Na,K pump abolishes the prevalence of the β-effect.

Furthermore, the ischemia brought on by coronary spasm causes a release of nickel from the myocardium, while exogenous Ni ions in quite comparable amounts are known to induce coronary constriction.[132] We can thus envisage a vicious circle in which ischemia caused by spasm, atherogenic coronary stenosis, or thrombosis entails alterations which in their turn stabilize the spasm, turning it into contracture, and all this results in protracted ischemia leading to coronary necrosis.

On the other hand, the adrenergic effect of stress accompanying ischemia is responded to by activated endothelial synthesis of PGs, and first of all prostacyclin, which is an endogenous vasodilator and antiaggregative agent; this can prevent the formation of the above vicious circle and the ischemic damage. Another natural vasodilatory and consequently anti-ischemic agent is the endothelial relaxing factor.[134] Interestingly, this appears to be the mechanism of the vasodilatory effect of such a major anti-ischemic pharmacological factor as nitrates, as nitroglycerin was found to induce PG biosynthesis.[135]

The fourth pathogenetic mechanism by which stress aggravates ischemic damage involves such a component of the stress reaction as hyperventilation, which naturally leads to increased blood oxygen tension and hypocapnic alkalosis. These shifts in their turn attenuate the coronary blood flow[136] and augment the tonicity of coronary arteries (through enhanced access of calcium to the binding sites on myofibrillar troponin in the vascular muscle cells) followed by their contracture.[137] Clinicophysiological studies demonstrate that hyperventilation and attending hypocapnic alkalosis in IHD patients entail a 15% decrease in coronary flow[138] as well as attacks of angina[139] that can be abolished with a calcium blocker diltiazem, which does not change the coronary blood gas composition. This again points to the central role of excess calcium in the mechanisms of damage.

The fifth pathogenetic mechanism is that catecholamines promote blood coagulation and formation of thrombi,[140] whereby the blood platelets release potent vasoactive compounds, and in particular thromboxane A_2[141] and 5-hydroxytryptamine (serotonin) and histamine, which augment the spasm dangerously combining with thrombosis. This is most likely to happen in those coronary arterial regions where there are initial atherosclerotic alterations.[142]

Shepherd and Vanhoutte[13] have shown that normally the intact endothelium releases prostacyclin to inhibit platelet aggregation and monoamine oxidase to decompose serotonin and other monoamines. Thus the action of the PG system is not only vasodilatory, but also antithrombotic, which is definitely seen in experimental studies of the blood flow through stenosed coronary arteries. The partial narrowing of the coronary artery may result in gradual cyclic attenuation of coronary flow in dogs, these oscillations being due to platelet aggregation and disaggregation.[143] This only happens when coronary constriction is accompanied by elevation in blood thromboxane, while in other cases it can only be elicited by large doses of indomethacin, which inhibits PG synthesis.[144] Conversely, administration of prostacyclin in all cases abolishes the flow oscillations in the constricted coronary artery and thereby prevents thrombosis. So the question of whether or not there is risk of persistent spasm, thrombosis, and finally myocardial infarction is determined by the state of such a "regional" stress-limiting system as PGs.

The sixth pathogenetic mechanism has been recently elucidated and consists in that protracted stress reaction lowers the resistance to hypoxia and reoxygenation.

Our experiments together with Belkina and Matsievskii were aimed at evaluating the cardiac contractile function, its work, and coronary bed resistance during normoxia, ischemia, and reoxygenation in control animals and in those that had undergone EPS 2 h prior to testing. The left ventricular and the carotid pressure were recorded in parallel, and the stroke volume and cardiac output were determined with the use of an ultrasonic flow sensor.[145]

Table 8 demonstrates that the stress itself did not cause appreciable changes in the contractile function or in the total peripheral resistance. Substantial differences between control and poststress animals were found in reoxygenation: the developed ventricular pressure, the mean carotid pressure, and the cardiac output at the 30th min of reoxygenation proved to be significantly lower upon stress, so that the external cardiac work was threefold less. There is thus no doubt that EPS markedly aggravates the impairment of the cardiac contractile function in reoxygenation.

The seventh mechanism stems from the adrenergic mobilization of the cardiac function in stress which, combined with the regulatory increased vascular resistance, causes heart overloading and may aggravate the ischemic damage not only in spasm or thrombosis, but in simple atherosclerotic stenosis.

At first glance this seems to be contradictory with the coronary vasodilation due to the main β-adrenergic effect of stress and to activation of the local adenosinergic and PG systems. Mudge et al.[23] explained that in presistent stenosis of a large coronary artery a surplus load cannot be compensated for by regulatory dilation of the downstream region of the coronary bed because of the lack of a sufficient volume of incoming blood to distend the vessels. Such an interpretation, albeit not exhaustive, is nevertheless in full agreement with the data of Verrier et al.[146] concerning the effect of coronary artery stenosis on the behavioral stress in dogs. When the dogs were enraged by taking away food, in the absence of coronary stenosis this enhanced the coronary arterial flow by 147% and lowered the coronary resistance by 38%; in mechanical stenosis with a special cuff there was no appreciable change in the coronary flow, whereas the coronary vascular resistance increased by 33%, indicating a stress-induced vasoconstriction.

Notwithstanding all the danger of ischemia brought about by stenosing atherosclerosis, spasm, thrombosis, or a stress-induced combination of these factors, it should be borne in mind that the organism possesses both immediate and long-term mechanisms for limiting the cardiac overload and ischemia. An immediate response of this kind is attenuation of the circulatory function in adjustment to the lower capabilities of the damaged heart,[147] when cardiovascular reflexes (1) decrease the arterial bed resistance and relieve the cardiac load, and (2) cause partial storing of blood. This of course can only be effective at rest and diminished basal metabolism. Long-term compensation for ischemia is ensured by proliferation of intracardiac and extracardiac collaterals[148] involving enhanced nucleic acid and protein synthesis.[149] In essence *the course of ischemic disease in great measure reflects the dynamic balance between the stenosing atheroma formation and the growth of collaterals. In many cases this latter compensating factor proves no less effective than aortic-coronary shunting and ensures clinical compensation or subcompensation.*

It is noteworthy that, besides medicinal agents causing adenosine accumulation (dipyridamole, etc.), the development of the coronary bed and specifically collaterals can be efficiently induced without drugs, and first and foremost with adaptation to intermittent hypoxia, which will be further dealt with in detail.

The eighth and quite important mechanism by which the stress reaction (caused exogenously or by myocardial infarction) can upset the circulation and entail not only cardiac, but also brain ischemia is the profound impairment of vascular contractile function and tonicity. We made a study of two aspects of such disturbances: (1) impaired contractility of

TABLE 8
Effect of EPS on the Cardiac Contractile Function in Transient Ischemia and Subsequent Reperfusion

Indices	Series	Before ischemia	Ischemia 1 min	Ischemia 30 min	Reperfusion 1 min	Reperfusion 30 min
Left ventricular developed pressure (mmHg)	Control	116 ± 4.4	87 ± 4.1	83 ± 2.5	81 ± 3.5	72 ± 5.6
	EPS	107 ± 6.3	73 ± 6.4	64 ± 5.2	63 ± 5.5	49 ± 6.3
Heart rate (min^{-1})	Control	388 ± 15	383 ± 17	379 ± 17	368 ± 14	349 ± 18
	EPS	415 ± 16	300 ± 15	418 ± 18	384 ± 19	310 ± 18
Mean carotid pressure (mmHg)	Control	77 ± 4.7	60 ± 4.2	54 ± 3.9	51 ± 4.1	45 ± 4.0
	EPS	67 ± 6.8	54 ± 5.1	37 ± 1.3	38 ± 3.1	31 ± 3.0
Cardiac output (ml/min)	Control	34 ± 2.9	41 ± 3.4	33 ± 2.9	27 ± 2.5	20 ± 2.7
	EPS	37 ± 3.2	43 ± 3.0	35 ± 3.9	25 ± 3.2	11 ± 1.3
Total peripheral resistance ($dyn{\cdot}s{\cdot}cm^{-3}$)	Control	3174 ± 309	1950 ± 181	2181 ± 214	2517 ± 230	3286 ± 340
	EPS	2717 ± 432	1674 ± 180	1599 ± 190	2025 ± 304	3799 ± 234
Cardiac external work (J/min)	Control	0.35 ± 0.03	0.33 ± 0.02	0.23 ± 0.01	0.18 ± 0.02	0.12 ± 0.02
	EPS	0.33 ± 0.03	0.31 ± 0.03	0.18 ± 0.02	0.14 ± 0.02	0.04 ± 0.01

Note: Control, n = 10; EPS, n = 7.

the capacity vessels attending stress or infarction and leading to excessive storing of blood and diminished blood inflow to the heart, minute volume, and arterial pressure,[150] and (2) impaired endothelium-dependent contraction and relaxation of aorta which, though being a conducting vessel, nevertheless roughly reflects the ability of the coronary vessels to respond by contraction to catecholamines and by relaxation to the endothelium-derived factor.[151]

The first part of work was carried out on the portal vein representing one of the main reservoirs for blood in the organism. It was found that normally the rate of spontaneous contractions of the portal vein were 4.4 ± 0.4 min^{-1}, developed tension 122 ± 24 mg, IFS 192 ± 15 mg/min per mg wt (''intensity of the functioning of structures'' calculated as the product of developed tension by contraction rate divided by vein mass), tension buildup velocity 48 ± 7.7 mg/s, and relaxation velocity 67 ± 17 mg/s. Upon EPS all contractile parameters were markedly lowered: developed tension 8-fold, tension buildup and relaxation velocities 4.4- and 6-fold, respectively, and IFS 6-fold. Thus the depression of the portal vein contractile activity (exemplified in Figure 11) in EPS was much more pronounced than that of the heart.[152]

Further, it was found that the dependence of developed tension on the stretching load is not appreciably altered, suggesting that the relation between actin and myosin is not impaired in stress. This, together with the high stability of the myofibrillar proteins even in prolonged ischemia,[153] argues against the stress damage to the vascular smooth-muscle contractile machinery as such and makes it most plausible that the observed depression of contractility of the portal vein is due to hindered access of calcium or energy provision.

This is supported by the greater sensitivity of the isolated portal vein preparations from poststress animals to a lack of calcium or glucose. Indeed, 7 min after a calcium stepdown in the supplied fluid the IFS decreased by 36% as compared to only 13% in the control; this is likely to result from impaired ability of the sarcolemmal and SR membranes in the portal vein myocytes to take up and retain calcium. When glucose was removed from the solution, the decreases in the rate and tension of contractions in poststress preparations were also more pronounced than in controls; this can be explained by the activation of glycolysis and glycogenolysis by excess catecholamines in stress which exhausts the glycogen stores in the portal vein.

The most dramatic differences in the reaction of the portal vein preparations from control and poststress animals were observed when the temperature was changed in the range 28 to

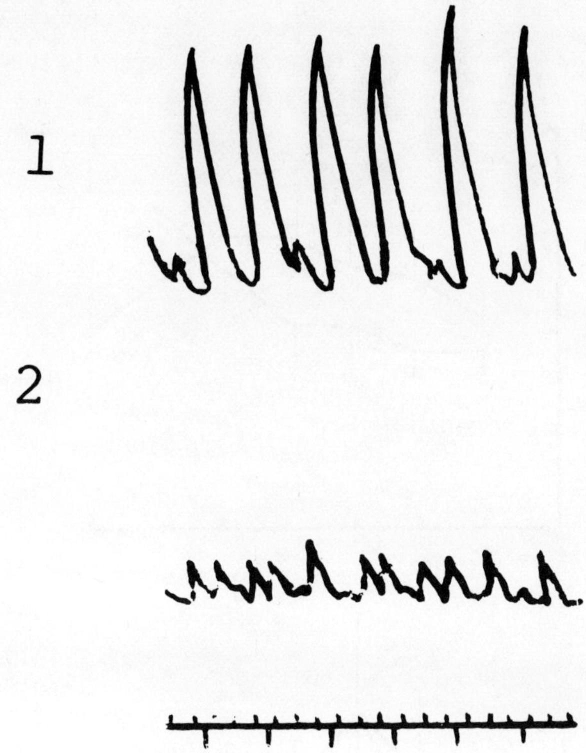

FIGURE 11. Effect of EPS on portal vein contractility. Spontaneous phasic contractions of preparations from (1) a control rat and (2) a rat subjected to EPS.

35°C. Figure 12A shows that with increasing temperature the contraction rate reflecting the automatism of the natural vein pacemakers[154] clearly increases in the control, but tends to decrease upon stress; the IFS (Figure 12B) only slightly declined in the control, but fell fivefold upon stress. It should be emphasized that all experiments had to be carried out at subphysiological temperatures because at 37.7°C the poststress preparations, unlike the controls, display no spontaneous contractile activity.

The tonic response of the portal vein preparations to 6×10^{-7} g/ml norepinephrine upon EPS proved to be ten times less. Hence the lesser ability of norepinephrine to cause tonic contraction and thereby to decrease the volume of the portal bed would affect the efficiency of sympathoadrenal mobilization of the blood stored in the portal vessels.

In the aggregate the above demonstrates that *EPS affects the portal vein muscle in such a way as to diminish its contractile activity and adrenoreactivity; this may be involved in overfilling of the portal bed, arterial hypovolemia, and collaptoid effects in severe stress or myocardial infarction.*

In the second part of our work, studying the effects of stress and infarction on contraction and relaxation of the isolated ring of the thoracic aorta, we took account of the fact that the intact endothelium of arterial vessels is essential for regulation of their reactivity.[134] Endothelial damage in various conditions such as atherosclerosis,[155] hypertension,[156] toxic catecholamine concentrations,[157] or anoxia[158] can weaken or even invert the process of the endothelium-dependent vascular relaxation, which may result in enhanced peripheral resistance to the blood flow and coronary spasm.[159]

On the other hand, it is known that acute myocardial infarction is often attended by a marked drop in vascular tone and arterial pressure, up to collapse and cardiogenic shock. We therefore tried to find out whether or not these clinically important events, besides the neurohumoral factors, might involve augmented endothelium-dependent relaxation.

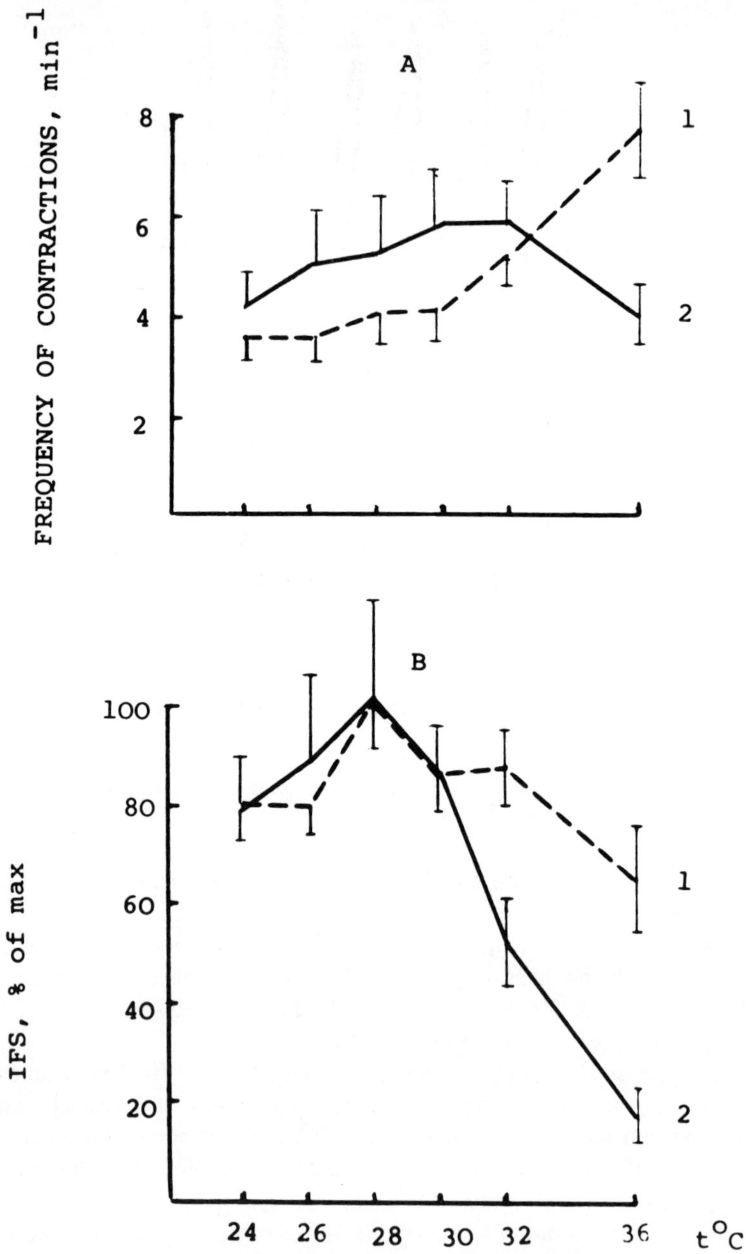

FIGURE 12. Dependence of the contraction rate (A) and intensity of functioning of the structures (B) of the portal vein on the temperature of the perfusing solution. IFS is expressed as percentage of that at 28°C. (1) Control, (2) EPS.

The force of contraction developed by the aorta with intact endothelium in response to different norepinephrine concentrations was not appreciably altered by stress or myocardial infarction. Removal of the endothelium, as could have been expected, resulted in increased response to norepinephrine which was much more pronounced after EPS and infarction (Figure 13).

A similar pattern is observed in the effects of EPS and infarction on the velocity of aortic contraction. The contractile reaction to the α-adrenergic agonists has two components:

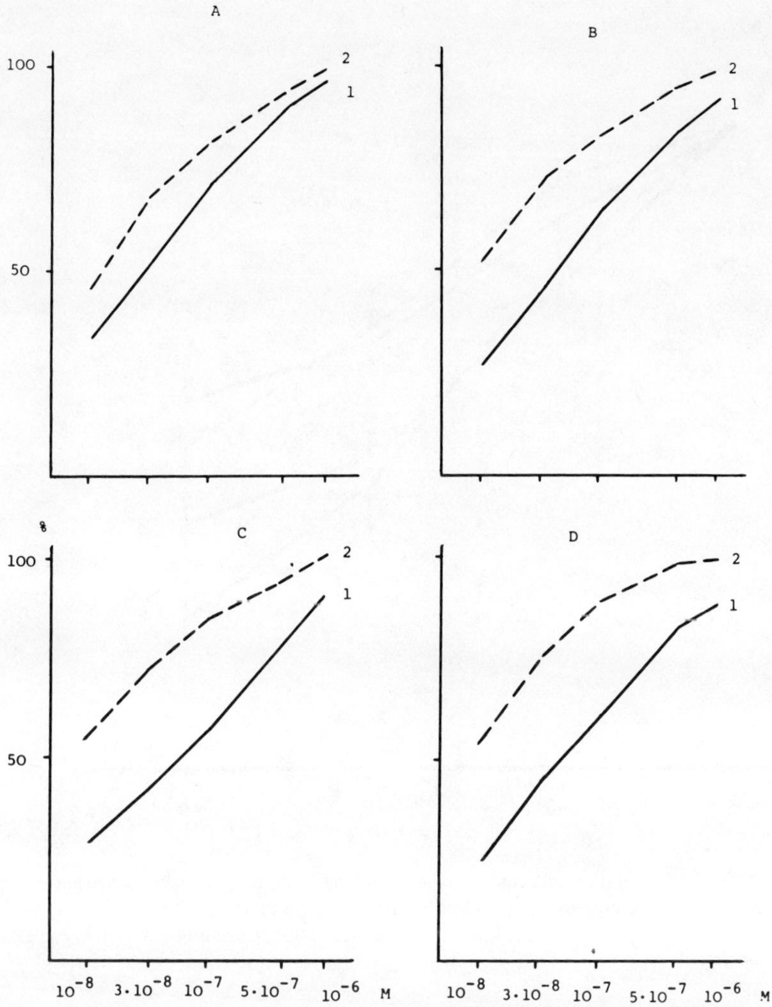

FIGURE 13. Effect of EPS and experimental myocardial infarction on the norepinephrine-induced contraction of isolated rat aorta. (A) Control, (B) sham operation, (C) EPS, (D) myocardial infarction. (1) Intact preparation, (2) preparation with removed endothelium. Abscissa, norepinephrine concentration, *M*; ordinate, contraction force, percent (100% assigned to contraction of the de-endothelized preparation at the highest norepinephrine concentration).

a rapid phasic and a slow tonic one.[160,161] The velocity of the tonic response remained practically the same in all series and at all acting concentrations, and also was not affected by removal of the endothelium. As to the phasic response, its velocity upon stress and infarction is decreased by 15 to 20% in preparations with intact endothelium; upon removal of the endothelium, the velocity of response to norepinephrine increased much more after stress and infarction: e.g., by 74 and 88%, respectively, at 10^{-7} *M* norepinephrine, as compared to 28% in the control.

These facts agree with the idea that the endothelium produces an inhibitory effect on the velocity and force of the catecholamine-induced aortic contraction.[162] Furthermore, our data suggest that this inhibitory influence of the endothelium is augmented in infarction and EPS.

To test this we studied the effects of stress and myocardial infarction on the acetylcholine-

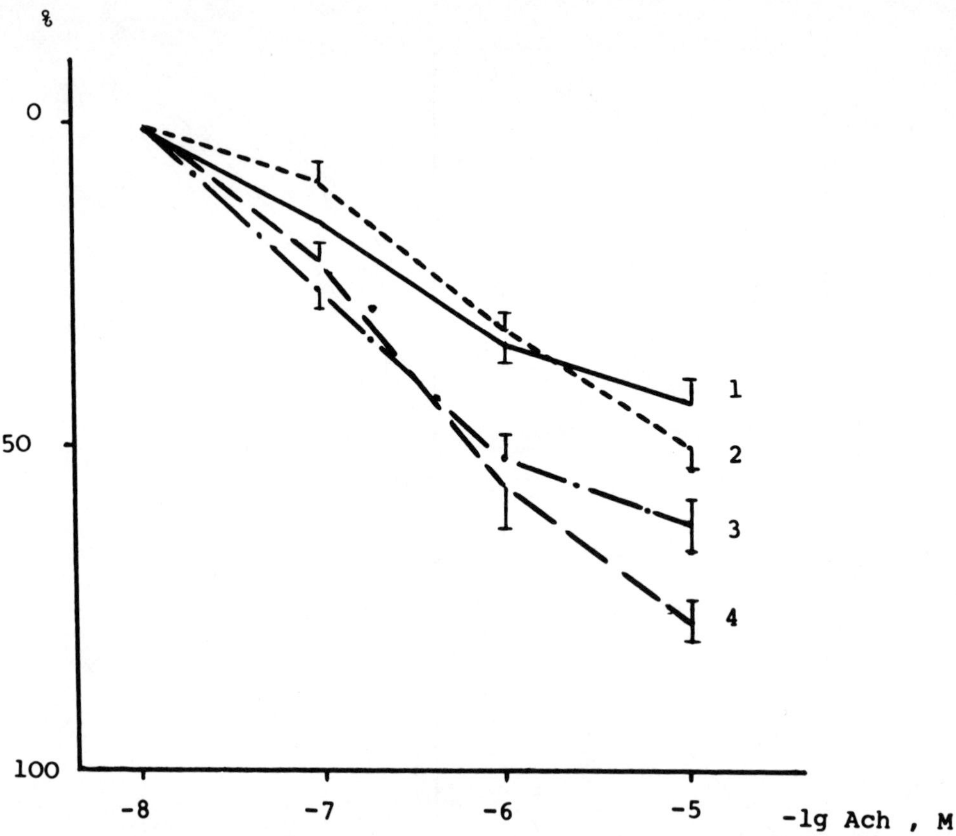

FIGURE 14. Effect of EPS and experimental myocardial infarction on the endothelium-dependent relaxation of isolated rat aorta caused by acetylcholine. (1) Control, (2) sham operation, (3) EPS, (4) myocardial infarction. Abscissa, acetylcholine concentration, *M*; ordinate, extent of relaxation, percent of contraction caused by $5 \cdot 10^{-7}$ *M* norepinephrine.

induced aortic relaxation which directly characterizes the function of the intact endothelium.[162] Figure 14 shows that aortic preparations from animals that had undergone infarction and EPS were relaxed by acetylcholine in a significantly greater degree than those from control or sham-operated animals. Preparations without endothelium did not relax in response to acetylcholine.

Thus, *experimental myocardial infarction and EPS potentiate the relaxing influence of the endothelium on the vascular smooth muscle, which is manifest in attenuation of norepinephrine induced contraction as well as in acetylcholine-induced relaxation.*

It is essential that the alterations brought on by experimental myocardial infarction are similar to those after EPS, which points to the stress origin of such shifts. This is also supported by the fact that thoracotomy — surgical stress — although not enhancing the endothelium-dependent relaxation, still causes similar, albeit much smaller, changes in the contractile parameters (Figure 14). Again, Webb et al.[163] have recently shown that psychosocial stress in mice augments the endothelium-dependent vascular relaxation.

Further, Table 9 demonstrates that in animals with experimental myocardial infarction the drop in arterial pressure coincides in time with the enhancement of the endothelium-dependent relaxation, and vice versa, the restitution of blood pressure is simultaneous with the reduction of the endothelial function; again, one can see that in all groups there is a high negative correlation between these indices. Hence the enhancement of the endothelium-dependent vascular smooth muscle relaxation that we have found in myocardial infarction

TABLE 9
Correlation Between Arterial Pressure and Endothelium-Dependent Relaxation

Conditions	Arterial pressure (mmHg)	Relaxation (% of contraction force)	Correlation coefficient
Control	109 ± 1.0	49 ± 4.6	−0.87
Infarction, 3 h	73 ± 1.4[a]	71 ± 0.7[a]	−0.93
Infarction, 24 h	99 ± 6.5	49 ± 8.2	−0.78
Sham operation, 3 h	112 ± 2.3	50 ± 3.2	−0.78
Sham operation, 24 h	108 ± 1.6	39 ± 3.9	−0.56

[a] $p < 0.01$ as compared to the control.

and EPS can, among other factors, be involved in the drop in blood pressure typical of infarction and heavy stress.

In assessing the probable mechanism of the enhanced endothelial influence on the vascular smooth muscle, it should be recalled that stress entails activation of LPO and phospholipases, and increases the blood levels of free fatty acids.[152] A number of free-radical oxidation products induce the release of the endothelium-derived relaxing factor (EDRF) or potentiate its release by endothelium-linked vasodilators.[164] The free fatty acids amplify the endothelium-dependent relaxation; conversely, the latter is hindered by phospholipase inhibitors.[165] The metabolism of arachidonic acid, which is considered an EDRF precursor,[165,166] is increased by catecholamines.[167] However, the significance of each of these factors for the enhancement of relaxation in stress is yet to be elucidated.

Regardless of its mechanism, the EDRF-mediated relaxation is indisputably important in the regulation of vascular tone. Until recently, impairment of this endothelial function has only been regarded as a possible cause of increased vascular resistance and coronary spasm.[159] In our experiments the situation is quite the opposite: activation of the endothelium-dependent relaxation overcomes the constrictive action of catecholamines on the aortal smooth muscle with an ensuing arterial-pressure drop in EPS and infarction. *This may be involved in collaptoid conditions and cardiogenic shock developing in infarction and other stressful situations;* this suggestion, of course, requires thorough testing, in particular, of the behavior of arterioles which mainly determine the peripheral resistance.

All these data once again emphasize the danger brought by the combination of ischemia and stress. On the other hand, it cannot be overlooked that these disturbances to the vascular walls of the venous and arterial bed are but transient and disappear rather soon (within 1 to 3 d). This reversibility, which we have seen to be typical of the most various stress damages, apparently arises from activation of the central stress-limiting systems that restrict the very stress reaction in duration, as well as of the local stress-limiting systems: the adenosinergic one which blocks calcium entry into the vascular smooth-muscle cells,[168,169] the antioxidant one which suppresses lipid peroxidation, etc.

All the above-considered mechanisms through which an excessive or protracted stress reaction is intertwined with the pathogenesis of ischemic heart disease are summarized by the scheme in Figure 15. One can see that the detrimental factors (in essence, the manifold effects of the stress reaction) can as well be actualized in exogenously evoked stress and in endogenous stress secondary to and caused by ischemic pain in the heart and fear of death.

The gloomy side of the concept is that the fatal vicious circle ought to close both in severe exogenous stress causing ischemia and in ischemia causing a strong and protracted stress reaction. This is, however, not really so. Many millions of people go through trying stresses and do not respond with ischemia, and millions of people with ischemia for many years remain active members of the society, and not infrequently sustain considerable stress

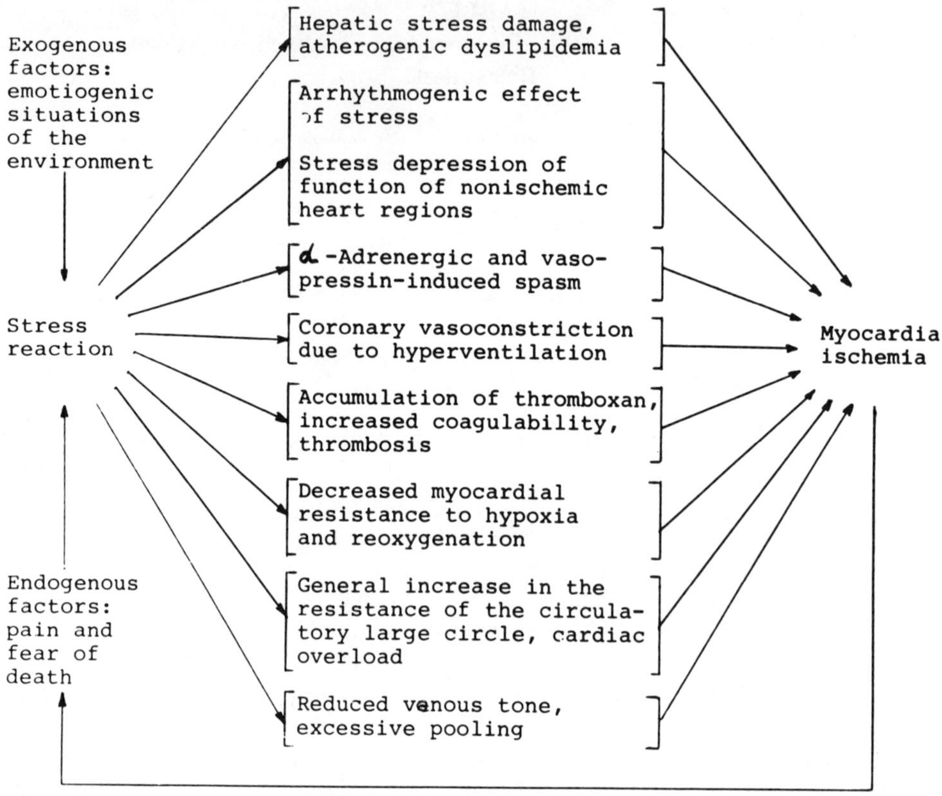

FIGURE 15. Role of stress in ischemic myocardial damage. For explanations see text.

loads, though not without unfavorable consequences. This paradox is especially vivid with the environmental stress reactions. Indeed, the role of biosocial stress in the pathogenesis of mental disorders, duodenal and gastric ulcers, grave bile-duct dyskinesia, skin diseases, malignant tumors, and finally ischemic heart disease dealt with here, is quite well known. Moreover, the pathological role of the stress reaction is such a popular idea as prevents many researchers from appreciating the paramount circumstance that most people and animals encountering the so-called hopeless situations do not die, but acquire a certain resistance to them.

We shall concentrate on the mechanism of this admirable resistance later when considering the stress-limiting systems. Here it must again be emphasized that *the stress reaction is really quite important for the onset, course, and outcome of the ischemic disease.* To understand the principles of its therapy it is essential to clearly realize the relation of ischemic and stress factors at every stage of its development. This is especially significant in recognizing the mechanisms of arrhythmias, sudden death, and *in approaching correctly the major question of the differentiation between the primary ischemic disease, which evolves as the direct result of stenosing coronary atherosclerosis, and the stress arrhythmic heart disease, which evolves first of all as the result of primary stress damage.*

V. RELATION BETWEEN STRESS REACTION AND ISCHEMIA IN THE PATHOGENESIS OF ARRHYTHMIAS AND SUDDEN CARDIAC DEATH

The modern definition of sudden cardiac death is the death of an apparently healthy normal person ensuing from a cardiac attack within an hour from its onset. In point of fact, various epidemiological studies demonstrate that in half of the cases or more the death comes in the first 10 to 15 min from the beginning of the attack. The ECG, when recorded, in most cases reveals cardiac fibrillation.[170] In the U.S. the annual toll of sudden death was estimated at 220,000 to 280,000 in the early 1980s;[171] it is no less common in other developed countries and on the whole constitutes one of the main causes of mortality and a major health problem in the modern world.

Since coronary atherosclerosis is quite widespread, and according to many epidemiological studies[172,173] the sudden death and the coronary disease share the risk factors, a rather common viewpoint is that sudden death is the direct result of the progression of coronary arterial atherosclerosis. However, the vast experience of modern resuscitation shows that in many cases the timely use of defibrillation and other proper means restores the rhythmic activity of the heart and preserves life without recurrence of fibrillation for quite some time.[170]

On the other hand, quite a number of researchers maintain that in most pecple who die a sudden cardiac death, despite more or less pronounced coronary sclerosis, there is no thrombosis of the coronary arteries, myocardial necrosis, or other organic damage of the cardiac muscle that could itself be the cause of death.[170,174]

It is such contradictory results that have made most topical the question of to what extent atherosclerosis as such can cause fibrillation and sudden death, and what part therein can be played by other aggravating factors such as stress.

A quantitative analysis of Thomas et al.[175] shows that pronounced coronary stenosis (75% in one or two arteries) is found with the same frequency in a group of IHD and sudden death and in a control group of those who died of unrelated causes, so that *even advanced atherosclerosis can hardly be regarded as the cause of fibrillation and sudden cardiac death.* Furthermore, about half of the cases of sudden death display none of such reliable hallmarks of ischemia as thrombosis of the coronary vessels or myocardial infarction. Indeed, a comparative study of 868 autopsies carried out in 5 research centers in the U.S. demonstrates that in sudden cardiac death the incidence of a fresh thrombus obstructing a large coronary vessel is from 17 to 46%.[176] In full conformity with this, it has been shown that in many cases fibrillation and sudden cardiac death are not associated with myocardial infarction, and that acute myocardial infarction is reliably found only in 13 to 40% of cases of sudden cardiac death within 6 h from the onset of attack.[177,178]

Nevertheless, there is a standpoint that the myocardial infarction is not found in sudden cardiac death only because the pathoanatomist is dealing with the early stage of ischemic alterations that are not revealed with routine methods. Indeed, obvious macroscopic alterations typical of myocardial infarction take 18 to 24 h to develop, whereas with histological techniques it can be diagnosed in 8 to 12 h of myocardial ischemia. A shorter ischemia preceding death is most difficult to discern;[176] yet a macroscopic test with nitro tetrazolium blue detects an early stage of infarction in 52% of cases of sudden cardiac death,[179] while the microscopic test detects ischemic damage in 46%.[180] These indices are unlikely to change much in the future. In fact, patients who develop an infarction after resuscitation from sudden cardiac death are now known to differ paradoxically in prognosis from those who have no infarction. Recurrence of fibrillation in resuscitated patients who "have got their infarction" is far rarer than in those who have none (2% vs. 22%, respectively). Hence a large necrotic region in the myocardium is associated with a much smaller probability of arrhythmias.[176] To complicate the matters still more, we can recall the rather old but none the less significant work of Enos et al.,[181] who found pronounced atherosclerosis of coronary vessels among U.S. soldiers who had fought in Korea, i.e., in healthy young men. Of those killed in action (mean age 22.1) 10% had coronary artery stenosis exceeding 70%. *All this means that marked atherosclerosis or even ischemic damage in the form of infarction by themselves are often not at all sufficient to cause fibrillation and sudden cardiac death.*

On the other hand, we have seen that there are many cases of sudden cardiac death in the absence of any atherosclerotic or ischemic alterations. In other words, *people may live with pronounced atherosclerosis, and people may suddenly die without any atherosclerosis. Hence, besides stenosing atherosclerosis and attending ischemia there must some other etiological, triggering factor.*

Stress can be such a trigger, as demonstrated by Myers and Dewar,[182] who analyzed the circumstances preceding sudden death in 100 men under 70 with coronary atherosclerosis proved at necropsy. It was found that 23% of the deceased had experienced severe emotional stress within 30 min before death, 40% within the last day, and 22 to 23% had been under stress for 6 months or more.

At present there is extensive epidemiological evidence available that shows that biosocial stress in great measure predetermines the mortality from heart fibrillation and sudden cardiac death in masked and overt coronary disease, whereas alleviation of this "stress pressure" has an opposite effect. Thus a study of 17,500 Whitehall employees having coronary atherosclerosis (age 40 to 64) showed that in the group occupying the lowest positions the cardiac mortality was 3.6 times higher than among those of the same age, but close to the top.[183] This result could have been simply and plausibly explained by the effect of stress on the development of coronary atherosclerosis. However, the most impressive point of this work is that age, blood pressure, smoking, height-weight ratio, glucose tolerance, and plasma cholesterol could only account for a minor portion of this drastically increased cardiac mortality. *The major determinant of mortality was the low social status and attending chronic biosocial stress pressure.*

These facts put in the forefront the question by what mechanisms the stress can provoke arrhythmic and ischemic cardiac responses in IHD, and how much it contributes to these often fatal events. To get some insight into this problem, in our already mentioned study with Khalfen and Lyamina we compared the response of adrenergic regulation and cardiac function to the stress load and to the standard VEL in healthy subjects and in patients with IHD of different severity.

As follows from Table 10, epinephrine excretion at rest in IHD with functional class I-II angina is 40% higher as compared to the healthy subjects, and under stress its relative increase is about the same; thus the blood epinephrine concentration is higher in IHD patients.

Norepinephrine concentration in IHD declines by 22% at rest, but drastically increases under stress (by 90 to 102% vs. 24% in healthy subjects, $p < 0.001$). It is noteworthy that in IHD with class I-II angina the epinephrine/norepinephrine ratio at rest is already elevated to 0.89 to 0.91, i.e., actually to or above the stress level, and does not appreciably change under stress.

Table 10 further shows that dopamine excertion in IHD is decreased significantly and proportionately to the severity of the disease. Indeed, it is a 31% decrease in class I-II angina, 37% in class III-IV angina, and 50% in IHD with previous myocardial infarction. Accordingly, the physiologically important ratio dopamine/(epinephrine + norepinephrine) is 30 to 40% lower both at rest and under stress.

It should be borne in mind that first, dopamine is the precursor of epinephrine and norepinephrine in catecholamine synthesis, and may accumulate in stress owing to reduced activity of the limiting enzyme β-dopamine hydroxylase,[184] and second, dopamine is the mediator of a separate dopaminergic system whose neurons are widely represented in the brain and the spinal cord.[185,186] Dopamine restricts the adrenergic activity at the central level,[187] and accordingly the density of dopamine receptors in the brain is higher in rats that are more resistant to stress.[188] Activation of dopamine receptors by dopamine agonists has also been shown to prevent ulceration of the gastric mucosa in stress.[189]

The dopamine deficiency in IHD patients at rest and under stress, and progression of this deficiency with progressing IHD severity are in our opinion one of the explanations of the enhanced vulnerability of such patients to stress situations.

TABLE 10
Adrenergic Responses (ng/min) to Stress Load in Healthy Subjects and IHD Patients

Group	Epinephrine		Norepinephrine		E/NE		Dopamine		Dopamine/E + NE	
	Before load	After load	Before load	After load	Before load	After load	Before load	After load	Before load	After load
Healthy (n = 21)	3.60±0.70	6.50±0.81	6.30±0.81	7.71±0.83	0.57±0.06	0.74±0.09	292±18	372±22	29.6±1.8	26.0±1.6
IHD (n = 72)	4.06±0.91	6.82±0.92	4.46±0.81	8.22±0.82	0.91±0.08	0.88±0.08	194±18	276±19	22.7±1.2	19.6±1.1
Angina pectoris class I-II (n = 26)	5.04±0.90	9.01±0.92	4.99±0.83	9.79±0.86	1.01±0.06	0.92±0.08	202±21	254±30	20.1±1.1	18.8±1.1
Angina pectoris class III-IV (n = 25)	3.80±0.75	6.08±0.84	4.57±0.73	7.69±0.61	0.83±0.05	0.79±0.05	186±18	245±21	22.2±1.2	17.6±1.1
IHD with previous myocardial infarction (n = 21)	3.20±0.63	4.99±0.73	3.72±0.68	6.93±0.69	0.85±0.05	0.72±0.06	148±16	216±18	21.3±1.2	18.1±1.2

Under physical load the minor shifts in dopamine excretion did not reach statistical significance. Epinephrine excretion in all forms of IHD except those with myocardial infarction increased 1.5- to 2-fold, while norepinephrine excretion decreased to the same extent; therefore under physical load the change in the epinephrine/norepinephrine ratio was similar to though smaller than that under stress load.

In the aggregate these data demonstrate that IHD is attended with such potentially arrhythmogenic alterations in the adrenergic regulation as elevated epinephrine/norepinephrine ratio and lowered dopamine/epinephrine + norepinephrine ratio, which are more pronounced under stress than under physical load.

The physical tolerance was lowered in IHD patients(maximal load 109 ± 11 W as compared to 201 ± 15 W for healthy subjects). At the same time, increases in the Katz index (HR × APs/100) under SL and VEL were about the same in IHD patients and healthy controls. This decreased efficiency of cardiac performance has been demonstrated in a number of works. Further, the increases in the contraction and relaxation velocities are two to three times less in IHD patients, so that under both types of load the IHD patients display depression of the contraction and relaxation indices.

The use of the relaxation index in this form has been first proposed in the mid-1970s,[190] and its pronounced decrease under load or high catecholamine concentrations reflects the impairment of membrane calcium transporting mechanisms which have been demonstrated in both stress-induced and ischemic cardiac damage. It is of interest in this context that in IHD patients under stress both indices were depressed proportionately to increased excretion (and therefore blood concentration) of epinephrine.

On the whole, this means that the enhanced adrenergic effect, along with alterations in the cardiac muscle itself, is involved in the depression of contraction and relaxation indices in IHD patients under stress load.

Table 11 demonstrates the detectability of ischemic and arrhythmic reactions in IHD with the use of stress and physical loads. The ischemic reaction is revealed in 64% of cases with VEL and in only 29.5% with SL; however, out of 27 patients with an ischemic response to SL only 8 responded to VEL. Hence the SL revealed 19 additional cases of ischemic response, and the total percentage of patients with documented myocardial ischemia increased to 84.8%.

The practical significance of this fact is obvious, and makes expedient a combination of both tests for a fuller diagnosis of IHD. The theoretical aspect is that the pathogenesis of ischemic attacks may differ among coronary patients: in some of them the attacks are provoked by enhanced cardiac function, whereas in others by the adrenergic effect on the pathologically altered heart.

Table 11 further shows that the physical load elicited potential arrhythmias only in 8% of IHD patients, while the SL was effective in 22%. Moreover, of 7 patients responding arrhythmically to VEL, 5 also responded to SL. In sum, the detectability of rhythm and conduction disorders with the two tests was about 24%.

The fact that the stress load is a more efficient means of revealing arrhythmias in IHD, besides being practically important, also unambiguously testifies that enhanced adrenergic action on the heart is more likely to provoke arrhythmias in IHD patients than surplus physical load.

In full conformity with this, the SL eliciting arrhythmias in IHD in most cases increases the Katz index only by 30 to 40% whereas the maximal VEL, which increases this index twofold to threefold, quite rarely causes such disturbances. In essence this means that in stress the elevated catecholamine concentration evokes arrhythmias not through increased cardiac function (which is not large enough to cause relative hypoxia), but directly affecting the electric stability of the heart.

Interestingly, the ischemic responses to SL, unlike those to VEL, were also independent

TABLE 11
Detection of Ischemic and Arrhythmic Reactions with Physical Load (VEL) and Stress Load (SL) in IHD Patients (n = 92)

	Detectability (%)
Ischemic response to:	
VEL	64
SL	29.5
VEL and/or SL	84.8
Arrhythmic response to:	
VEL	8
SL	22
VEL and/or SL	23.9

of increased cardiac function. At maximal physical load the various forms of ischemic reaction in 91% of all IHD cases were observed after the Katz index (mainly reflecting the cardiac oxygen consumption) had increased by more than 75%; under the SL 89% of ischemic reactions took place before a 75% increase in the Katz index.

Thus, the greater cardiac vulnerability to the arrhythmogenic and ischemic effects of stress observed in this work may be due to the enhanced adrenergic component of the stress reaction, to the lower efficiency of the stress-limiting systems, and of course to profound alterations in the heart itself. As a result, in IHD patients a moderate stress is more likely to cause an arrhythmogenic effect than the maximal tolerable physical load; this effect appears to be realized not through enhanced cardiac function, but by direct action of catecholamines and other stress hormones on the heart, as has been postulated earlier.

Taken together with the data on primary stress cardiac damage (Chapter 1) and primary stress arrhythmias (the beginning of this chapter), the above signifies that in cardiac disease the detrimental factors — ischemic caused by stenosing atherosclerosis, and excessive stress reaction caused by defects in stress-limiting systems — may result in arrhythmias and cardiac fibrillation in three ways:

1. Primary ischemic cardiac damage and its arrhythmogenic effect
2. Primary stress cardiac damage and its arrhythmogenic effect in the absence of stenosing coronary sclerosis and ischemia
3. Combined arrhythmogenic effects of ischemia and stress

The first variant is conventional, well studied, and comprehensively presented in the literature. The second one is substantiated by the above experimental and clinical data. Finally, the third one appears to occur at the later stages of stenosing coronary sclerosis, and can only be understood on the basis of clear notion of the first two. Therefore, in summing up this chapter it is reasonable to first compare the ischemic and the stress damage to the heart and only then to consider how their combination can bring on arrhythmias, fibrillation, and sudden cardiac death. The data available on the primary stress damage to the heart show that this phenomenon is profoundly different in its etiology, pathogenesis, and clinical manifestations from what is usually implied by the term "ischemic disease". Indeed, stenosing coronary sclerosis causing myocardial ischemia is now well known to be itself the sequela of genetical defects in or alimentary overloading of the hepatic mechanisms for metabolic elimination of cholesterol. This idea has been supported by the studies of Anichkov[191] on experimental alimentary atherosclerosis and by the works of Brown and Goldstein,[112] who found a hepatic system of receptors removing LDLP from the blood, and convincingly proved by dietary and other measures for preventing coronary disease.

TABLE 12
Differentiation Between Ischemic Heart Disease and Stress Arrhythmic Heart Disease

	Ischemic heart disease	Stress arrhythmic heart disease
1. Etiology	Defects in cholesterol-eliminating systems	Defects in stress-limiting systems
2. Key pathogenetic link	Senosing coronary sclerosis → myocardial ischemia	Excessive stress reaction → stress damage to the heart
3. Ischemic response to physical load	Marked "ischemic" ECG changes and cardiac pains	Absent
4. Arrhythmic response to physical load	Rare at peak load	Absent or occurs after load
5. Ischemic response to stress load	Occurs in about one third of cases	Absent
6. Arrhythmic response to stress load	Rare (about 10% of cases)	Frequent
7. Arrhythmias at rest	Secondary, ischemia-linked, abolishable with vasodilators	Primary, without ischemia, vasodilators poorly effective
8. Myocardial infarcts	Vast, early	Microfocal, late
9. Therapy with sedatives, neuroleptics, tranquilizers, adrenoblockers	Partly effective, restricts secondary stress reaction to ischemia	Quite effective, restricts primary stress reaction
10. Prophylaxis by adaptation to hypoxia, physical load, etc.	Partly effective	Quite effective

As to the stress damage to the heart, it is a result of exceedingly long and strong stress reactions, and can be more or less completely prevented by adaptation to short stress exposures which activate the modulatory stress-limiting systems of the organism. These systems — opioidergic, GABA-ergic, serotoninergic, as well as antioxidant, adenosinergic, and PG ones — have already been briefly mentioned and will be dealt with in detail in Chapters 4 and 5. Notably, it is the genetic or acquired deficiency of the central and the cellular systems of protection from stress, and not secondary ischemia caused by stress spasm and thrombosis, that is in many cases the basis of stress arrhythmias, blocks, and cardiopathies.

The set of distinctions between the ischemic heart disease and the stress arrhythmic heart disease listed in Table 12 is proposed as a working hypothesis with a clear understanding that at a certain stage of the process stress and ischemia are deeply intertwined. The main justification of this concept is not only the profound and to my mind undebatable differences in the etiology and the pathogenesis of these two conditions, but also the fact that their prognosis, prophylaxis, and therapy are also different in many aspects of clinical importance.

While differentiating the etiology, pathogenesis, and clinics of these two processes, we should at the same time bear in mind their pronounced mutual potentiation, for which three basic mechanisms can be discerned.

First, the stress by direct noncoronarogenic damage to the conduction system and contractile myocardium can give rise to multiple zones of depolarization and conduction defects. This stress-induced enhancement of the electric heterogeneity of the heart is aggravated by interruption of intercellular contacts by excess calcium and adds to the depolarization foci and numerous conduction blocks caused by ischemia. As a result, the cardiac electric stability, which we have seen to be only relative even in apparently healthy people, turns out to be deeply impaired and brings on grave arrhythmias, fibrillation, and cardiac arrest.

The second and more conventional mechanism is that under certain conditions the stress can be conducive to further development of coronary sclerosis, coronary spasm, and coronary thrombosis, thereby deepening the ischemia and leading to acute myocardial infarction which in its turn is complicated with arrhythmias and cardiac fibrillation.

The third mechanism is that the ischemic focus or the infarct causes pain and fear, i.e., gives rise to a stress reaction which, as we have seen, damages the nonischemic myocardial regions, increases the load on the heart, and may directly aggravate the ischemia.

The major issue from these three possibilities is that *prevention, restriction, or abolishment of a stress attack on the heart can be highly effective in protecting the heart not only from arrhythmias, but also from ischemia induced or aggravated by stress.* On the basis of this general concept we shall in subsequent chapters turn to the main subject of this book, that is, to nondrug protection of the heart from stress and ischemia with the use of adaptation to environmental factors which causes a stable enhancement of the power and efficiency of the stress-limiting and antihypoxic systems of the organism.

REFERENCES

1. **Laughlin, M.,** An analysis of the risk of human cardiac damage during +G(Z) stress: a review, *Aviat. Space Environ. Med.,* 53, 423, 1982.
2. **Korteweg, G., Boeles, T., and Tencate, J.,** Influence of stimulation of some subcortical areas on electrocardiogram, *J. Neurophysiol.,* 20, 100, 1957.
3. **Lown, B., Verrier, R. L., and Corbalan, R.,** Psychologic stress and threshold for repetitive ventricular response, *Science,* 143, 834, 1973.
4. **Lown, B., Verrier, R. L., and Rabinowitz, S. H.,** Neural and psychologic mechanisms and the problem of sudden cardiac death, *Am. J. Cardiol.,* 39, 890, 1977.
5. **Lown, B. and De Silva, R.,** Role of psychologic stress and autonomic nervous system changes in provocation of ventricular premature complex, *Am. J. Cardiol.,* 41, 979, 1978.
6. **Blatt, C. M., Rabinowitz, S. H., and Lown, B.,** Central serotonergic agents raise the repetitive extrasystole threshold of the vulnerable period of the canine ventricular myocardium, *Circ. Res.,* 44, 723, 1979.
7. **Brodsky, M., Wu, D., and Denes, D. P.,** Arrhythmias documented by 24 hour continuous electrocardiographic monitoring, *Clin. J. Cardiol.,* 39, 390, 1977.
8. **Bjerregaard, P.,** Prevalence of cardiac arrhythmias in healthy subjects, in *Cardiac Arrhythmias in the Active Population,* Chumberlain, D. A. and Kulbertus, H., Eds., Mölndad, Sweden, 980, 24.
9. **Meerson, F. Z., Belkina, L. M., Sazontova, T. G., Saltykova, V. A., and Arkhipenko, Yu. V.,** The role of lipid peroxidation in pathogenesis of arrhythmias and prevention of cardiac fibrillation with antioxidants, *Basic Res. Cardiol.,* 82, 123, 1987.
10. **Verrier, R. L. and Lown, B.,** Sympathetic-parasympathetic interactions and ventricular electrical stability, in *Neural Mechanisms in Cardiac Arrhythmias,* Schwartz, P. T., Brown, H. M., Malliani, A., and Zanchetti, A., Eds., Raven Press, New York, 1985, 75.
11. **Verrier, R. L. and Hagestaad, E. L.,** Neural mechanisms in cardiac arrhythmias, in *Mechanism and Treatment of Cardiac Arrhythmias,* Reiser, H. J. and Horowitz, L. N., Eds., Urban and Schwarzenberg, Baltimore, 1985, 76.
12. **Vatner, S. F. and Hintze, T. H.,** Mechanism of constriction of large coronary arteries by β-adrenergic receptor blockade, *Circ. Res.,* 53, 389, 1983.
13. **Shepherd, J. T. and Vanhoutte, P. M.,** Spasm of the coronary arteries: causes and consequences (the scientist's viewpoint), *Mayo Clin. Proc.,* 60, 33, 1985.
14. **Rosen, M. R.,** Mechanisms for arrhythmias, *Am. J. Cardiol.,* 61, 2A, 1988.
15. **Rona, G., Chappel, C. I., Balazs, T., and Gaudry, R.,** An infarct-like myocardial lesion and other toxic manifestations produced by isoproterenol in the rat, *Arch. Pathol.,* 67, 443, 1959.
16. **Waldenström, A. P., Hjalmarson, A. C., and Thornell, L. E.,** A possible role of noradrenaline in the development of myocardial infarction, *Am. Heart J.,* 95, 43, 1978.
17. **Timmermans, P. B. W. M., Chin, A. T., and Thoolen, M. J. M. C.,** Calcium handling in vasoconstriction to stimulation of $alpha_1$- and $alpha_2$-adrenoreceptors, *Can. J. Physiol. Pharmacol.,* 65, 1649, 1987.
18. **Michell, R. H.,** Inositol lipid breakdown as a step in alpha-adrenergic stimulus — response coupling, *Clin. Sci.,* 68 (Suppl. 10), 43s, 1985.
19. **Suematsu, E., Hirata, M., Hashimoto, T., and Khriyama, H.,** Inositol-1,4,5-triphosphate releases Ca^{2+} from intracellular store sites in skinned single cells of porcine coronary artery, *Biochem. Biophys. Res. Commun.,* 120, 481, 1984.
20. **Jackson, E. K.,** Role of adenosine in noradrenergic neurotransmission in spontaneously hypertensive rats, *Am. H. Physiol.,* 253, H909, 1987.

21. **Thandroyen, F. T., Flint, N. S., Worthington, M. G., and Opie, L. H.,** Arrhythmogenic action of alpha-1-adrenoreceptor stimulation in isolated non-ligated rat heart, *J. Mol. Cell. Cardiol.*, 17 (Suppl. 3), N13, 1985.
22. **Murray, P. A. and Vatner, S. F.,** α-Adrenoreceptor attenuation of the coronary vascular response to severe exercise in the conscious dog, *Circ. Res.*, 45, 654, 1979.
23. **Mudge, G. H., Grossman, W., Mills, R. M., Lesch, M., and Braunwald, E.,** Reflex increase in coronary vascular resistance in patients with ischemic heart disease, *N. Engl. J. Med.*, 295, 1333, 1976.
24. **Robertson, R. M., Wood, A. J. J., Vaughn, W. K., and Robertson, D.,** Exacerbation of vasotonic angina pectoris by propranolol, *Circulation*, 65, 281, 1982.
25. **Bristow, M. R., Kantrowitz, N. E., Ginsburg, R., and Fowler, M. B.,** β-Adrenergic function in heart muscle disease and heart failure, *J. Mol. Cell. Cardiol.*, 17 (Suppl. 2), 41, 1985.
26. **Chierchia, S., Brunelli, C., Simonetti, I., Lazzari, M., and Maseri, A.,** Sequence of events in angina at rest: primary reduction in coronary flow, *Circulation*, 61, 759, 1980.
27. **Deanfield, J. E., Maseri, A., Selwyn, A. P., Ribeiro, P., Chierchia, S., Krikler, S., and Morgan, M.,** Myocardial ischemia during daily life in patients with stable angina: its relation to symptoms and heart rate changes, *Lancet*, 2, 756, 1983.
28. **Maseri, A., L'Abbate, A., Chierchia, S., Parodi, O., Severi, S., Biagini, A., Distante, A., Marzilli, M., and Ballestra, A. M.,** Significance of spasm in the pathogenesis of ischemic heart disease, *Am. J. Cardiol.*, 44, 788, 1979.
29. **Raizner, A. E., Chahine, R. A., Ishimori, T., Verani, M. S., Zacca, N., Jamal, N., Miller, R. R., and Luchi, R. J.,** Provocation of coronary artery spasm by the cold pressor test. Hemodynamic, arteriographic and quantitative angiographic observations, *Circulation*, 62, 925, 1980.
30. **Lown, B.,** Verbal conditioning of angina pectoris during exercise testing, *Am. J. Cardiol.*, 40, 630, 1977.
31. **Verrier, R. L. and Lown, B.,** Influence of neural stability during acute myocardial ischemia and infarction, in management of ventricular tachycardia: role of mexiletine, in *International Congress Series*, No. 458, Sandoe, E., Julian, D. G., and Bell, J. W., Eds., Excerpta Medica, Amsterdam, 1978, 94.
32. **Levy, M. N. and Blattberg, B.,** Effect of vagal stimulation on the overflow of norepinephrine into the coronary sinus during cardiac sympathetic nerve stimulation in the dog, *Circ. Res.*, 38, 81, 1976.
33. **Watanabe, A. M., Lindemann, J. P., Jones, L. R., Besch, H. R., and Bailey, J. C.,** Biochemical mechanisms mediating neural control of the heart, in *Disturbances in Neurogenic Control of Circulation*, Abboud, F. M., Fozzard, J. P., Gilmore, J. P., and Reis, D. J., Eds., American Physiological Society, Bethesda, MD, 1981, 189.
34. **Zigmond, M. and Harvey, J.,** Resistance to central norepinephrine depletion and decreased mortality in rats chronically exposed to electric foot shock, *J. Neuro-Visc. Relat.*, 31, 373, 1970.
35. **Meerson, F. Z., Gorina, M. S., Zeland, A. M., and Giber, L. M.,** Influence of emotional pain stress on the contractile function and adrenoreactivity of the cardiac muscle (in Russian), *Byull. Eksp. Biol. Med.*, 11, 528, 1979.
36. **Engel, G. L.,** Psychologic stress, vasodepressor (vasovagal) syncope and sudden death, *Ann. Int. Med.*, 89, 403, 1978.
37. **Corley, K. C., Shiel, F. O., Mauck, H. P., and Creenhoot, J.,** Electrocardiographic and cardiac morphological changes associated with environmental stress in squirrel monkeys, *Psychosom. Med.*, 35, 361, 1973.
38. **Corley, K. C., Mauck, H. P., and Shiel, F. O.,** Cardiac responses associated with yoked-chair shock avoidance in squirrel monkey, *Psychophysiology*, 12, 439, 1975.
39. **Corley, K. C., Shiel, F. O., Mauck, H. P., Clark, L. S., and Barber, J. H.,** Myocardial degeneration and cardiac arrest in squirrel monkeys. Physiological and psychological correlates, *Psychophysiology*, 14, 322, 1977.
40. **Johansson, G., Jonsson, L., Lannek, L., Blomgren, L., Lindberg, P., and Poupa, O.,** Severe stress-cardiopathy in pigs, *Am. Heart J.*, 87, 451, 1974.
41. **Hofer, M. A.,** Cardiac and respiratory function during sudden prolonged immobility in wild rodents, *Psychosom. Med.*, 32, 633, 1970.
42. **Meerson, F. Z., Radzievskii, S. A., Giber, L. M., Kogan, A. Kh., Rozhitskaya, I. I., Volovinskaya, O. I., and Pshennikova, M. G.,** Heart damage in emotional stress and prophylaxis of this phenomenon by prior adaptation to altitude hypoxia (in Russian), *Dokl. Akad. Nauk SSSR*, 237, 977, 1977.
43. **Smetnev, A. S., Shevchenko, N. M., and Grosu, A. A.,** Sinus node dysfunction syndrome (in Russian), *Kardiologiya*, 2, 5, 1988.
44. **Djiane, K., Egre, A., and Bory, M.,** L'enregistrement electrocardiographique continu des 50 subjects normal, in *Troubles des Rythme et Electrostimulation*, Puel, P., Ed., Toulouse, 1977, 161.
45. **Clarke, J. M., Hamer, G., and Shelton, J. P.,** The rhythm of the normal human heart, *Lancet*, 2, 508, 1976.
46. **Engel, U. R. and Burckhardt, D.,** Häufigkeit und Art von Herzrhythmussförungen sowie EKG. — Veränderungen bei Jungendlichen Herzgesunden Probemden, *Schweiz. Med. Wochenschr.*, 105, 1467, 1975.

47. **Von Dietz, A. and Kirchhoff, H. W.,** Die Variationsbreite von Herzrhythmussförmgen bei Herzgesunden, *Z. Kardiol.,* 62, 289, 1973.
48. **Meerson, F. Z. and Bukina, T. A.,** Nonischemic cardiac rhythm disorders in pilots, in *Abstr. III Sci.-Pract. Conf. Medical Provision for Flight Safety and Medical Flight Testing* (in Russian), Gosud. NII Grazhd. Aviatsii, Moscow, 1987, 19.
49. **Meerson, F. Z. and Bukina, T. N.,** On detection of latent nonischemic arrhythmias in pilots with stress load, in *Problems of Clinical Medicine in Civil Aviation* (in Russian), Natradze, D. A. and Gel'man, B. L., Eds., Gosud. NII Grazhd. Aviatsii, Moscow, 1988, 70.
50. **Karvasarskii, B. D.,** *Neuroses* (in Russian), Meditsina, Moscow, 1980.
51. **Berezin, F. B., Miroshnikov, M. N., and Rozhanets, R. V.,** *The Method of Many-Sided Examination of the Personality in Clinical Medicine and Psychohygiene* (in Russian), Nauka, Moscow, 1976.
52. **Skibitskii, V. V.,** Effect of phenibut and eglonil on the frequency of paroxysms of tachoarrhythmia and central hemodynamics in patients with neurocirculatory dystonia (in Russian), *Vrach. Delo,* 8, 22, 1983.
53. **Smetnev, A. S., Bunin, Yu. A., Firstova, M. I., Malyshev, Yu. M., Klembovskii, A. A., Nargizyan, A. B., and Asymbekova, E. U.,** The state of myocardial blood flow in patients with various forms of supraventricular cardiac rhythm disturbances (in Russian), *Kardiologiya,* 3, 39, 1985.
54. **Lombardi, F., Malfatto, G., Belloni, A., and Garimoldi, M.,** Effect of sympathetic activation on ventricular ectopic beats in subjects with and without evidence of organic heart disease, *Eur. Heart J.,* 8, 1065, 1987.
55. **Smetnev, A. S., Bunin, Yu. A., Firstova, M. I., Smirnov, I. E., Markov, Kh. M., Savchenko, A. P., and Asymbekova, E. U.,** Content of endogenous prostanoids in patients with supraventricular cardiac rhythm disturbances (in Russian), *Kardiologiya,* 6, 18, 1984.
56. **Neglia, D., Levorato, D., Berti, S., Marzilli, M., Pelosi, G., Marcassa, C., Bongiorni, M. G., L'Abbate, A., and Contini, C.,** Diagnosi e caratterizzazione funzionale di iniziale danno myocardica in pazienti con aritmie condiache, *Cardiologia,* 32, 713, 1987.
57. **Lowler, K. A.,** Cardiovascular and electrodermal response pattern in heart rate reactive individuals during psychological stress, *Psychophysiology,* 17, 467, 1980.
58. **Sokolov, E. I. and Belova, E. V.,** *Emotions and Cardiac Pathology* (in Russian), Nauka, Moscow, 1983.
59. **Sidorenko, G. I. and Kachesova, T. A.,** A novel psychophysiological "information test" and its possible use in cardiology (in Russian), *Kardiologiya,* 8, 63, 1984.
60. **Sidorenko, B. A. and Revenko, V. N.,** Use of the psychoemotional test in patients with ischemic heart disease (in Russian), *Kardiologiya,* 5, 80, 1984.
61. **Kvantaliani, T. G., Kavtaradze, V. G., and Mamaladze, G. T.,** Complex use of psychological and physical load tests in the dynamics of ischemic heart disease (in Russian), *Kardiologiya,* 6, 68, 1981.
62. **Rizhinashvili, Z. A., Golitsyn, S. P., Khramelashvili, V. V., and Smetnev, A. S.,** Use of psycho-emotional test in patients with different cardiovascular diseases (in Russian), *Kardiologiya,* 6, 34, 1987.
63. **Aslan, S., Nelson, L., Carrathers, M., and Lader, M.,** Stress and age effects on catecholamines in normal subjects, *J. Psychosom. Res.,* 25, 33, 1981.
64. **Green, J. R., Korovetz, M. J., Shanklin, D. R., De Vito, J. J., and Taylor, W. J.,** Sudden unexpected death in three generations, *Arch. Intern. Med.,* 124, 359, 1969.
65. **McRae, J. R., Wagner, G. S., Rogers, M. C., and Canen, R. V.,** Paroxysmal familial ventricular fibrillation, *J. Pediatr.,* 84, 515, 1974.
66. **Lown, B.,** Sudden cardiac death: biobehavioral perspective, *Circulation,* 76 (Suppl., pt I), 186, 1987.
67. **Rozenberg, V. D. and Nepomnyaschikh, L. M.,** *Coronarography in Pathological Morphology* (in Russian), Meditsina, Novosibirsk, 1987.
68. **Davies, M. S., Anderson, R. H., and Becker, A. E.,** *The Conduction of the Heart,* Butterworths, London, 1983.
69. **Cebelin, M. S. and Hirsh, C. S.,** Human stress cardiomyopathy. Myocardial lesions in victims of homicidal assaults without internal injuries, *Hum. Pathol.,* 11, 123, 1980.
70. **Wolf, S.,** Behavioral aspects of cardiac arrhythmia and sudden death, *Circulation,* 76, pt 2, I-174, 1987.
71. **Meerson, F. Z. and Pshennikova, M. G.,** *Adaptation to Stress Situations and Physical Loads* (in Russian), Meditsina, Moscow, 1988.
72. **Vlay, S. C.,** Ventricular tachycardia — fibrillation on the first day of medical school, *Am. J. Cardiol.,* 57, 483, 1986.
73. **Wellens, H. J. J., Vermeulen, A., and Durrer, D.,** Ventricular fibrillation occurring on arousal from sleep by auditory stimuli, *Circulation,* 46, 661, 1972.
74. **McLaran, C. J., Gersh, B. J., Sugrue, D. D., Hammill, S. C., Zinsmeister, A. R., Wood, D. L., Holmes, D. R., and Osborn, M. J.,** Out of hospital cardiac arrest in patients without clinically significant coronary artery disease electrophysiological and survival characteristics with those in similar patients who have clinically significant coronary artery disease, *Br. Heart J.,* 58, 583, 1987.
75. **Belhassen, B., Shapira, I., Shoshani, D., Paredes, A., Miller, H., and Laniado, S.,** Idiopathic ventricular fibrillation: inducibility and beneficial effects of class I antiarrhythmic agents, *Circulation,* 75, 809, 1987.

76. **Baron, R. and Kirscher, R.,** Sudden night-time death among South East Asians, *Lancet,* 1, 764, 1983.
77. **Hayashi, M., Murata, M., and Saton, M.,** Sudden nocturnal death in young males from ventricular flatter, *Jpn. Heart J.,* 26, 585, 1985.
78. **Helsing, K. J. and Szklo, M.,** Mortality after bereavement, *Am. J. Epidemiol.,* 114, 41, 1981.
79. **Helsing, K. J., Szklo, M., and Comstock, G. W.,** Factors associated with mortality after widowhood, *Am. J. Public Health,* 71, 802, 1981.
80. **Rabkin, S. W., Mathewson, F. A. L., and Tate, R. B.,** Chronobiology of cardiac sudden death in men, *J.A.M.A.,* 44, 1357, 1980.
81. **Kubler, W.,** The conduction and cardiac sympathetic systems: metabolic aspects, *J. Am. Coll. Cardiol.,* 5 (Suppl. 6), 157B, 1985.
82. **Bailey, J. C., Kovach, R. J., and Rardon, D. P.,** Anatomical, biochemical and electrophysiologic evidence for parasympathetic innervation of the ventricle, in *Mechanisms and Treatment of Cardiac Arrhythmias,* Reiser, H. J. and Horowitz, L. N., Eds., Urban and Schwarzenberg, Baltimore, 1985, 57.
83. **Panagia, V., Pierce, G. N., Dhalla, K. S., Ganguly, P. K., Beamish, R. E., and Dhalla, N. S.,** Adaptive changes in subcellular calcium transport during catecholamine-induced cardiomyopathy, *J. Mol. Cell. Cardiol.,* 17, 411, 1985.
84. **Salem, B. I., Haikal, M., Zambrano, A., Bollis, A., and Gowda, S.,** Acute myocardial infarction with normal coronary arteries: clinical and angiographic profiles with ergonovine testing, *Tex. Heart Inst. J.,* 12, 1, 1985.
85. Abstracts for the IX Congress of the International Society for Heart Research, New Delhi, India, 28 Sept. to 2 Oct. 1982.
86. Abstracts for the X Congress of the International Society for Heart Research, Moscow, USSR, 23 to 28 Sept. 1980.
87. Conference on Behavioral Medicine and Cardiovascular Disease, Sea Island, Georgia, 3 to 7 Feb. 1985, *Circulation,* 76, pt 2, suppl., 1987.
88. **Hearse, D. J.,** The protection of the ischaemic myocardium: the state of the art, in The 3rd Symp. of Soviet Section of the International Society for Heart Research, Baku, 5 to 8 Oct. 1986.
89. **Kloner, R. A. and Braunwald, E.,** Observations on experimental myocardial ischaemia, *Cardiovasc. Res.,* 14, 371, 1980.
90. *Handbook of Cardiology* (in Russian), Chazov, E. I., Ed., Meditsina, Moscow, 1982.
91. **Opie, L. H., Nathan, D., and Lubbe, W. F.,** Biochemical aspects of arrhythmogenesis and ventricular fibrillation, *Am. J. Cardiol.,* 43, 131, 1979.
92. **Meerson, F. Z.,** *Pathogenesis and Prevention of Stress and Ischemic Damage to the Heart* (in Russian), Meditsina, Moscow, 1984.
93. **Wit, A.-L.,** Cardiac arrhythmias — electrophysiological mechanisms, in *Mechanisms and Treatment of Cardiac Arrhythmias,* Reiser, H. J. and Horowitz, L. N., Eds., Urban and Schwarzenberg, Baltimore, 1985, 11.
94. **Tret'yakova, K. A.,** A study of the cholesterol biosynthesis in rats upon adrenal cortex stimulation with ACTH (in Russian), *Probl. Endokrinol.,* 5, 87, 1966.
95. **Khomulo, P. S.,** On the significance of prolonged strain of the nervous system in development of atherosclerosis in dogs (in Russian), *Dokl. Akad. Nauk SSSR,* 152, 727, 1963.
96. **Khomulo, P. S.,** Neurogenic atherosclerosis and the mechanism of its development (in Russian), *Kardiologiya,* 5, 140, 1974.
97. **Barats, S. S. and Mel'nikova, Z. M.,** Hypertensive disease and coronary atherosclerosis among workers of the Uralmash Plant (in Russian), *Sov. Med.,* 8, 13, 1962.
98. **Gol'dberg, V. A.,** Role of occupational factors and nutrition in the epidemiology of coronary atherosclerosis, in *Incidence of Hypertensive Disease and Coronary Atherosclerosis, and Living Conditions* (in Russian), Myasnikov, A. A. and Ryvkina, I. A., Eds., Meditsina, Leningrad, 1964, 53.
99. **Clarkson, T. B., Kaplan, J. R., Adams, M. R., and Manuck, S. B.,** Psychosocial influence on the pathogenesis of atherosclerosis among nonhuman primates, *Circulation,* 76, pt 2, suppl., I-29, 1987.
100. **Meerson, F. Z., Tverdokhlib, V. P., Ozerova, I. N., Tvorogova, M. T., and Olfer'eva, A. M.,** Influence of emotional pain stress on the lipid level and cholesterol esterification in rat blood (in Russian), *Patol. Fiziol. Eksp. Ter.,* 4, 27, 1987.
101. **Desiderato, O., Mackinnon, J. R., and Hissom, H. J.,** Development of gastric ulcers in rats following stress termination, *Comp. Physiol. Psychol.,* 87, 208, 1974.
102. **Klimov, A. N.,** Causes and conditions of development of atherosclerosis, in *Preventive Cardiology* (in Russian), Kositskii, G. I., Ed., Meditsina, Moscow, 1977, 260.
103. **Miller, G. and Miller, N. E.,** Plasma high-density lipoprotein concentration and development of ischaemic heart disease, *Lancet,* 1, 16, 1975.
104. **Klimov, A. N., Nagornev, V. A., Zubzhigskii, Yu. N., and Denisenko, A. D.,** in *Biochemical Bases of the Pathogenesis of Atherosclerosis* (in Russian), Klimov, A. N., Ed., Meditsina, Leningrad, 1980, 46.
105. **Titov, V. N., Rudnev, V. I., and Tvorogova, M. G.,** Experimental substantiation of the antiatherogenic effect of high-density lipoproteins (in Russian), *Kardiologiya,* 5, 103, 1981.

106. **Gerasimova, E. N. and Perova, N. V.,** Self-regulation of the functional state of high-density lipoproteins and its disturbance in hypoalphacholesterolemia (in Russian), *Vopr. Med. Khim.*, 1, 32, 1985.
107. **Glomset, J. and Norum, K. R.,** The metabolic role of lecithin: cholesterol acyltransferase: perspectives from pathology, *Adv. Lipid Res.*, 11, 1, 1973.
108. **Simon, J. and Boyer, J.,** Production of lecithin:cholesterol acyltransferase by the isolated perfused rat liver, *Biochim. Biophys. Acta,* 218, 549, 1970.
109. **Stokke, K. and Norum, K.,** Determination of lecithin:cholesterol acyltransferase in human blood plasma, *Scand. J. Clin. Lab. Invest.*, 27, 21, 1971.
110. **Ridgway, N. and Dolphin, P.,** Serum activity and hepatic secretion of lecithin:cholesterol acyltransferase in experimental hypothyroidism and hypercholesterolemia, *J. Lipid Res.*, 26, 1300, 1985.
111. **Meerson, F. Z., Tverdokhlib, V. P., Nikonorov, A. A., Filippov, V. K., Frolov, V. A., and Afonina, S. N.,** Role of suppression of hepatic cholesterol 7-α-hydroxylase activity in the evolvement of atherogenic stress dyslipidemia (in Russian), *Kardiologiya,* 9, 85, 1988.
112. **Brown, M. S. and Goldstein, D. L.,** How low-density lipoprotein receptors affect cholesterol metabolism and development of atherosclerosis (in Russian), *V Mire Nauki* (trans. *Scientific American),* 1, 27, 1985.
113. **Satinsky, J., Kosowsky, B., and Lown, B.,** Ventricular fibrillation induced by hypothalamic stimulation during coronary occlusion (Abst.), *Circulation,* suppl. 2, pt II, 60, 1971.
114. **Verrier, R. L. and Lown, B.,** Behavioral stress and cardiac arrhythmias, *Annu. Rev. Physiol.*, 46, 155, 1984.
115. **Lown, B. and Verrier, R.,** Neural activity and ventricular fibrillation, *N. Engl. J. Med.*, 294, 1165, 1976.
116. **Leriche, R., Hermann, L., and Fontaine, R.,** Ligature de la coronarie gauche et fonction chez l'animal intact, *C. R. Seances Soc. Biol. Paris,* 107, 545, 1931.
117. **Verrier, R., Thompson, P., and Lown, B.,** Ventricular vulnerability during sympathetic stimulation: role of heart rate and blood pressure, *Cardiovasc. Res.*, 8, 602, 1974.
118. **Dorofeev, G. I., Shanin, Yu. N., Efimov, N. V., and Ivashkin, V. T.,** Diagnostic and prognostic significance of cyclic nucleotide determination in cardiac rhythm disturbances (in Russian), *Voen.-Med. Zh.*, 2, 59, 1985.
119. **Knight, R. I., Hillyard, S. A., Woods, D. L., and Neville, H. J.,** The effect of frontal and temporal-parietal lesions on the auditory evoked potential in man, *Electroencephalogr. Clin. Neurophysiol.*, 50, 112, 1980.
120. **Skinner, J. and Jingling, C.,** Central gating mechanism that regulates event-related potentials and behavior: a neural model for attention, in *Progress in Clinical Neurophyisology,* Desmedt, J. E., Ed., S. Karger, Basel, 1977, 70.
121. **Skinner, J.,** Psychosocial stress and sudden cardiac death: brain mechanisms, in *Stress and Heart Disease,* Beamish, R. E., Singal, P. K., and Dhalla, N., Eds., Kluwer Academic, Boston, 1985, 44.
122. **Ukhtomskii, A. A.,** *The Dominant* (in Russian), Nauka, Moscow-Leningrad, 1966.
123. **Kryzhanovskii, G. N.,** *Determinant Structures in Nervous System Pathology: Generator Mechanisms of Neuropathological Syndromes* (in Russian), Meditsina, Moscow, 1980.
124. **Hoffman, B. and Cranefield, P.,** The physiological basis of cardiac arrhythmias, *Am. J. Med.*, 37, 670, 1964.
125. **Wit, A. and Rosen, M.,** Pathophysiologic mechanisms of cardiac arrhythmias, *Am. Heart J.*, 106, 798, 1983.
126. **El-Sherif, N., Mehrá, R., Gough, W., and Zeiler, R.,** Ventricular activation patterns of spontaneous and induced ventricular rhythmus in canine one-day-old myocardial infarction, *Circ. Res.*, 51, 152, 1982.
127. **Meerson, F. Z.,** Stress damage to nonischemic divisions of the heart in experimental infarction and its prevention, *Clin. Cardiol.*, 6, 163, 1983.
128. **Adelstein, R. S. and Sellers, J. R.,** Effects of calcium on vascular smooth muscle contraction, *Am. J. Cardiol.*, 59, 48, 1987.
129. **Feigl, E. O.,** Sympathetic control of coronary circulation, *Circ. Res.*, 37, 88, 1975.
130. **Hamilton, C. A. and Reid, J. L.,** α_1-Adrenoceptor desensitization, *Eur. J. Pharmacol.*, 152, 179, 1988.
131. **Simons, M. and Downing, S. E.,** Coronary vasoconstriction and catecholamine cardiomyopathy, *Am. Heart J.*, 109, 297, 1985.
132. **Rubanyi, G., Kalabay, L., Pataki, Yu., and Hajda, K.,** Nickel-induced vasoconstriction in the isolated canine coronary artery by a tonic Ca^{2+} activation mechanism, *Acta Physiol. Hung.*, 59, 155, 1982.
133. **Van Nueten, J. M. and Vanhoutte, P. M.,** Effect of the Ca^{2+} antagonist lidoflasine on normoxic and anoxic contraction of canine coronary artery smooth muscle, *Eur. J. Pharmacol.*, 64, 173, 1980.
134. **Furchgott, R. F. and Zawadzki, J. V.,** The obligatory role of endothelial cells in the relaxation of arterial smooth muscle by acetyl choline, *Nature,* 288, 373, 1980.
135. **Morcillio, E., Reid, P., and Dubin, N.,** Myocardial prostaglandin E release by nitroglycerin and modification by indomethacin, *Am. J. Cardiol.*, 45, 53, 1980.
136. **Rowe, G., Gastillo, C., and Crumptont, C.,** Effect of hyperventilation on systemic and coronary hemodynamics, *Am. Heart J.*, 63, 67, 1962.

137. **Fleckenstein, A., Nakayama, K., Fleckenstein-Grün, G., and Byon, J.,** Interaction of hydrogen ions, calcium antagonistic drugs with excitation-contraction coupling of vascular smooth muscle, in *Ionic Action on Vascular Smooth Muscle,* Betz, E., Ed., Springer-Verlag, Berlin, 1976, 117.
138. **Nowlin, J., Troyer, W., Collins, W., et al.,** The association of nocturnal angina pectoris with dreaming, *Ann. Intern. Med.,* 63, 1040, 1965.
139. **Groves, B., Marcus, F., Ewy, G., and Phibbs, B.,** Coronary arterial spasm in variant angina pectoris produced by hyperventilation and valsava — documented by coronary arteriography, in *Coronary Artery Medicine and Surgery,* Horman, J. C., Ed., Appleton-Century-Crofts, New York, 1975, 311.
140. **Haft, J., Fain, R., and Levitas, L.,** Intravascular platelet aggregation in the heart induced by stress, *Circulation,* 47, 353, 1973.
141. **Ellis, E., Oelz, O., and Roberts, L.,** Coronary arterial smooth muscle contraction by a substance released from platelets evidence that it is thromboxane A_2, *Science,* 193, 1135, 1976.
142. **Ginsburg, R., Bristow, M. R., Davis, K., Dibiase, A., and Billingham, M. F.,** Quantitative pharmacologic responses of normal and atherosclerotic isolated human epicardial coronary arteries, *Circulation,* 69, 430, 1984.
143. **Folts, J., Crowell, E., and Rowe, G.,** Platelet aggregation in partially obstructed vessels and its elimination with aspirin, *Circulation,* 54, 365, 1976.
144. **Tada, M., Ezumi, K., and Yamagushi, M.,** Reduction of prostacyclin synthesis as a possible cause of transient flow reduction in partially constricted canine coronary artery, *J. Mol. Cell. Cardiol.,* 16, 1137, 1984.
145. **Matsievskii, D. D.,** Telemetric measurement of blood flow with ultrasound (in Russian), *Byull. Eksp. Biol. Med.,* 9, 119, 1970.
146. **Verrier, R. L., Hagestad, E. L., and Lown, B.,** Behaviorally induced coronary vasoconstriction in dogs with critical coronary artery stenosis, *Fed. Proc. Fed. Am. Soc. Exp. Biol.,* 43, 1003, 1984.
147. **Meerson, F. Z.,** *The Failing Heart: Adaptation and Deadaptation,* Raven Press, New York, 1983.
148. **Millard, R. W.,** Induction of the functional coronary collaterals in the swine heart, *Basic Res. Cardiol.,* 76, 468, 1981.
149. **Meerson, F. Z.,** *The General Mechanism of Adaptation and Prophylaxis* (in Russian), Nauka, Moscow, 1973.
150. **Manukhina, E. B.,** The portal vein and its contractile function in norm and pathology (in Russian), *Usp. Fiziol. Nauk,* 3, 45, 1988.
151. **Meerson, F. Z., Manukhina, E. B., Lapshin, A. V., and Ustinova, E. E.,** Relation of the endothelium-dependent relaxation of aorta and the arterial pressure in myocardial infarction in the rat (in Russian), *Byull. Eksp. Biol. Med.,* 7, 21, 1989.
152. **Meerson, F. Z.,** *Adaptation, Stress and Prophylaxis,* Springer-Verlag, Berlin, 1984.
153. **Katz, A. M. and Maxwell, J. B.,** Actin from heart muscle: sulfhydryl groups, *Circ. Res.,* 14, 345, 1964.
154. **Hinghofer-Szalkay, H., Kenner, T., and Estelberger, W.,** Special analysis of spontaneous contraction of the isolated portal vein of rat, *Pfluegers Arch.,* 364, 157, 1976.
155. **Sreeharan, N., Yayakody, R. L., Senerathe, M. P. J., Thomson, A. B. R., and Kappagoda, C. T.,** Endothelium-dependent relaxation and experimental atherosclerosis in the rabbit aorta, *Can. J. Pharm.,* 604, 1451, 1986.
156. **Lockette, W., Otsuka, Y., and Carretero, O.,** The loss of endothelium-dependent relaxation in hypertension, *Hypertension,* 8, 61, 1986.
157. **Makhmudov, R. M., Mamedov, Ya. D., Dolgov, V. V., and Repin, V. S.,** Quantitative evaluation by scanning electron microscopy of endothelial lesion in rabbit aorta perfused with catecholamines (in Russian), *Cor Vasa,* 27, 456, 1985.
158. **De Mey, J. G. and Vanhoutte, P. M.,** Anoxia and endothelium dependent reactivity of the canine femoral artery, *J. Physiol.,* 335, 65, 1983.
159. **Vanhoutte, P. M.,** Could the absence or malfunction of vascular endothelium precipitate the occurrence of vasospasm?, *J. Mol. Cell. Cardiol.,* 18, 679, 1986.
160. **Fleckenstein-Grun, G.,** Role of transmembrane Ca^{2+} supply in phasic and tonic activation of vascular smooth muscle, vasodilatation efficacy of calcium antagonists, in *Membranes and Muscle,* Proc. Int. Symp., Berman, M. C., Gevers, W., and Opie, L., Eds., IRL Press, Oxford, 1985, 6, 235.
161. **Furchgott, R. F.,** Role of endothelium in responses of vascular smooth muscle, *Circ. Res.,* 53, 557, 1983.
162. **Malta, E., Schini, V., and Miller, R. C.,** Effect of endothelium on basal and α-adrenoceptor stimulated calcium fluxes in rat aorta, *Naunyn-Schmiedebergs Arch. Pharmacol.,* 334, 63, 1986.
163. **Webb, R. C., Vander, A. J., and Henry, J. P.,** Increased vasodilator responses to acetylcholine in psychological hypertensive mice, *Hypertension,* 9, 268, 1987.
164. **Rubanyi, G. M. and Vanhoutte, P. M.,** Oxygen-derived free radicals, endothelium and responsiveness of vascular smooth muscle, *Am. J. Physiol.,* 250, H815, 1986.

165. **Mullane, K. M. and Pinto, A.,** Endothelium, arachidonic acid, and coronary vascular tone, *Fed. Proc. Fed. Am. Soc. Exp. Biol.*, 46, 54, 1987.
166. **Forstermann, U.,** Properties and mechanisms of production and action of endothelium-derived relaxing factor, *J. Cardiovasc. Pharmacol.*, 8 (Suppl. 10), S45, 1986.
167. **Wennmalm, A.,** Prostaglandin-mediated inhibition of noradrenaline release, *Prostaglandins*, 15, 113, 1978.
168. **Dutta, P., Jones, A. W., and Mustafa, S. J.,** Uptake and efflux of calcium by canine coronary arteries and the action of adenosine, *Basic Res. Cardiol.*, 79, 519, 1984.
169. **Fenton, R. A., Bruttig, S. P., Rubio, R., and Berne, R. M.,** Effect of adenosine on calcium uptake by intact and cultured vascular smooth muscle, *Am. J. Physiol.*, 242, H797, 1982.
170. **Lown, B., De Silva, R., Reich, P., and Murawski, B.,** Psychophysiologic factors in sudden cardiac death, *Am. J. Psychiatr.*, 137, 1325, 1980.
171. **Jenkins, C.,** The epidemiology of sudden cardiac death: incidence, clinical features, biomedical and psychological risk factors, in *Stress and Heart Disease*, Beamish, R. E., Singal, P. K., and Dhalla, N. S., Eds., Kluwer Academic, Boston, 1985, 17.
172. **Kuller, L. H., Talbott, E. O., and Robinson, C.,** Environmental and psychosocial determinants of sudden death, *Circulation*, 76, II, 177, 1987.
173. **Myerburg, R. F.,** Sudden cardiac death: epidemiology, causes and mechanisms, *Cardiology*, 74 (Suppl. 2), 2, 1987.
174. **Friedman, M., Manwaring, J., and Rosenman, R.,** Instantaneous and sudden death: clinical and pathological differentiation in coronary artery disease, *JAMA*, 224, 1319, 1973.
175. **Thomas, A. C., Davies, M. J., and Popple, A. W.,** A pathologist view of sudden cardiac death, *Dev. Cardiovasc. Med.*, 4, 34, 1980.
176. **Lie, J. T. and Titus, J. L.,** Pathology of the myocardium and the conduction system in sudden coronary death, *Circulation*, 52 (Suppl. 3), 41, 1975.
177. **Januscevičus, S. I. and Milasauskene, M. A.,** Recording cases of sudden out-of-hospital death of acute myocardial infarction and acute coronary failure, and its significance for improving control of ischemic disease (in Russian), *Kardiologiya*, 1, 22, 1976.
178. **Mazur, N. A. and Zhukov, V. N.,** Sudden death of acute coronary failure (in Russian), *Kardiologiya*, 1, 27, 1976.
179. **Östergaard, K.,** Heart-autopsy findings in cases of sudden death, *Acta Pathol. Microbiol. Scand.*, Sect. A, 86, 279, 1978.
180. **Alexandru, E. and Dobresku, G.,** Histochemical and histoenzymic researches in coronary sudden death, *Morphol. Embryol.*, 24, 229, 1978.
181. **Enos, W. F., Holmes, R. H., and Beuer, J.,** Coronary disease among U.S. soldiers killed in action in Korea, *JAMA*, 152, 1090, 1953.
182. **Myers, A. and Dewar, H. A.,** Circumstances attending 100 sudden deaths from coronary artery disease with coroner's necropsies, *Br. Heart J.*, 37, 1133, 1975.
183. **Rose, G. and Marmot, M. G.,** Social class and coronary heart disease, *Br. Heart J.*, 45, 13, 1981.
184. **Meerson, F. Z., Malyshev, V. V., Manukhina, E. B., and Petrova, V. A.,** Effect of stress and the antioxidant ionol on catecholamine biosynthesis and dopamine content in the heart and adrenal glands (in Russian), *Byull. Eksp. Biol. Med.*, 12, 663, 1987.
185. **Ungerstedt, U.,** Stereotaxic mapping of the monoamine pathways in the rat brain, *Acta Physiol. Scand.*, Suppl. 367, 1, 1971.
186. **Lindvall, O. and Björklund, A.,** The organization of the descending catecholamine neuron systems in the rat brain as revealed by the glyoxylic acid fluorescence method, *Acta Physiol. Scand.*, Suppl. 412, 48, 1974.
187. **Doda, M. and Gyorgy, L.,** Dopaminergic inhibition of sympathetic activity in the cat, *Pol. J. Pharmacol.*, 37, 397, 1985.
188. **Varfolomeev, S. O.,** *Physiology and Biochemistry of Mediator Processes* (in Russian), 1, 58, 1985.
189. **Hernandez, D. E., Adcock, J. W., Stanley, D. A., and Prange, A. J.,** Involvement of dopamine in stress gastric ulceration, *Dig. Dis. Sci.*, 30, 380, 1985.
190. **Meerson, F. Z. and Kapel'ko, V. I.,** Role of interconnection between cardiac muscle contractile function intensity and relaxation velocity and heart adaptation to high load (in Russian), *Kardiologiya*, 7, 43, 1974.
191. **Anichkov, N. N.,** Main results of studies carried out at the Department of Pathological Anatomy, Institute of Experimental Medicine (AMS USSR) on the problem of atherosclerosis (in Russian), *Vestn. Akad. Med. Nauk SSSR*, 11, 29, 1961.

Chapter 3

ADAPTATION TO STRESS AND ITS CARDIOPROTECTIVE EFFECT IN STRESS, ISCHEMIC, AND REPERFUSION DAMAGE

I. INTRODUCTION

Adaptation to stress is a state achieved as a result of repeated exposure to moderate stress, and manifests itself in that a hopeless emotiogenic situation or other strong stress factors (that before impaired the animal or human behavior and caused real damage to the organism) lose their destructive effects. In this chapter we shall consecutively consider the very phenomenon of adaptation and its neuroendocrine mechanisms, the adaptive protection from cardiac stress damage, and finally, the chief place will be occupied by the cardioprotective influence of adaptation in ischemic and reperfusion damages, infarction, and postinfarction cardiosclerosis, with the main attention being paid to its antiarrhythmic effect.

II. ADAPTATION TO STRESS AND ITS MAIN NEUROHUMORAL MECHANISMS

The process of adaptation to stress situations has for millenia been empirically used in training for military and other occupations requiring stability in extreme situations, i.e., maintaining an expedient behavioral stereotype despite imminent hazards. Yet as a scientific problem adaptation to stress became a subject of study only about 25 to 30 years ago.

To date, reiteration of brief nondamaging stress exposures has been shown to enhance the organismic resistance to severe stress exposures and to prevent stress damage to the heart and other organs. Thus, prior adaptation of rats to stress efficiently prevents or restricts the disturbances caused by heavy stress to myocardial structure, contractile function, metabolism,[1-3] and cardiac electric stability, as well as the arrhythmogenic effect of stress.[4,5] It also prevents gastric stress ulceration, impairment of portal vein contractility,[6] stress anorexia,[7] the oncogenic effect of stress,[8] and mortality from severe electric-pain exposures.[9] Adaptation to stress has also proved to enhance the organismic resistance not only to stress, but also to a broad spectrum of other detrimental factors. It prevents or restricts the ischemic and reperfusion damage to cardiac contractility and electric stability (i.e., it is an antiarrhythmic factor which we shall further consider in more detail) as well as direct chemical injury to internal organs[10] and radiation injury,[11] enhances cold tolerance,[12] etc.

It can be thought that the protective action of adaptation is underlain by neurohormonal and cellular regulatory changes developing in the organism with repeated exposures to stress, and (1) restricting the intensity and duration of the stress reaction itself and (2) enhancing the resistance of the target organs to stress hormones and mediators.

Indeed, in response to heavy stress the adapted animals develop either no or only minor stress reaction. This has been convincingly proved for the major links of the stress reaction: the adrenergic and the hypophysial-adrenal ones.[3,13,14] In rats adapted to brief emotional pain stress (EPS), a severe 6-h EPS did not change the corticosterone levels in the adrenal glands and plasma, whereas in nonadapted animals they increased twofold to threefold.[3]

Besides, such adaptation significantly attenuated the catecholamine "discharge" into the blood and completely prevented the decline of epinephrine in the adrenal glands and norepinephrine in the heart consistently observed under stress in nonadapted animals.[3,15]

Adaptation to stress also restricts the duration of the stress reaction as evidenced by the shorter poststress eosinopenia,[3] which is directly associated with the blood level of corticosteroids.

Thus, adaptation to stress results in abatement of the stress reaction. What are the mechanisms of this phenomenon? A natural suggestion is that in the course of adaptation the stress-effecting systems become less powerful, whereby the stress reaction to the detrimental factor proves weaker. Diverse experimental studies have shown that this is not so. On the contrary, adaptation turned out to enhance the potential capacity of the stress-effecting systems. This first of all applies to the leading stress-effecting system, the sympathoadrenal one, and has been convincingly proved for catecholamine biosynthesis in the adrenal glands in adaptation to immobilization stress, in the classical work of Kvetnansky et al.[16] During such adaptation, enhanced adrenal secretion of catecholamines was accompanied by a more than threefold increase in adrenal tyrosine hydroxylase activity within the first week of daily immobilization episodes. Further on, repeated stress exposures for 6 weeks did not alter this index: a high plateau of enzyme activity and catecholamine synthesis has been established, ensuring stable adrenal hyperfunction. After the end of adaptation the enzyme activity returned to normal within 2 weeks. It is essential that the increased tyrosine hydroxylase activity corresponds to the enhanced catecholamine content in the adrenal glands. Therefore, adaptation augments the physiological resources of this important stress-effecting organ. It is also noteworthy that such adaptation is associated with increased potential ability of the brain adrenergic centers to synthesize and release catecholamines.[17] Thus, adaptation to stress is attended by generalized enhancement of the physiological power of the stress-effecting adrenergic system.

It further turned out that the lack of blood corticosteroid elevation in response to heavy stress in adapted animals, i.e., "fading" of the adrenocortical link of the stress reaction, also does not result from exhaustion of the functional resources of the adrenal cortex. On the opposite, injected ACTH causes a much greater elevation of blood corticosterone in stress-adapted than in nonadapted animals.[18] This is important evidence that adaptation involves (1) increased power of the adrenocortical link of the stress-effecting sympathoadrenal system and (2) altered organismic reaction to stress at the central level, i.e., at the level of releasing factors and ACTH. It is at this level that some mechanisms are actuated by adaptation and, despite the stress, hinder the output of releasing factors and tropic hormones, and prevent increased secretion of stress hormones and mediators (in this case corticosterone).

Study of the adaptation to stress also revealed that the abatement of the stress reaction in adapted animals combines with a peculiar decline in the sensitivity of the target organs to stress mediators and hormones: a phenomenon of desensitization. In recent years this has been demonstrated as a decreased number of β-adrenoreceptors and lower catecholamine sensitivity of the adenylate cyclase system the brain and peripheral tissues,[5] and as a decreased number of cytoplasmic receptors for corticosteroids in cardiomyocytes.[19] The decreased number and efficiency of adrenoreceptors appears to be an essential element of enhanced resistance of executive organs to stress damage.

On the whole, *there are three main features characteristic of adaptation to stress: (1) increased power of the stress-effecting systems; (2) smaller extent of their activation, i.e., fading of the stress reaction; (3) enhanced resistance of executive organs and tissues to stress hormones and mediators, an important place in which is occupied by receptor desensitization.* Hence adaptation gives rise to a paradoxical situation: despite the increased potential of the stress-effecting systems, the stress reaction either does not occur at all or is substantially attenuated.

There are further two essential particulars of adaptation to stress situations. First, the process takes place under conditions when no way out of the situation can be found by external behavioral adaptation, and represents a kind of internal adaptation to an apparently hopeless situation — a probable physiological equivalent of what in common parlance is called patience or endurance. Second, checked excitation of the stress-effecting systems (i.e., reduced concentrations of catecholamines acting on the target organs) combines with desensitization to diminish the stress damage to internal organs. A concept thus emerges that some mechanisms inhibiting the stress-effecting systems in repeated or protracted stress situations are the mechanisms of endurance and of natural prophylaxis of stress damage.

Several years ago we put forward a hypothesis[20] that an *essential element of adaptation to environmental stress is activation of central regulatory mechanisms that, during the action of emotional pain or like stimuli, hinder the output of releasing factors and thereby of-catecholamines and corticosterone. In the brain, certain neuronal systems synthesize and release mediators: GABA, dopamine, serotonin, glycine, opioid, and other peptides, which interact with the stress-effecting systems to modulate their activity; they can be thought to restrict the stress reaction. No less important regulatory systems — adenine nucleotides, prostaglandins, and antioxidants — operate at the periphery to control the effects of catecholamines and other stress factors and thereby to prevent stress damage.*

We have designated these central and peripheral mechanisms as stress-limiting modulatory systems.

The function of the stress-limiting systems can be supposed to have become coupled in the course of evolution to the function of the stress-effecting systems, and accordingly their functional capacity should be augmented in the repetitive exposures to stress. This restricts the stress reaction and provides for the protective effects of adaptation to stress, which can as well include protection from diverse environmental factors whose action can be blocked by the metabolites of the stress-limiting systems.

This concept was the basis of using adaptation to brief stress exposures, or metabolites of the stress-limiting systems, for prevention and experimental therapy of not only stress damages, but also diseases in which stress is pathogenetically important.

To assess the validity of this approach and of the very concept of the stress-limiting systems, we shall further consider some facts characterizing the state of these systems in the stress reaction and their adaptation role.

1. *The stress reaction is consistently coupled with activation of biosynthesis and release into the blood of the metabolites of central and peripheral stress-limiting systems.* Thus, in acute stress beta-endorphin and ACTH are discharged into the blood from the pituitary body in equimolar amounts.[21,22] It is essential that such coupling between the stress-effecting and the opioidergic systems is quite tight, since it is genetically determined by ACTH and beta-endorphin being synthesized in the pituitary cells as a common polypeptide precursor, the pro-opiocortin comprising, besides ACTH, alpha-, beta-, and gamma-melanotropins as well as beta-lipotropin. As a result, in response to the hypothalamic corticotropin-releasing factor there is a concomitant release of ACTH and beta-endorphin from the anterior pituitary into the blood. The second stage of coupling takes place at the regulatory level and consists in that corticosterone produced in response to ACTH suppresses, through the negative feedback mechanism, the pituitary synthesis of ACTH and endorphins.[21-23]

The significance of the coupled mobilization of the opioid peptide system in activation of the stress-effecting systems will be later considered in fuller detail. Here it would suffice to say that opioid peptides are intimately linked functionally both with the stress-effecting adrenergic system and with the stress-limiting serotonergic and dopaminergic systems, and modulate them all: specifically, opioid peptides restrict the effects of adrenergic activation and potentiate the effects of the serotonergic system.

Activation of the peripheral stress-limiting systems is also coupled to the stress reaction; this has been most comprehensively studied for prostaglandins which control the adrenergic effect at the level of target organs (see Chapter 5).

Thus, the coupling of the stress-effecting and the stress-limiting systems is indeed a general mechanism of the timely restriction of the stress reaction.

2. *Adaptation to repeated stress episodes is attended by enhanced biosynthesis and accumulation of the stress-limiting metabolites in certain brain regions and on the periphery.*

Thus, in adaptation to short immobilization episodes the content of leu- and met-enkephalins and beta-endorphin in the structures of the striate body and hypothalamus rises by 70 to 100%, and the adrenal content of leu- and met-enkephalins increases 2 to 2.5 times on average.[24] Similarly, the hypothalamic content of met-enkephalin in the course of electroconvulsive treatment rises by about 60%, the maximum coinciding in time with the evolvement of the antidepressive effect of electroconvulsive therapy.[25]

At present, data are available that show that adaptation to repeated stress is accompanied by enhanced levels of and synthetic capacity for serotonin and dopamine in some structures of the hypothalamus, the midbrain, and the medulla oblongata.[26,27]

It is yet difficult to fully appreciate the significance of such adaptive shifts since the specific interlinks between the regulatory systems are not yet clear enough. However, some facets are already conceivable. In particular, elevated dopamine appears to be important for the protective effect of adaptation, since stimulation of the presynaptic dopaminergic receptors on the sympathetic terminals suppresses norepinephrine release and thereby restricts the adrenergic effects of the stress reaction, e.g., prevents stress gastric ulceration and causes hypotension and bradycardia.[28] It is also known that at the brain level norepinephrine and dopamine act as a stimulator and an inhibitor, respectively, of ACTH secretion, especially in the amygdaloid central nucleus and anterior and lateral hypothalamus.[29] This favors a suggestion that elevated dopamine should restrict such a component of the stress reaction as the output of the corticotropin-releasing factor.

On the whole, a picture gradually emerging is one of *coordinated steady-state activation of the central stress-limiting systems in adaptation to stress with a resulting protective effect.*

3. *Adaptation to stressful situations has been shown to involve increased activity of the stress-limiting systems directly protecting the cell membranes from stress-induced and other damages.* An example is the increase in the activity of antioxidant enzymes, catalase and superoxide dismutase (SOD), in the myocardium by 38 and 16%, respectively.[30] Accordingly, the resistance of spontaneously contracting isolated auricles to the arrhythmogenic action of a chemical inducer of free-radical oxidation, H_2O_2, proves to be twofold to threefold greater in adapted animals.[31] Likewise, adaptation to a permanent minimal restraint gradually, in 7 d, results in a threefold activation of prostaglandin synthesis in the fundus of the rat stomach. Thereupon, concentrated solutions of ethanol, mannitol, or hydrochloric acid, which, on direct contact used to injure about 95% of the mucosal surface, practically lose their detrimental effect. This protective action of adaptation is completely abolished by an inhibitor of prostaglandin synthesis, indomethacin.[10]

Thus, there are grounds for speaking about the adaptive enhancement of the efficiency of direct cytoprotective action of the stress-limiting systems operating at the level of executive organs, which are highly likely to attenuate the adrenoreactivity and responsiveness to corticosteroids and to be thus involved in the desensitization mechanism.

4. *Metabolites and activators of the stress-limiting systems, viz regulatory peptides, GHBA, prostaglandins, antioxidants, as well as synthetic analogs of these compounds, successfully prevent stress damage to internal organs, i.e., act like adaptation to stress.*

Studies in our laboratory have shown that administration of beta-endorphin, GHBA, delta-peptide and its cyclic derivative, and natural and synthetic antioxidants consistently prevent stress damage to the heart, stomach, and brain, as well as stress depression of some important links of antitumor immunity.[32] In other words, the listed chemical agents act similarly to prior adaptation to repeated stress situations.

This implies that studying the central and peripheral mechanisms limiting the stress reaction and involved in adaptation to stress is not only theoretically important, but also allows the stress-limiting metabolites and their synthetic analogs to be used to prevent and abolish stress disorders as well as noninfectious diseases in which stress plays a pathogenetic role.

Accordingly, we shall first consider the cardioprotective effects of adaptation to stress, and then the opportunities of pharmacological heart protection with metabolites of the stress-limiting systems.

III. ADAPTIVE PROTECTION OF THE HEART FROM STRESS DAMAGE AND ATHEROGENIC DYSLIPIDEMIA

Our first work on prevention of stress damage to the myocardial contractile function[33] has shown that the disturbances of right atrial extensibility and contractility upon emotional pain stress (described in detail in Chapter 1) are preventable with a course of adaptation to brief immobilization stresses imposed by fixing the animals in the supine position for 15 min to 1 h daily.

Curves in Figure 1 demonstrate the dynamics of contractility during atrial stretching. It can be seen that by itself the adaptation achieved with not very numerous spaced stress episodes does not at all depress the myocardial contractility parameters; on the contrary, for adapted animals the curves of extensibility, developed tension, and the Starling curves lie somewhat higher than the control ones.

As in previous studies,[34] stress causes depression of myocardial extensibility, its peculiar rigidity (Figure 1A), depression of developed tension (Figure 1B), and marked depression of the Starling curve (Figure 1C). Prior adaptation counteracted this complex of disturbances to the atrial contractile function (its effect is denoted by the shaded zone in the figures), as well as the stress-induced decline in the integrative index of the myocardial contractile function — IFS (i.e., specific work per unit myocardial mass).

Thus, a rationally dosed adaptation to stress allows complete prevention of the depression of myocardial contractility in prolonged stress.

Further studies[35] showed that the same holds true for the ventricles of the isolated heart. Thus, a work with isometrically contracting hearts from control, adapted, and stressed animals was carried out according to Fallen et al.[36] and included, besides measuring the left ventricular developed and diastolic pressure, determination of the diastolic defect — an integrative index of impairment of diastolic relaxation (calculated as the integral diastolic pressure over the time when it exceeded the zero line.)

As known from our previous experiments,[20] the diastolic defect increases with increasing Ca^{2+} concentration in the perfusing liquid, increasing contraction frequency, and decreasing temperature which hinders the action of the cation pumps. In other words, this index in great measure depends on the membrane mechanisms of calcium transport.

Table 1 demonstrates that in hearts isolated from animals that had undergone immobilization stress, at stimulation frequencies of 120 and 300 min^{-1} there was a reduction in developed pressure (43 and 50 mmHg vs. respectively 80 and 97 mmHg in the controls). To the imposed rate of 300 min^{-1} these hearts responded by incomplete relaxation — the diastolic defect not observed in the control. The poststress hearts could not adopt a higher contraction rate.

Adaptation to repeated brief stress exposures did not itself affect the contractile function, but prevented the above defects in the hearts of animals subjected to stress after adaptation.

Thus, adaptation to brief stress episodes prevents the stress-induced depression of ventricular contractility and the diastolic defect which is a manifestation of impaired mechanisms of calcium homeostasis in the cardiac muscle.

This latter fact was the first to lead us to a suggestion confirmed in further studies that adaptation to stress somehow enhances the function of the cell mechanisms for calcium transport in the heart (see Chapter 6).

Hence it becomes understandable that prior adaptation to stress also prevented the main stress disturbances of the cardiac electric stability such as lowering of the fibrillation threshold

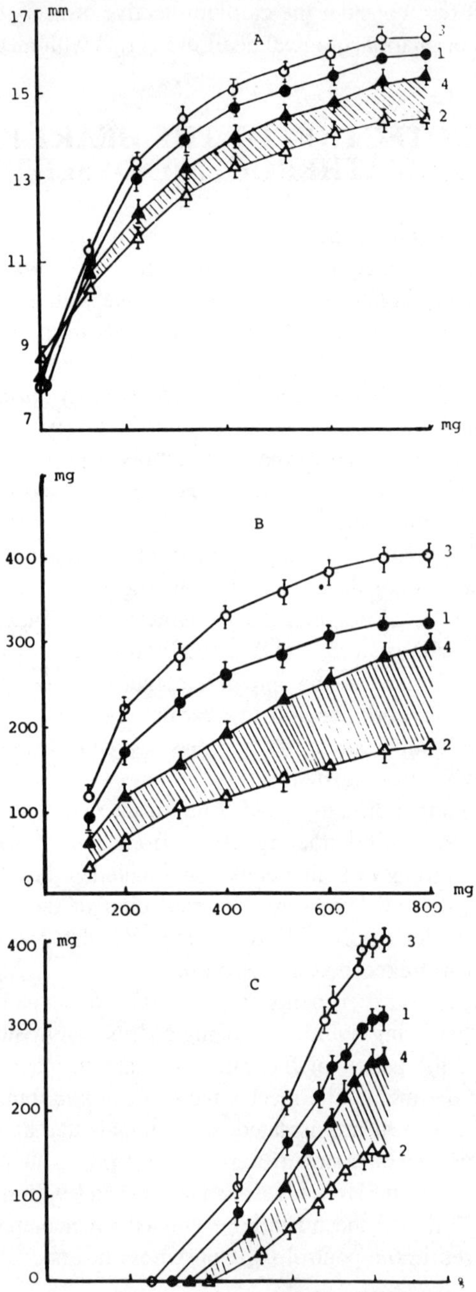

FIGURE 1. Effect of prior adaptation to short stresses on (A) extensibility, (B) developed tension, and (C) Starling curve of rat right auricle in prolonged stress. The abscissae are (A,B) load at rest, mg; (C) atrial length, percent of L_{max}. The ordinates are (A) atrial length, mm; (B,C) developed tension, mg. (1) Control, (2) stress, (3) adaptation, (4) adaptation plus stress.

and decreasing resistance of the sinus node to the impeding influence of the vagus nerve. The data presented in Table 2 and Figure 2 depict the results of these experiments. Table 2 shows that the marked fall in the fibrillation threshold caused by a 10-h immobilization stress is completely prevented with prior adaptation. The protective effect of adaptation is also clearly observed in respect of the vagal inhibition of the heart automatism (Figure 2).

TABLE 1
Impairment of Myocardial Contractile Function After Immobilization Stress at Different Imposed Contraction Frequencies

		Contraction frequency (min^{-1})			
Indices	**Series**	**120**	**300**	**400**	**500**
Developed pressure	Control	80 ± 2.5	97 ± 3.8	115 ± 4.5	106 ± 3.9
	Stress	43 ± 1.6	50 ± 2.5	—	—
	Adaptation	85 ± 3.1	105 ± 4.8	98 ± 4.0	90 ± 3.2
	Adaptation + stress	78 ± 2.6	108 ± 4.5	103 ± 4.2	73 ± 1.9
	p_{1-2}	<0.001	<0.001		
	p_{2-4}	<0.001	<0.001		
Diastolic defect	Control	0	0	26.5 ± 2.3	53.2 ± 3.7
	Stress	0	18.6 ± 1.9	—	—
	Adaptation	0	0	31.2 ± 3.0	59.6 ± 4.0
	Adaptation + stress	0	0	36.0 ± 2.8	63.8 ± 5.2
Diastolic pressure	Control	4.3 ± 0.40	±	6.9 ± 0.53	12.2 ± 1.03
	Stress	4.8 ± 0.32	8.1 ± 0.55	—	—
	Adaptation	6.1 ± 0.55	4.5 ± 0.33	11.7 ± 0.87	19.3 ± 1.07
	Adaptation + stress	5.8 ± 0.44	3.9 ± 0.24	11.1 ± 0.75	26.8 ± 1.56
	p_{1-2}	>0.05	<0.001		
	p_{2-4}	>0.05	<0.001		

TABLE 2
Effect of Prior Adaptation to Short Stress Exposures on the Fibrillation Threshold After Prolonged Stress

Series	**Heart rate (min^{-1})**	**Ventricular fibrillation threshold (mA)**
Control (n = 12)	445 ± 7	7.4 ± 0.3
Stress (n = 10)	446 ± 8	3.8 ± 0.2[a]
Adaptation (n = 12)	436 ± 8	7.9 ± 0.7
Adaptation + stress (n = 12)	443 ± 8	7.9 ± 0.5

[a] $p < 0.01$ compared to the control.

Thus, upon stimulation of the vagus nerve with a triple-threshold current the heart rate in control animals drops over twofold. The negative chronotropic effect of the vagus nerve is significantly enhanced upon prolonged stress: 12 h after, the contraction rate drops by a factor of 3.3. Adaptation itself markedly attenuates the negative vagal effect, the heart rate decreasing only by 25%, and thereby fully compensates for its poststress enhancement so that the heart rate in adapted animals subjected to stress drops not more than in the control. Thus, *gradual and not very long adaptation to brief stress episodes preventing stress disturbances of the cardiac function also abolishes the poststress decline in the cardiac fibrillation threshold and counteracts the poststress decrease in the resistance of sinus node automatism to vagal inhibition.*

The cardioprotective effect of adaptation, initially proved for the stress disorders in the cardiac contractile function and electric stability, soon got a direct explanation in that adaptation was found to prevent the complex of metabolic and structural alterations described in detail in Chapter 1 of this book under the term of primary cardiac stress damage.

The data of our work[35] presented in Table 3 show the release of enzymes from the isolated hearts into the perfusate, and demonstrate that though the adaptation itself tends to increase somewhat the release of myocardial enzymes, nevertheless with a high degree of reliability it attenuates the marked (twofold to threefold) enhancement of their leakage

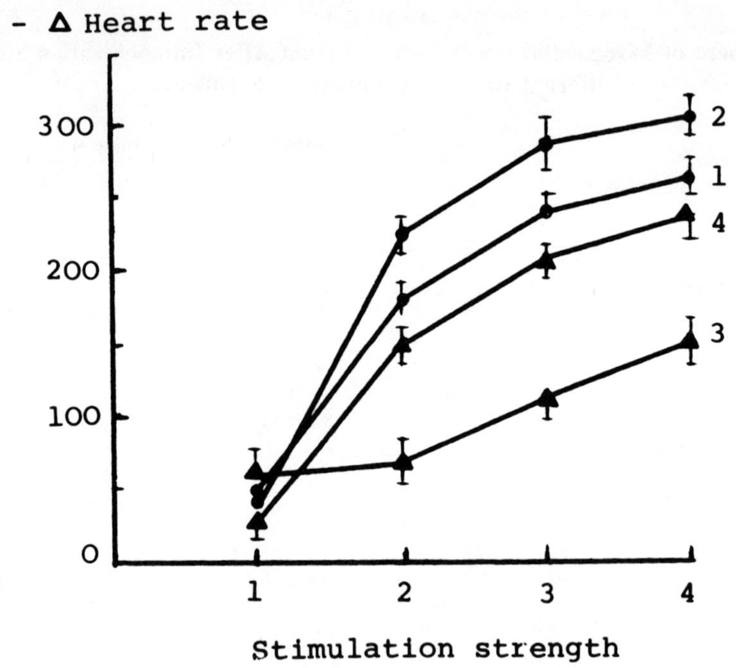

FIGURE 2. Effect of prior adaptation to short stress exposures on the negative chronotropic effect of vagal stimulation. The abscissa is strength of vagal stimulation, multiples of threshold current. The ordinate is the decrease in heart rate, min^{-1}. (1) Control, (2) stress, (3) adaptation, (4) adaptation plus stress.

TABLE 3
Effect of Stress and Adaptation on Enzyme Activity in the Perfusate of Isolated Rat Hearts (U/h·g myocardium)

Series	AST[a]	MDH[b]	LDH[c]	RNase
Control	18.9 ± 1.38	1.53 ± 0.12	10.2 ± 1.02	1279 ± 132
Stress	52.9 ± 4.97	4.32 ± 0.40	22.5 ± 1.78	4043 ± 312
Adaptation	25.7 ± 2.95	1.88 ± 0.20	12.5 ± 1.07	1582 ± 122
Adaptation + stress	35.2 ± 3.17	2.25 ± 0.23	14.7 ± 1.22	2182 ± 163
$p_{1\text{-}2}$	<0.001	<0.001	<0.001	<0.001
$p_{1\text{-}4}$	<0.001	<0.05	<0.05	<0.05
$p_{2\text{-}4}$	<0.01	<0.001	<0.001	<0.001

[a] Aspartate transaminase.
[b] Malate dehydrogenase.
[c] Lactate dehydrogenase.

induced by stress. This prompts an idea that adaptation somehow stabilizes the plasma membrane, diminishing its injury in stress. In full conformity with this are the data of Table 4, obtained with hearts instantly transferred into liquid nitrogen from adapted and nonadapted animals that had undergone stress.

Table 4 shows that the stress-induced activation of lipid peroxidation, described earlier and manifesting itself as a threefold rise in the myocardial content of hydroperoxides and Schiff bases, is largely prevented by adaptation; the same holds true for mobilization of glycogen store typical of stress.

Notably, the cardioprotective effect of adaptation turned out to be not an exclusive

TABLE 4
Effect of Immobilization Stress and Adaptation to Short Stress Exposures on Glycogen Content and Lipid Peroxidation in Rat Hearts

Series	Glycogen (mg/100 g tissue)	Lipid hydroperoxides (nmol/mg lipid)	Schiff bases (U/mg lipid)
Control	548 ± 53	5.1 ± 0.33	3.69 ± 0.19
Stress	317 ± 29	18.9 ± 1.22	9.72 ± 0.75
Adaptation	450 ± 36	6.7 ± 0.81	4.53 ± 0.40
Adaptation + stress	412 ± 32	7.4 ± 0.89	4.86 ± 0.33
p_{1-2}	<0.001	<0.001	<0.001
p_{1-4}	<0.05	<0.05	<0.02
p_{2-4}	<0.02	<0.001	<0.001

feature of immobilization stress, but was also fully reproducible in adaptation to short emotional pain episodes, which gave protection from prolonged (6-h) EPS.

Thus in our study with Malyshev and Lifant'ev we adapted the animals to short episodes of EPS (the anxiety neurosis model according to Desiderato described in Chapter 1; 12 seanccs of 40 min each every other day) and then subjected the adapted and nonadapted animals to a 6-h EPS. As already indicated in Chapter 1, upon such stress exposure the maximal disturbances of the main parameters of myocardial energy metabolism develop 45 h later.

Table 5 unambiguously demonstrates that, as in earlier experiments, EPS deeply impaired mitochondrial oxidation and oxidative phosphorylation with the NAD-linked substrate glutamate. Adaptation completely prevented these alterations as well as the stress-induced decline in myocardial glycogen. In the same work it was also found that adaptation prevented the microfocal myofibrillar contractural injury typical of stress, and accumulation of technetium pyrophosphate usually observed in poststress myocardium.

Further studies demonstrated that besides the heart this adaptational protection encompasses other internal organs including the liver, whose stress-induced deterioration has been explicitly shown (Chapter 1) to be decisive in atherogenic dyslipidemia. Table 6 shows that gradual adaptation to brief immobilization stresses, while not affecting the overall plasma cholesterol content, at the same time prevents or substantially attenuates the stress-induced dyslipidemia: 2 h after stress the atherogenicity index in adapted animals remains at the control value, and after 1 d its rise is only half that in nonadapted animals. Hence the adaptation naturally coupled with activation of the organismic stress-limiting systems is really protective against stress atherogenic dyslipidemia.

In considering this pronounced protective effect of adaptation, it was important to elucidate which particular stress-limiting systems play the main part in it. Since activated lipid peroxidation in vital organs is known to be a chief pathogenetic link of stress damage (Chapter 1), we supposed that a prominent role in the antistress effect of adaptation is played by the antioxidant systems. Therefore, instead of adaptation we tried to prevent stress dyslipidemia with the antioxidant ionol (butylated hydroxytoluene), which was administered at 20 mg/kg daily for 3 d before stress. As evident in Table 6, prior administration of ionol produces approximately the same preventive effect as prior adaptation to stress.

The significance of these results is underscored by the fact that they are quite in line with the recent data[37] obtained in a survey of an organized contingent of young persons that had experienced a complex of such stressful influences as separation from the family, breaking the life stereotypes, entering a new community, and physical work. Therewith these people developed pronounced atherogenic dyslipidemia as manifest by increased low-density lipoprotein cholesterol and atherogenicity index; only 3 months later, upon prolonged adaptation to stress situations, these phenomena gradually wore off.

TABLE 5
Effect of Emotional Pain Stress (EPS) on Oxidative Phosphorylation of Cardiac Mitochondria and Myocardial Glycogen Content in Rats Not Adapted and Optimally Adapted to Stress

	Respiration and phosphorylation indices				
Series (n = 12 each)	**O / t**	**RC**	**ADP / O**	**ADP / t**	**Glycogen content (m*M*)**
Control	253 ± 23	2.86 ± 0.2	1.95 ± 0.1	522 ± 41	5.5 ± 0.26
Adaptation	269 ± 21	3.17 ± 0.3	1.97 ± 0.2	532 ± 45	6.1 ± 0.41
EPS, 45 h after	162 ± 14[a]	1.70 ± 0.1[b]	1.30 ± 0.2[c]	276 ± 39[b]	2.1 ± 0.15[b]
Adaptation + EPS, 45 h after	254 ± 27	2.92 ± 0.3	1.94 ± 0.2	521 ± 42	6.0 ± 0.38

[a] $p < 0.01$.
[b] $P < 0.001$.
[c] $p < 0.05$.

TABLE 6
Effect of Emotional Pain Stress, Adaptation to Stress, and Antioxidant on Serum Lipids and Atherogenicity Index

	Cholesterol			
Series	**Total**	**HDLP[a]**	**Triglycerides**	**Atherogenicity index**
Control (n = 9)	70.8 ± 3.5	52.6 ± 2.8	52.8 ± 4.2	0.35
EPS, 2 h after (n = 10)	66.4 ± 2.0	43.6 ± 2.1	46.3 ± 2.7	0.52
EPS, 24 h after (n = 9)	58.6 ± 4.5	22.7 ± 1.7	40.8 ± 3.2	1.60
Adaptation (n = 9)	65.4 ± 6.8	48.4 ± 3.2	20.2 ± 3.4	0.35
Adaptation + EPS 2 h after (n = 8)	55.8 ± 6.2	42.7 ± 3.1	10.2 ± 1.4	0.30
Adaptation + EPS 24 h after (n = 8)	55.4 ± 5.6	32.7 ± 4.1	8.8 ± 1.0	0.70
Ionol (n = 8)	68.2 ± 5.8	50.2 ± 3.8	50.8 ± 6.9	0.36
Ionol + EPS, 2 h after (n = 9)	70.2 ± 4.0	50.4 ± 4.8	44.2 ± 6.1	0.39
Ionol + EPS, 24 h after (n = 8)	65.8 ± 1.3	34.7 ± 3.1	34.0 ± 5.6	0.80

[a] HDLP = High-density lipoproteins.

Thus, the stress dyslipidemia and its prevention with adaptation shown above are not just experimental observations, but natural events in humans, so the possibility of preventing such disorders with prior adaptation to stress or with synthetic antioxidants acquires much practical importance.

In full agreement with the above results, Table 7 shows that the changes characteristic of hepatic stress damage — accumulation of malonic dialdehyde (MDA), inactivation of SOD in the liver, and marked elevation of the specific hepatic enzyme fructose 1,6-diphosphate aldolase in the blood — are attenuated by prior adaptation to brief stresses or by ionol to about the same extent as the stress-induced dyslipidemia. It is interesting that by themselves (i.e., in nonstressed animals) both factors increase SOD activity in the liver and thereby create a certain "safety margin" against excessive lipid peroxidation and damage to the central organ of cholesterol metabolism. The latter fact is in line with our data obtained for peroxidation in liver homogenates induced with Fe^{2+}/ascorbate (Figure 3): MDA accumulation was substantially greater in preparations from poststress nonadapted animals, whereas prior adaptation as such markedly attenuated MDA formation and largely counter-

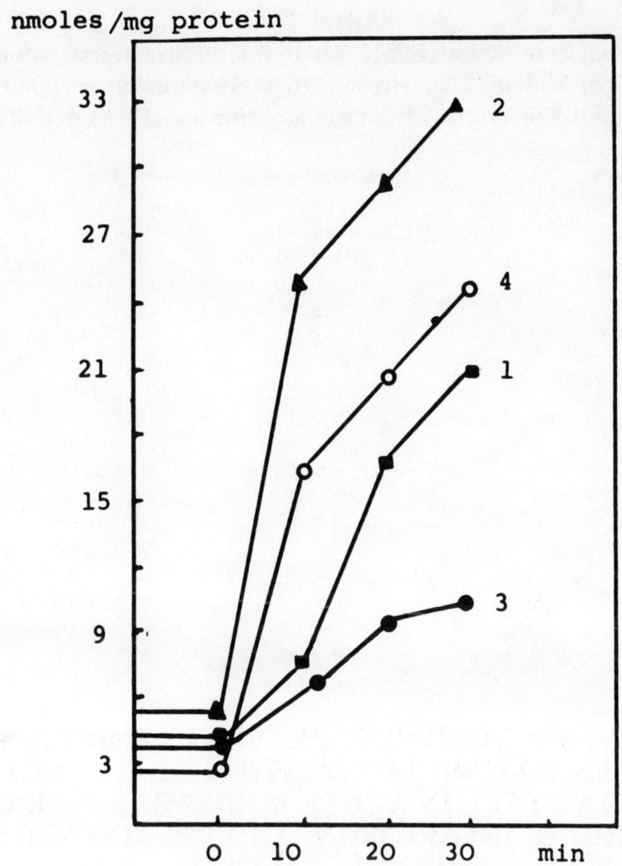

FIGURE 3. Effect of adaptation to short stresses and of prolonged EPS on induction of lipid peroxidation in liver with Fe/ascorbate. The abscissa is time after induction in minutes. The ordinate is malonic dialdehyde content in nanomoles per milligram protein. (1) Control, (2) EPS, (3) adaptation, (4) adaptation plus EPS.

acted the stress induction of peroxidation, most probably owing to enhanced activity of antioxidant systems.

Further, it was confirmed that hepatic stress damage involves inactivation of cholesterol 7-α-hydroxylase, and this is preventable with prior adaptation.

On the whole, adaptation to short stresses can prevent not only myocardial stress damage, but also hepatic stress damage and thereby atherogenic dyslipidemia, which is a weighty pathogenetic factor of coronary sclerosis and ischemic heart disease.

The importance of these data is determined by the fact that the stress reaction participates virtually in all pathogenetic links of ischemic disease (see Figure 8 in Chapter 2). Hence, adaptation that protects the organism from stress damage must also protect the heart from ischemic damage.

TABLE 7
Effect of Emotional Pain Stress (EPS), Adaptation to Stress, and Antioxidant on Hepatic Content of Malonic Dialdehyde (MDA), Hepatic Superoxide Dismutase (SOD) Activity, and Fructose 1,6-Diphosphate Aldolase (FDA) Activity in Blood

Series	MDA (nmol/g prot.)	SOD (U/g prot.)	FDA (U/ml)
Control N = 9	300 ± 30	64.6 ± 7.3	124 ± 80
EPS, 2 h after (n = 8)	640 ± 50	30.8 ± 2.0	316 ± 20
	$p_{1-2}<0.001$	$p_{1-2}<0.001$	$p_{1-2}<0.001$
EPS, 24 h after (n = 8)	370 ± 20	50.3 ± 3.9	282 ± 20
	$p_{1-3}>0.05$	$p_{1-3}>0.05$	$p_{1-3}<0.001$
Adaptation (n = 10)	340 ± 10	93.8 ± 4.3	140 ± 10
	$p_{1-4}<0.05$	$p_{1-4}<0.01$	$p_{1-4}<0.05$
Adaptation + EPS 2 h after (n = 8)	370 ± 40	85.5 ± 5.6	176 ± 22
	$p_{2-5}<0.001$	$p_{2-5}<0.001$	$p_{2-5}<0.001$
	$p_{4-5}>0.05$	$p_{4-5}>0.05$	$p_{4-5}>0.05$
Adaptation + EPS 24 h after (n = 7)	290 ± 10	80.6 ± 6.4	—
	$p_{4-6}>0.05$	$p_{4-6}>0.05$	
Ionol (n = 9)	330 ± 20	96.2 ± 4.1	100 ± 20
		$p_{1-7}<0.01$	
Ionol + EPS, 2 hr after (n = 8)	350 ± 20	78.1 ± 3.8	120 ± 80
	$p_{2-8}<0.001$	$p_{2-8}<0.001$	$p_{2-8}<0.001$
Ionol + EPS, 24 h after (n = 8)	290 ± 10	68.1 ± 2.6	—
	$p_{1-9}>0.05$	$p_{1-9}>0.05$	

IV. ADAPTATION TO STRESS PREVENTS AND ABOLISHES DISTURBANCES TO CARDIAC CONTRACTILE FUNCTION AND ELECTRIC STABILITY IN ACUTE ISCHEMIA, REPERFUSION, MYOCARDIAL INFARCTION, AND POSTINFARCTION CARDIOSCLEROSIS

With a view to using adaptation as a cardioprotector against stress, it was deemed expedient to ascertain first how adaptation affects the cardiac contractile function and tolerance to load and hypoxia in the whole organism.

Together with Belkina we studied the rat heart contractile function *in situ* by electromanometric recording of the left ventricular pressure at physiological rest and under load imposed with aortic clamping.

The main results presented in Figure 4 bring out two issues. First, adaptation to short immobilization stresses did not appreciably alter the left ventricular contractile function at relative physiological rest; there was only a tendency to decreasing developed pressure, contraction rate, and relaxation velocity. Second and most important, the adaptation substantially enhanced the heart resistance to maximal load: at the 5th second of aortic clamping all contractile parameters were practically similar in control and adapted animals, and at the 25th second the depression of the contractile function was pronounced in the controls, but insignificant in the adapted rats. As a result, the adapted animals exceeded the controls in developed pressure by 43%, in IFS by 77%, in contraction velocity by 80%, and in relaxation velocity by 43%. It is noteworthy that the higher contractile function in adapted animals was retained with the diastolic pressure decreased almost by 40%, and therefore can hardly be attributed to a more effective operation of such self-regulatory mechanisms as the Starling mechanism.

It should be borne in mind that adaptation to repeated stress consistently entails steady-state activation of catecholamine synthesis in the brain and adrenal glands, i.e., in the long run, increased power of the sympathoadrenal system. It can therefore be thought that one of the factors providing for the maintenance of cardiac function under maximal load in

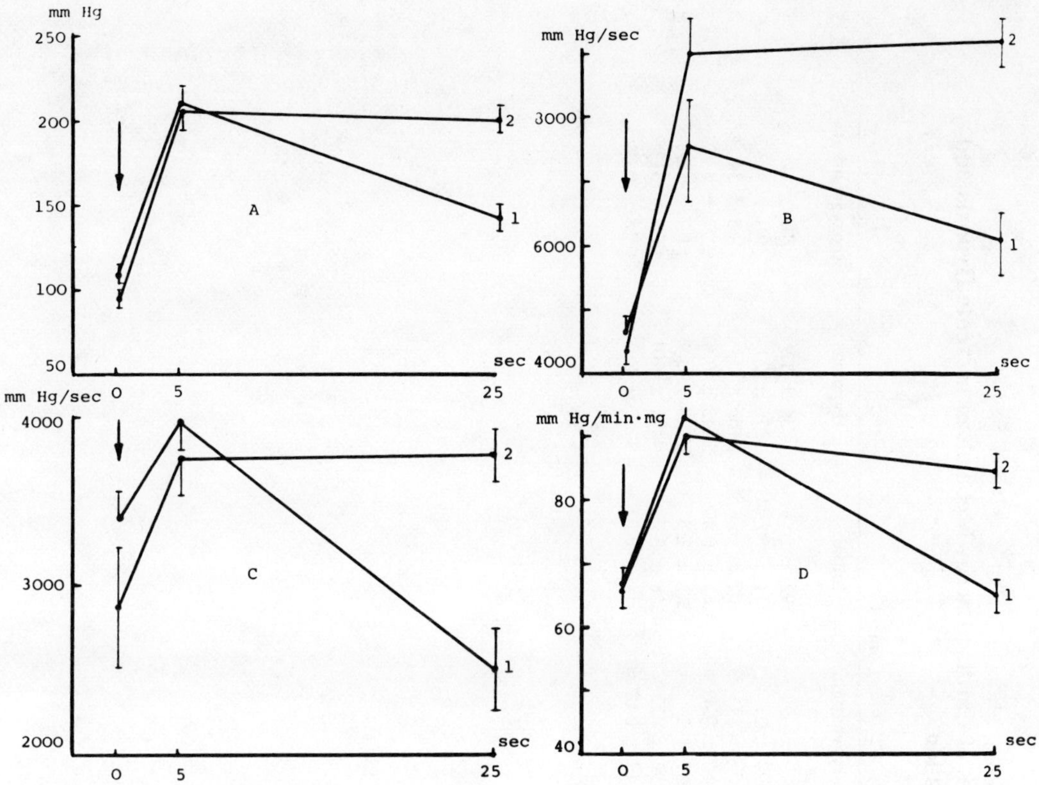

FIGURE 4. Effect of adaptation to short stress exposures on the rat left ventricular contractile function upon aortic clamping. The abscissa is time after clamping in seconds. The ordinates are (A) developed pressure, mmHg; (B) maximal pressure buildup rate, mmHg/s; (C) maximal pressure drop rate, mmHg/s; (D) IFS, mmHg/min·mg. (1) Control, (2) adaptation.

adapted animals is the more stable positive inotropic influence of the adrenergic system on the heart. There is, however, no doubt that a no less important part in the protective adaptational effect can be played by increased myocardial resistance to hypoxia; so at the next step of our study we considered the effect of adaptation to stress on cardiac resistance to hypoxic hypoxia in rats created *in situ* by switching off the respiration apparatus.

In this work carried out together with Golubeva and Kopylov, we used the following criteria: creatine phosphate (CP) content and creatine phosphokinase (CPK) activity, adenine nucleotide content, glycogen content, and phosphorylase activity. In the course of the acute experiment, after stabilization of the cardiac contractile function the apparatus for controlled respiration was switched off for 4 min to create hypoxic hypoxia; then it was switched back on for reoxygenation. For biochemical studies the hearts were instantly frozen in liquid nitrogen with the Wollenberger forceps (1) before hypoxia, in stable function; (2) at the end of the fourth minute of hypoxia, in depressed contractile function; and (3) at the end of the fifth minute of reoxygenation, when the function was to some extent restored.

The data in Table 8 show that, as in earlier published works, in control nonadapted animals hypoxia decreased the ATP content by more than 30%, CP by an order of magnitude and glycogen almost threefold, whereas lactate more than doubled. Concurrently, CPK reliably declined by 16% and there was a tendency to a decrease in total phosphorylase. In reoxygenation the CP and ATP levels were restituted to about 80% of initial values, and glycogen and lactate did not reverse at all; CPK remained at the hypoxic level, while phosphorylase continued to decrease and finally fell by more than 20%. Thus, the most

TABLE 8
Effect of Adaptation to Short Stress Exposures on The Indices of Cardiac Energy Metabolism in Acute Hypoxia and Reoxygenation

	Control					
Indices	Initial	Hypoxia	Reoxygenation	Initial	Hypoxia	Reoxygenation
CP (μmol/100 g tissue)	614 ± 42	60 ± 15	479 ± 49	592 ± 30	56 ± 12	703 ± 42[a]
ATP (μmol/100 g tissue)	412 ± 28	284 ± 17	328 ± 21	411 ± 30	276 ± 29	401 ± 42[a]
Glycogen (mg/100 g tissue)	408 ± 29	142 ± 16	153 ± 17	502 ± 76	166 ± 38	165 ± 34
Lactate (μmol/100 g tissue)	1.55 ± 0.11	3.84 ± 0.29	3.40 ± 0.41	1.61 ± 0.40	3.45 ± 0.67	2.77 ± 0.70
CPK (mmol/min·100 g tissue)	54.4 ± 1.8	46.0 ± 1.0	47.7 ± 2.1	52.2 ± 2.5	52.9 ± 2.9[a]	51.7 ± 1.5
Total phosphorylase (A + B)	4002 ± 134	3528 ± 231	3192 ± 272	4668 ± 347	4401 ± 401[a]	4328 ± 313[a]
Phosphorylase A/(A + B) ratio	0.18 ± 0.02	0.31 ± 0.03	0.17 ± 0.02	0.18 ± 0.02	0.37 ± 0.04	0.18 ± 0.04

[a] Difference from respective controls statistically significant; n = 9 ÷ 16 in different series.

interesting feature of the results in control animals is the moderate but persistent decline in vital enzymes of energy metabolism — CPK and phosphorylase — which is not abolished in reoxygenation.

Animals adapted to stress displayed the same complex of disturbances of energy metabolism typical of acute hypoxia (decreasing ATP, CP, and glycogen, increasing lactate), but no hypoxic decline in CPK and phosphorylase. Still more marked differences revealed themselves in reoxygenation: the adapted animals maintained both enzymic activities and achieved complete recovery of ATP and superrecovery of CP.

Physiological experiments showed that hypoxic hypoxia depresses the cardiac contractile function in both control and adapted animals. Yet it is evident in Figure 5A that by such an integral index as IFS the adapted animals at the end of the fourth minute of hypoxia exceed the controls almost by half ($p < 0.05$). Accordingly, they restored the contractile function in reoxygenation much sooner than did the controls and, as in the case of the CP content, with superrecovery by the end of reoxygenation. A similar pattern was observed for another important index, contraction velocity (Figure 5B).

Thus, adaptation to stress enhances the stability of vital energy-metabolic enzymes CPK and phosphorylase in hypoxia and reoxygenation, and accelerates the restitution of contractile function in reoxygenation after hypoxic hypoxia. The results is enhanced resistance of the cardiac muscle to loading and hypoxia.

On this basis we studied the effect of prior adaptation to short stresses on the impairment of contractile function usual in experimental myocardial infarction. It was found that upon myocardial infarction produced according to Selye et al.,[38] such important indices of left ventricular function as developed pressure, IFS, pressure buildup, and drop rates decreased at rest by 25 to 30%. In adapted animals the depression of these parameters did not reach statistical significance. This effect was maintained under maximal load on the heart created by complete clamping of the aorta for 30 s. At maximal load on the left ventricle with an infarct, the effect of prior adaptation proved more pronounced than with the normal heart. Indeed, at the 25th second of aortic clamping the contractile indices in adapted infarction animals exceeded those in nonadapted infarction animals by the following factors: left ventricular developed pressure, 2.8 ($p < 0.001$); IFS, 3.8 ($p < 0.01$); maximal pressure buildup and drop rates, 3.7 and 3.25, respectively ($p < 0.001$) (Figure 6).

There is thus no doubt that *prior adaptation to short stress episodes markedly restricts the impairment of left ventricular contractile function in experimental infarction and is an efficient protection against ischemic damage. This protective effect can be due to attenuation of the necrotic zone as well as to prevention of injury to nonischemic heart regions usual in infarction.* We studied both possibilities.

To assess the influence of adaptation on nonischemic regions, we measured the function of right auricles isolated from adapted and nonadapted animals with left ventricular infarction. The adaptation as such did not appreciably affect the right atrial contractile function, but substantially attenuated its depression caused by left ventricular infarction (described in detail in Chapter 2, Section IV). In fact, in nonadapted animals the ventricular infarction decreased the maximal values of atrial developed force and IFS 2 to 2.5-fold, whereas in adapted ones the decrease was less than one third. Thus, prior adaptation to short stresses certainly lessened the functional impairment of nonischemic myocardial regions in experimental infarction.

Further experiments presented in Chapter 6 have shown that adaptation to repeated stress is accompanied by another cardioprotective effect, namely attenuation of the necrotic zone in experimental myocardial infarction.

Hence it can be stated that *the protective effect of prior adaptation to stress in experimental infarction comprises two components: restriction of the stress damage to nonischemic heart regions, and cytoprotective action attenuating the necrotic volume of the myocardium.*

It must, however, by emphasized that the adaptational protection of the heart against

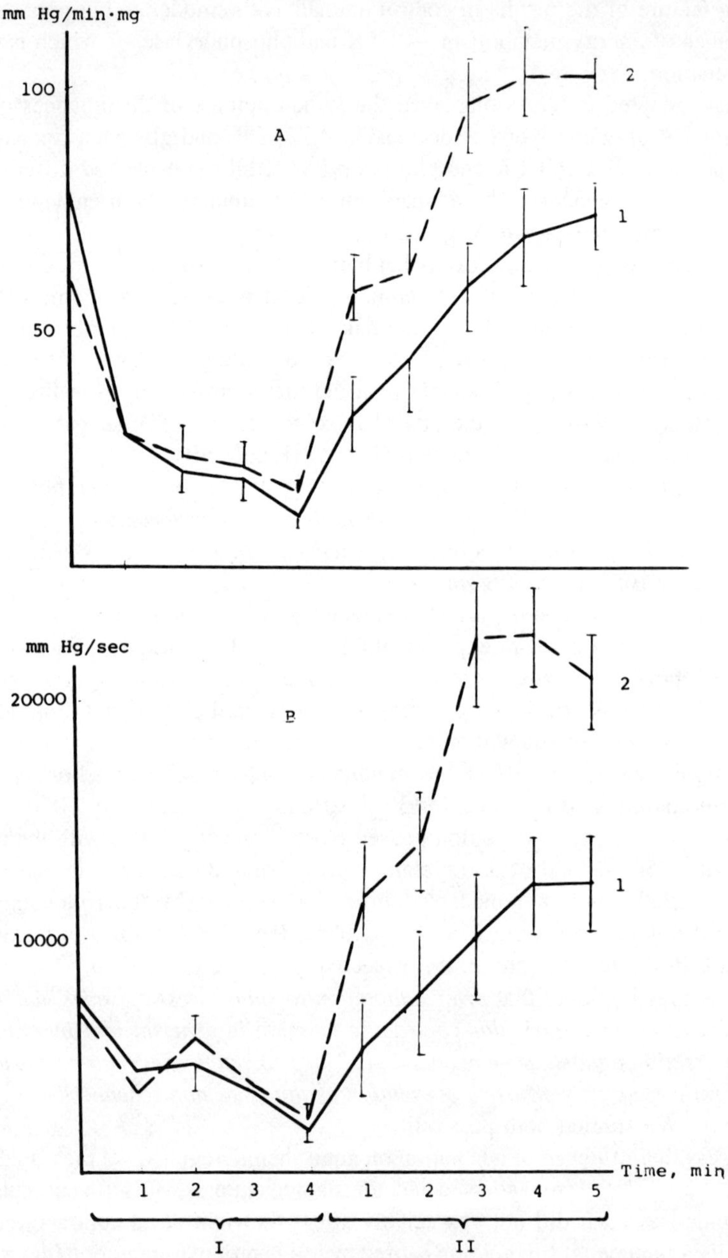

FIGURE 5. Effect of prior adaptation to stress on the dynamics of cardiac contractile function in anoxia and reoxygenation. The abscissa is time in minutes of (I) anoxia and (II) reoxygenation. The ordinates are (A) IFS, mmHg/min·mg; (B) maximal pressure buildup rate, mmHg/s. (1) Control, (2) adaptation.

ischemic damage cannot be reduced to mere restriction of necrosis. Such adaptation has been shown above to protect first and foremost against stress which always accompanies acute ischemia, reoxygenation, or myocardial infarction and has a profound arrhythmogenic action. In accord with this, our further studies demonstrate that adaptation to noninjurious short stress exposures furnishes a high degree of cardiac protection from arrhythmias common in acute ischemia, reperfusion, myocardial infarction, and postinfarction cardiosclerosis.[5]

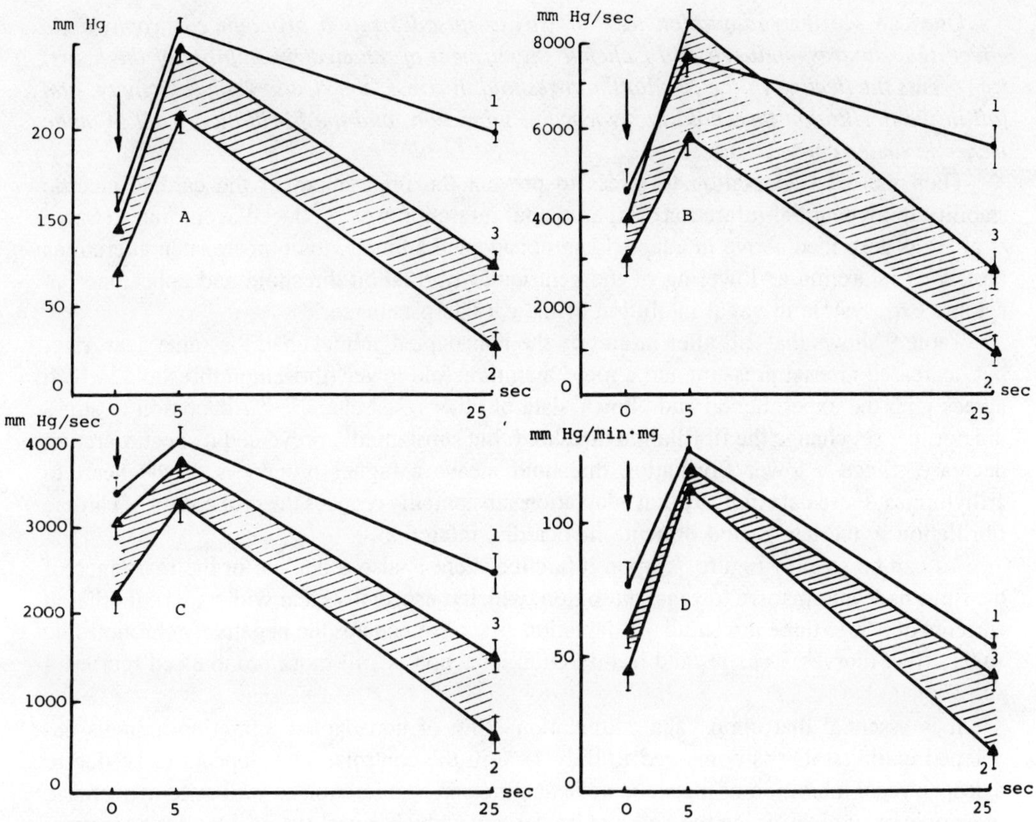

FIGURE 6. Effect of adaptation to stress on left ventricular contractile function of rat hearts with acute myocardial infarction upon aortic clamping. The abscissa is time after clamping in seconds. The ordinates are (A) developed pressure, mmHg; (B) maximal pressure buildup rate, mmHg/s; (C) maximal pressure drop rate, mmHg/s; (D) IFS, mmHg/min·mg. (1) Control, (2) infarction, (3) adaptation, (4) adaptation plus infarction. The shaded zone denotes the protective effect of adaptation.

Most of the data on impairment of the cardiac electric stability in response to coronary artery occlusion have been obtained under conditions quite far from natural (anesthesia, opened chest). Obviously, anesthesia would suppress the stress effect of ischemia, whereas thoracotomy would complicate it, which could make equivocal the evaluation of the effects of antistress factors on the cardiac electric stability. Therefore, we carried out our studies on the effect of acute ischemia on cardiac rhythm disorders and their prevention with closed-chest conscious animals using the technique of Lepran et al.,[48] which included two steps. First, under anesthesia a ligature was drawn under the left coronary artery and led out through a special cannula to just beneath the skin, but not tightened. Second, 3 to 5 d after these animals were fixed in the supine position while conscious, a skin incision was made and the ligature tightened on the coronary artery for 5 or 20 min. The incidence of various arrhythmias — fibrillation, ventricular tachycardia, and extrasystoles — and their overall duration were determined in control animals and those protected with adaptation to short stresses or with ionol.

In the first 5 min of ischemia, most of the controls (14 of 20) developed severe arrhythmias. In adapted animals, ventricular fibrillation was not observed at all, ventricular tachycardia only in 2, and extrasystole in 4 out of 20 rats. The difference was further deepened by the duration of arrhythmias in adapted animals being significantly less than in nonadapted ones. Thus the overall duration of arrhythmias was 541 s in the control, but only 36 s (i.e., 15 times less) in adapted rats.

One can see that *adaptation to short stress episodes has a pronounced prophylactic effect against stress-induced and ischemic impairment of the electric stability of the heart: it prevents the decline in the fibrillation threshold in stress, the rise in ectopic activity, and fall in the fibrillation threshold in myocardial infarction, and the fibrillation itself in acute ischemia under consciousness.*

Then we used adaptation to stress to prevent the impairment of the cardiac electric stability in myocardial infarction. Experimental infarction was produced according to Selye et al.,[38] as described above in adapted and nonadapted animals, to compare such alterations typical of infarction as lowering of the ventricular fibrillation threshold and appearance of ectopic extrasystole in vagal inhibition of the cardiac pacemaker.

Table 9 shows that 2 d after infarction the nonadapted animals had the same heart rate, but decreased arterial pressure and a more than threefold lower fibrillation threshold, which agrees with the experimental and clinical data of other researchers.[51,52] Adaptation to stress did not, per se, change the fibrillation threshold, but substantially prevented its postinfarction decrease. Since a lower fibrillation threshold means a higher proneness of the heart to arrhythmias, these data indicate that adaptation substantially reduces the probability of cardiac fibrillation in the late period of acute myocardial infarction.

As can be seen in Figure 7, upon infarction there is also a decline in the resistance of the sinus node automatism to vagal inhibition, which is especially clear with vagal stimulation currents of two to three thresholds. Adaptation as such attenuates the negatively chronotropic vagal effect (curves 3 vs. 1), and in infarction its action is still more pronounced (curves 4 vs. 2).

It is essential that upon vagal stimulation, 70% of nonadapted infarction animals developed extrasystoles as compared to only 18% in the controls. This appears to be due to a deeper vagal inhibition of the sinus node automatism in infarction as well as to appearance of ectopic excitation foci in the necrotic border zone which reveal themselves upon suppression of the normal pacemaker. Such phenomena have been observed by researchers[53,54] and vagal stimulation is used as a means of detecting the latent ectopic excitation foci.[53,55,56] Our experiments show that prior adaptation to stress lowers the cardiac ectopic activity in myocardial infarction; just 18% of adapted infarction animals developed extrasystoles. Moreover, the total number of extrasystoles in adapted animals with infarction was even less than in controls. It is known that ectopic activation not only leads to extrasystoles, but is also a necessary link of spontaneous fibrillation.[53] Hence, the adaptational suppression of ectopic automatism means a lower probability of cardiac arrhythmias and fibrillation in the postinfarction period.

Thus, *adaptation to short stresses prevents the postinfarction decline in the ventricular fibrillation threshold and appearance of ectopic excitation foci, increasing the sinus node resistance to vagal inhibition.*

This promising result naturally gave rise to a question whether or not such adaptation can abolish the already existing disturbances of the electric stability when the detrimental factors proper — stress and ischemia — have long ceased to act and there is only the result of infarction, namely vast postinfarction cardiosclerosis. Indeed, as long ago as 1959 Sumarokov[57] showed that doses of epinephrine that in most normal dogs cause only transient bradycardia, in animals with postinfarction cardiosclerosis evoke paroxysmal ventricular tachycardia and ventricular extrasystole. To solve this question, adaptation to short immobilization stresses was started 15 d after experimental myocardial infarction, when the postinfarct scar had already mostly formed in the left ventricle. Adaptation was carried on for 2 weeks and then (1 month after infarction) adapted and nonadapted animals were tested for the fibrillation threshold and ectopic cardiac activity in acute experiments. By that time the postinfarct scar in the left ventricular myocardium was clearly defined visually and its weight was about the same in both series, varying from 151 to 165 mg.

TABLE 9
Prevention of the Postinfarction Decline in Ventricular Fibrillation Threshold with Prior Adaptation to Short Stress Exposures

Series	Heart rate (min^{-1})	Arterial pressure Systolic	Arterial pressure Diastolic	Fibrillation threshold (mA)
Control (n = 11)	404 ± 13	1427 ± 7	87 ± 12	7.0 ± 0.4
Infarction (n = 10)	394 ± 17	90 ± 7	66 ± 11	2.1 ± 0.2
Adaptation (n = 11)	401 ± 11	124 ± 8	76 ± 5	7.2 ± 0.2
Adaptation plus infarction (n = 11)	384 ± 13	94 ± 6	68 ± 4	5.5 ± 0.3

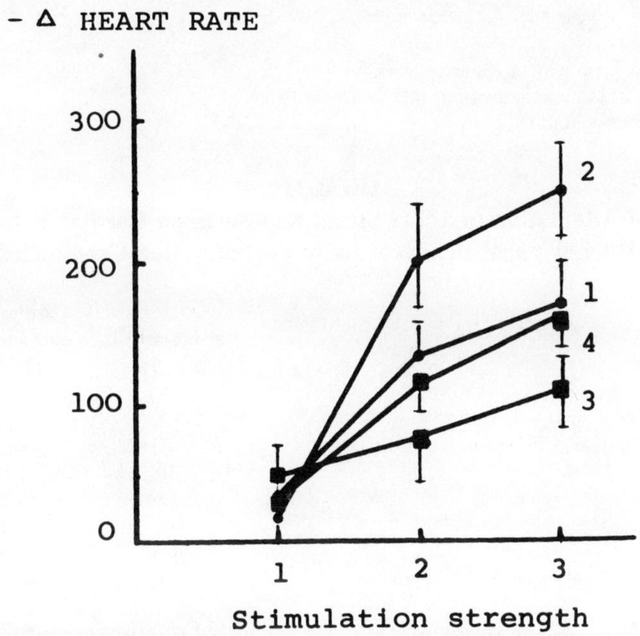

FIGURE 7. Effect of adaptation to stress on the negative chronotropic effect of vagal stimulation in acute myocardial infarction. The abscissa is strength of vagal stimulation, multiples of threshold current. The ordinate is the decrease in heart rate, min^{-1}. (1) Control, (2) infarction, (3) adaptation, (4) adaptation plus infarction.

Postinfarction cardiosclerosis did not appreciably change the heart rate, but in acute tests was consistently attended with the arterial systolic pressure lowered by 40 to 45 mmHg, i.e., more than by 25%. This pressure drop was not abolished by adaptation to stress. Further, postinfarction cardiosclerosis was consistently attended with a more than twofold decrease in the cardiac fibrillation threshold, which was completely abolished in adaptation.

Table 10 shows that cardiosclerosis increases somewhat the negatively chronotropic vagal effect, whereas adaptation to stress decreases it in both intact and cardiosclerotic animals by a factor of 1.5 to 2.3, thus more than completely overcoming the adverse influence of cardiosclerosis.

In these experiments, 30-s vagal stimulation could not elicit ectopic activity in adapted or nonadapted animals without cardiosclerosis. In nonadapted cardiosclerotic animals, extrasystoles are evoked already at threshold stimulation, with the cumulative number of extrasystoles over the four periods of stimulation (Table 11) amounting to 516, whereas adaptation to stress reduces this number more than threefold. This protective effect is certainly

TABLE 10
Effect of Adaptation to Short Stress Exposures on the Negative Chronotropic Effect (NCE) of the Vagus Nerve in Postinfarction Cardiosclerosis

Series[a]	Initial heart rate (min^{-1})	NCE (min^{-1})[b] at vagal stimulation, threshold units		
		1	2	4
Control	412 ± 9	38 ± 6	105 ± 20	151 ± 20
Cardiosclerosis	398 ± 12	40 ± 7	130 ± 20	194 ± 20
Adaptation	401 ± 9	33 ± 3	47 ± 9[c]	105 ± 14[c]
Cardiosclerosis + adaptation	358 ± 14	29 ± 4	55 ± 9[c]	96 ± 10[c]

[a] Each series comprised 11 animals.
[b] Expressed as decrease in the heart rate (beats per minute).
[c] $p < 0.05$ compared to the control.

TABLE 11
Effect of Adaptation to Short Stress Exposures on Cardiac Ectopic Activity During Vagal Bradycardia in Postinfarction Cardiosclerosis

	Cardiosclerosis (n = 11)	Cardiosclerosis plus adaptation (n = 11)
Total number of animals with extrasystoles	9	5
Number of extrasystoles in 30 s of vagal stimulation at:		
1 threshold	40	0
2 thresholds	65	1
3 thresholds	194	85
4 thresholds	262	80
Cumulative number of extrasystoles in group	561	166

Note: Control and adapted animals without cardiosclerosis had no extrasystoles during vagal stimulation in these experiments.

due to attenuated vagal action and probably to antiarrhythmic action of stress-limiting systems activated in adaptation.

Thus, *adaptation to stress abolishes the disturbances of cardiac electric stability (lowered fibrillation threshold and increased ectopic activity) characteristic of postinfarction cardiosclerosis.*

For appreciation of this result it is essential that the animals were taken into study 1 month after infarction. Hence, neither stress or ischemia could play any role in the observed disorders, and the beneficial effect of experimental therapy cannot be attributed to an anti-ischemic or antistress effect. The decreased fibrillation threshold and increased ectopic activity in postinfarction cardiosclerosis are due to the existence of a large enough connective-tissue scar in the left ventricular wall. It has been shown that in the scar and especially in its border zone there always are inclusions of cardiomyocytes that have survived acute ischemia and retain their bioelectric activity and near-normal histological structure; in recent studies these cells have been found to have lowered rest potential, decreased amplitude and upstroke velocity of the action potential (AP), and diversified alterations of the duration of AP and refractory phase.[58]

A priori, this complex of alterations can be supposed to constitute the basis of irregular conduction of excitation and to be thus involved in formation of reentry and cardiac fibrillation upon a premature impulse from an ectopic focus. In our experiments such an impulse was created by premature electric stimulation of the apex cordis, and the current necessary to cause reversible fibrillation in animals with postinfarction cardiosclerosis was half that in the control. The above interpretation is in complete accord with the results of clinicophysiological studies where the surviving cells of the border zone in postinfarction cardiosclerosis in humans were identified as the origin of ventricular tachycardia in chronic IHD patients.

In an epidemiological study of Wilhelmsson et al.,[59] people with rich stress experience had a reliably better life expectancy after myocardial infarction than people that had led a relatively peaceful life. Analogous data were earlier presented by Jenkins et al.,[60] who showed that people exhibiting a high emotional reaction to encountered situations have lower mortality from first and subsequent myocardial infarction than those with a moderate reaction. Of course, these clinical observations should be verified and extended. However, they are in line with the notion that rationally organized training to extremal situations such as the one acquired in military service lowers the probability of sudden cardiac failure.

On the whole, the body of facts available to date gives rise to at least two questions. First, can adaptation to small stresses be practically applied to heart protection?, and second, how does the phenomenon of adaptational protection change our theoretical notions of the mechanisms of arrhythmias and sudden death?

In solving the first of these questions, we tried to find out whether or not adaptation to such rough treatment as immobilization could be replaced with transauricular acupuncture, which is widely used on humans and is not associated with such great energy and structural expenditures as in the immobilization stress.

These studies[61] were carried out on Wistar male rats weighing 200 to 250 g; the animals were grouped in six series: (1) control; (2) a course of electroacupuncture (EA); (3) a 12-h immobilization stress; (4) stress after EA; (5) acute ischemia in left coronary artery occlusion; and (6) acute ischemia after EA. For EA, needles were introduced into the floor of both auricles near the external acoustic meatus, and pointed impulses (0.8 to 2 mA, 1.5 ms, 3 Hz) were delivered with a Jasper CS-504 electrostimulator for 20 min daily for 2.5 weeks. This dosage of electrostimulation approximated those used for reflexotherapy in humans. The immobilization stress was produced by fixing the animals by four limbs in the supine position for 12 h. Acute ischemia in conscious, closed-chest animals was produced according to Lepran et al.[48] All physiological and biochemical techniques have been described earlier. Catecholamine content in the adrenergic fibers of right ventricular myocardium was assayed by the luminometric method of Folck-Owman as modified by Krokhina.[62]

The transauricular EA used by us never elicited any pain reaction. Starting from the second or third exposure, the animals after 5 to 7 min of stimulation grew torpid and remained such for several minutes after the end of stimulation. During the seance the animals could be easily handled and laid on the back, i.e., there was no avoidance reflex or aggressive reaction.

The catecholamine content, phosphorylase A to total phosphorylase ratio, and glycogen content in the myocardium did not appreciably change after EA (Table 12), indicating the absence of a stress effect on the heart. The table further shows that immobilization stress, as in earlier works,[63] markedly decreased (by a factor of 2.5) the myocardial catecholamine content, with the ratio of active phosphorylase A to total phosphorylase increasing by half. Concurrent mobilization of glycogen decreased its myocardial content by one third. After the course of EA, which itself did not alter these indices, the effect of stress was different: the catecholamine content declined by not more than 25%, while the phosphorylase ratio and glycogen did not change significantly (Table 12).

The cardiac resistance to arrhythmogenic influences is known[64] to be inversely correlated with the phosphorylase ratio. The data of Table 13 agree with this nicely: the EA course as such only slightly raised the cardiac fibrillation threshold, but clearly attenuated its drop in

TABLE 12
Effect of Electroacupuncture (EA) on Catecholamine Content, Phosphorylase Activity, and Glycogen Content in Rat Heart During Stress

Series	Catecholamines, luminescence units	Phosphorylase A/(A + B) ratio	Glycogen (mg/ 100 g tissue)
Control	17.6 ± 1.57	0.43 ± 0.03	435 ± 14
	(n = 5)	(n = 7)	(n = 7)
EA	17.21 ± 1.41	0.45 ± 0.05	409 ± 14
	(n = 5)	(n = 10)	(n = 10)
Stress	7.0± 0.87	0.61 ± 0.04	290 ± 6
	(n = 5)	(n = 8)	(n = 8)
	$p_{1\text{-}3}$ <0.001	$p_{1\text{-}3}$ <0.01	$p_{1\text{-}3}$ <0.001
EA + stress	13.7 ± 1.00	0.47 ± 0.03	398 ± 23
	(n = 5)	(n = 10)	(n = 10)
	$p_{3\text{-}4}$ <0.001	$p_{3\text{-}4}$ <0.01	$p_{3\text{-}4}$ <0.01

TABLE 13
Prevention of the Stress Decline in Myocardial Fibrillation Threshold with a Course of Electroacupuncture (EA)

Series	Electric fibrillation threshold (mA)
Control (n = 10)	8.5 ± 0.5
EA (n = 9)	9.5 ± 1.5
	$p_{1\text{-}2}$ NS
Stress (n = 10)	3.3 ± 1.0
	$p_{1\text{-}3}$ <0.001
EA + stress (n = 8)	6.8 ± 0.8
	$p_{3\text{-}4}$ <0.001

stress. In other words, the EA course substantially alleviated the predisposition to arrhythmias usually created by the immobilization stress. Table 14 shows the effect of EA on the development of cardiac arrhythmias within 10 min of coronary occlusion in conscious animals. After EA there is a certain tendency to an increase in the latent period of arrhythmias, a more than fivefold decrease in the duration of ventricular tachycardia, and a more than threefold decrease in the overall duration of arrhythmias (mean values per animal).

Thus, a course of EA producing no defense reactions in animals or stress effects on the heart prevents activation of phosphorylase, mobilization of glycogen, markedly attenuates the drop of the cardiac fibrillation threshold in stress, and also substantially restricts the duration of arrhythmias in acute ischemia. Since in acute ischemia in conscious animals stress plays an important part in the development of arrhythmias, the data obtained prompt an idea that the cardioprotective antiarrhythmic action of EA is mostly due to its stress-limiting effect, i.e., depends on reflex activation of the stress-limiting systems.

This suggestion is supported by the fact that acupuncture causes accumulation of the GABA-ergic and opioidergic metabolites in the brain.[65-67] This makes promising further studies on the antiarrhythmic action of acupuncture in the clinic and on the stress-limiting systems as an important link in the therapeutic effect of this widely used method.

The adaptive activation of the stress-limiting systems and consequent adaptational protection of the heart against stress and ischemic damage and attendant impairment of cardiac electric stability, arrhythmias, and fibrillation are, in our opinion, important for further

TABLE 14
Effect of a Prior Course of Electroacupuncture (EA) on Arrhythmias in Coronary Artery Occlusion

Indices (mean per animal)	(v) Control (n = 11)	(vi) EA (n = 10)	$p_{v\text{-}vi}$
Latent period of arrhythmias, seconds	70 ± 29	130 ± 40	
Number of extrasystoles	24 ± 12	27 ± 7	
Ventricular tachycardia, seconds	62.3 ± 23.7	11.8 ± 8.9	<0.01
Ventricular fibrillation, seconds	34.2 ± 8.5	26.6 ± 6.6	
Total duration, seconds	114 ± 38.5	52.8 ± 10.8	<0.05

development of our understanding of the pathogenesis of arrhythmias, fibrillation, and sudden death.

Indeed, we could have already seen that people with definitely proved absence of ischemic disease may severely suffer and even die from neurogenic arrhythmias and cardiac fibrillation of stress origin, and on the other hand such dramatic cases are only few in the trials of life.

Further, considering the data on the epidemiology and pathologic anatomy of ischemic disease, we could see that with the same degree of atherogenic coronary sclerosis people may live and people may die of fibrillation and sudden death. It should be noted that arrhythmias can often be triggered (and thus the question of life or death decided) by environmental, biosocial, stressful situations. Even after an infarction has already formed, the development of fibrillation and the fatal outcome can be determined by the extent of stress reaction and its cardiotropic effect.

The fact that adaptation to stress (providing activation of stress-limiting systems) completely prevented in our experiments the impairment of cardiac electric stability in stress and infarction, abolished these phenomena in postinfarction cardiosclerosis, and substantially alleviated grave arrhythmias and fibrillation in acute ischemia, taken together with clinical data prompts an idea that the hereditary or ontogenetically acquired state of the stress-limiting systems in great measure predetermines the absence or occurence of arrhythmias and sudden death.

The concept of the relation of the stress-effecting and the stress-limiting systems in the pathogenesis of arrhythmias and fibrillation is to some extent reflected in the scheme of Figure 8. Under the influence of exogenous stress factors or afferent impulses from the ischemically damaged heart, in the higher divisions of the central nervous system (presumably in the frontal cortical lobes and in the adrenergic centers of the hypothalamus and medulla oblongata) there forms a stable enough system of excited centers which can once or repeatedly induce a strong adrenergic effect on the heart. This general layout is common for Schemes A and B, while their collation is an attempt to answer the eternal clinical question: why in most stress situations people have neither arrhythmias nor fibrillation, and furthermore, why fibrillation does not develop in most IHD patients and in most cases of acute ischemia? Figure 8A shows that such development of events is checked by activation of powerful stress-limiting systems, which is elaborately coupled with the stress reaction and prevents its injurious effects both at the central level (1) and in the heart proper (2). Clearly, such effective performance of the stress-limiting systems may be genetically determined or acquired through adaptation, as observed in our experiments. Figure 8B shows that such activation proves ineffectual in deficiency of the stress-limiting systems, either genetic or acquired because of prolonged stress exposure, intoxication, starvation, avitaminoses, etc. Then the cardiotropic detrimental effect of stress on the heart takes place by itself or combines with ischemia. It is such conditions that can most probably give rise to arrhythmias, fibrillation, and cardiac arrest.

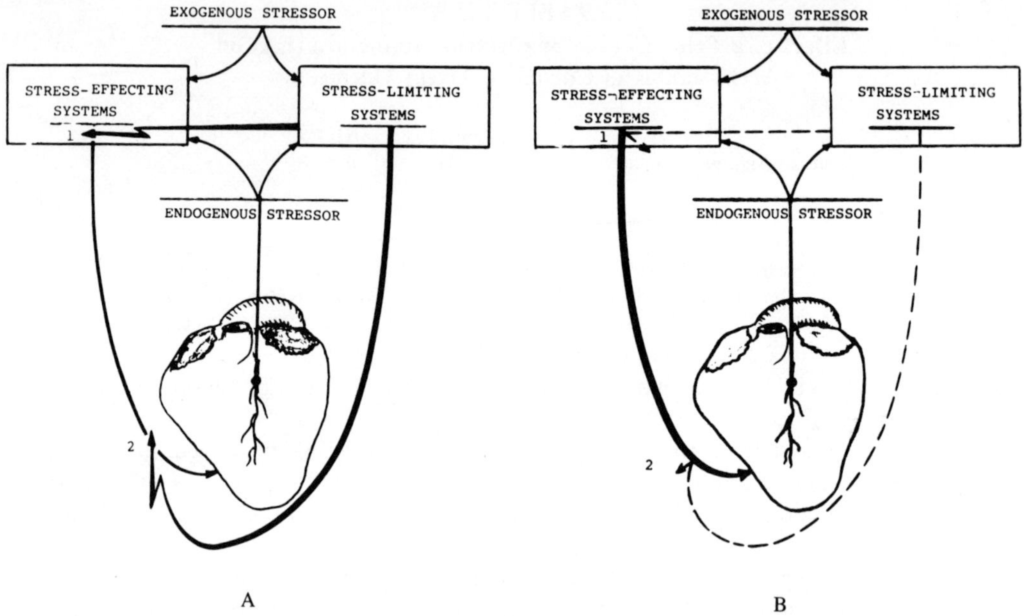

FIGURE 8. Adaptational increase in the physiological efficiency of stress-limiting systems prevents development of arrhythmias. (A) Organism with powerful stress-limiting systems. (B) Organism with deficient stress-limiting systems. (1) Central level of regulation; (2) cardiac self-regulation. For explanations see text.

It is easy to see that this working hypothesis is in accord with the real state of things presented in the preceding Chapter in detailed juxtaposition of stress arrhythmic heart disease and ischemic heart disease. Indeed, in stress arrhythmic disease the arrhythmias are clearly seen as neurogenically determined: they are readily elicited with stress load, but not with physical load, and develop despite intact coronary arteries in the absence of atherogenic dyslipidemia or coronary stenoses, i.e., in this case we are dealing with a selective pathology of the stress-limiting systems. Of course in this group there can also evolve secondary atherogenic dyslipidemia and coronary atherosclerosis owing to the above-considered atherogenic effect of stress.

In classical ischemic disease the situation is different. A primary defect in the cholesterol metabolism in the liver gives rise to atherogenic dyslipidemia with ensuing progressive coronary stenoses and ischemia which, depending on the state of the stress-limiting systems, may be aggravated by arrhythmias.

This is of course a most superficial description of the problem; to present a more specific concept of the stress-limiting systems, and to rationally use the mediators of these systems and their synthetic analogs as well as dosed adaptation for heart protection, a more concrete analysis is needed of the central and local stress-limiting systems and their place in the adaptational protection of the heart.

REFERENCES

1. **Meerson, F. Z., Dolgikh, T. V., Smolentseva, V. N., and Batrachenko, E. R.,** Prevention of disturbances to metabolism and function of the cardiac muscle in immobilization stress with prior adaptation to short stress exposures (in Russian), *Vopr. Med. Khim.,* 3, 41, 1985.
2. **Meerson, F. Z., Katkova, L. S., Kozlov, Yu. P., and Manukhina, E. B.,** Prevention of stress disturbances to the cardiac contractile function in prolonged stress with prior adaptation to short stress exposures (in Russian), *Byull. Eksp. Biol. Med.,* 12, 25, 1983.
3. **Meerson, F. Z., Malyshev, V. V., Ekimov, E. N., Petrova, V. A., and Lifant'ev, V. I.,** Effect of organismic adaptation to short stress exposures on the realization of stress reaction and disturbances to heart metabolism and contractile function caused by prolonged emotional pain stress (in Russian), *Vopr. Med. Khim.,* 1, 76, 1986.
4. **Meerson, F. Z., Belkina, L. M., Dyusenov, S. S., Ustinova, E. E., and Shabunina, E. V.,** Prevention of cardiac fibrillation with antioxidants and prior adaptation of animals to stress (in Russian), *Kardiologiya,* 8, 29, 1985.
5. **Meerson, F. Z. and Pshennikova, M. G.,** *Adaptation to Stress Situations and Physical Loads* (in Russian), Meditsina, Moscow, 1988.
6. **Manukhina, E. B., Katkova, L. S., and Meerson, F. Z.,** Comparative evaluation of the protective effect of adaptation to short stresses against damage to the heart and portal vein in prolonged stress (in Russian), *Byull. Eksp. Biol. Med.,* 8, 151, 1985.
7. **Stone, E. and Platt, J.,** Brain adrenergic receptors and resistance to stress, *Brain Res.,* 237, 405, 1982.
8. **Meerson, F. Z., Sukhikh, G. T., Katkova, L. S., and Van'ko, L. V.,** Prevention of depression of natural killer activity and myocardial contractile function in prolonged stress with prior adaptation to short stress exposures (in Russian), *Dokl. Akad. Nauk SSSR,* 247, 241, 1984.
9. **Zigmond, M. J. and Harvey, J.,** Resistance to central norepinephrine depletion and decreased mortality in rats chronically exposed to electric foot shock, *J. Neuro-Visc. Relat.,* 31, 373, 1970.
10. **Wallace, J. L. and Cohen, M. M.,** Gastric mucosal protection with chronic mild restraint: role of endogenous prostaglandins, *Am. J. Physiol.,* 247, G127, 1984.
11. **Gorizontov, P. D., Belousova, O. I., and Fedotova, M. I.,** *Stress and the Blood System* (in Russian), Meditsina, Moscow, 1983.
12. **Kuroshima, A., Habara, G., and Uehara, A.,** Cross adaptation between stress and cold in rats, *Pfluegers Arch.,* 402, 402, 1984.
13. **Mikulaj, L., Kvetnansky, R., Murgas, K., Parizkona, J., and Vencel, P.,** Catecholamines and corticosteroids in acute and repeated stress, in *Catecholamines and Stress,* Kopin, I. and Kvetnansky, R., Eds., Pergamon Press, New York, 1976, 445.
14. **Lishmanov, Yu. B., Trifonova, T. V., Tsibin, A. N., Maslova, L. V., and Dement'eva, L. A.,** Beta-endorphine and stress hormones of blood plasma in tension and adaptation (in Russian), *Byull. Eksp. Biol. Med.,* 4, 422, 1987.
15. **Pshennikova, M. G., Kuznetsova, B. A., Shimkovich, M. V., and Meerson, F. Z.,** Effect of adaptation to stress on the blood content of catecholamines and prostaglandins in acute stress (in Russian), in *Impairment of Regulatory Mechanisms and Their Correlation,* Proc. IVth All-Union Congr. Pathophysiol., Kishinev, in press.
16. **Kvetnansky, R., Weise, V., and Kopin, I. J.,** Elevation of adrenal tyrosine hydroxylase and phenylethanolamine-N-methyl transferase by related immobilization of rats, *Endocrinology,* 87, 744, 1970.
17. **Suthanthirorajan, N. and Subranmanyam, S.,** Influence of isolation stress on monoamine levels in discrete regions of the rat brain: correlation with behaviour, *Indian J. Physiol. Pharmacol.,* 27, 101, 1983.
18. **Mikulaj, L., Kvetnansky, R., and Murgas, K.,** Changes in adrenal response during intermittent and repeated stress, *Rev. Czech. Med.,* 20, 162, 1974.
19. **Eller, A., Nyakas, G., Szabo, G., and Endröczi, E.,** Corticosterone binding in myocardial tissue of rats after chronic stress and adrenalectomy, *Acta Physiol. Acad. Sci. Hung.,* 53, 205, 1981.
20. **Meerson, F. Z.,** *Adaptation, Stress, Prophylaxis* (in Russian), Nauka, Moscow, 1981.
21. **Dirksen, R., Wood, G., and Nijhuis, G.,** Mechanism of nalaxone therapy in the treatment of shock: a hypothesis, *Lancet,* 1, 607, 1981.
22. **Guillemin, R., Barge, Th., and Rossier, J.,** β-Endorphin and adrenocorticotropin are secreted concomitantly by the pituitary glands, *Science,* 197, 1367, 1977.
23. **Rossier, J., French, E., and Gros, C.,** Adrenalectomy, dexamethasone or stress alter opioid peptide level in rat anterior pituitary but not intermediate lobe of brain, *Life Sci.,* 25, 2105, 1979.
24. **Meerson, F. Z., Dmitriev, A. D., and Zayats, V. I.,** Prevention of impairment of the cardiac contractile function in experimental infarction with prior adaptation to stress and opioid peptides (in Russian), *Kardiologiya,* 9, 81, 1984.
25. **Hong, J. S., Gillin, J., Jang, H.-Y., and Costa, E.,** Repeated electroconvulsive shocks and the brain content of endorphines, *Brain Res.,* 177, 273, 1979.

26. **Anokhina, I. P., Yumatov, E. A., Ivanova, T. M., and Skotselyas, Yu. G.,** Biogenic amine content in different brain structures in rats adapted to chronic emotional stress (in Russian), *Zh. Vyssh. Nervn. Deyat. im. I. P. Pavlova,* 2, 348, 1985.
27. **Kvetnansky, R., Munco, A., Palkovits, M., and Mikulaj, L.,** Catecholamine in individual hypothalamic nuclei in stressed rats, in *Catecholamines and Stress,* Bratislava, 1975, 39.
28. **Schwartz, J.,** The dopaminergic system in the periphery, *J. Pharmacol.,* 15, 401, 1984.
29. **Beaulieu, S., Di Paolo, T., and Barden, N.,** Roles of the noradrenergic, dopaminergic and serotoninergic systems in the modulation of the ACTH response to stress by the amygdaloid central nucleus, *Can. J. Neurol. Sci.,* 12, 214, 1985.
30. **Meerson, F. Z., Pshennikova, M. G., Shabunina, E. V., Sazontova, T. G., and Belkina, L. M.,** Stress-limiting systems of the organism and prevention of cardiac fibrillation (in Russian), *Vestn. Akad. Med. Nauk SSSR,* 6, 47, 1987.
31. **Meerson, F. Z. and Katkova, L. S.,** Effect of prior adaptation to short stresses on the resistance of spontaneously contracting myocardium to a lipid peroxidation inducer (in Russian), *Byull. Eksp. Biol. Med.,* 12, 659, 1985.
32. **Meerson, F. Z., Dmitriev, A. D., Zayatz, V. I., and Manukhina, E. B.,** Prevention of disturbances of heart function in experimental infarction by adaptation to stressful activity: the role of opioid peptides in this phenomenon, in *Myocardial Metabolism,* Smirnov, V. N. and Katz, A. M., Eds., Academic Publishers, Harwood, 1987, 508.
33. **Meerson, F. Z., Katkova, L. S., Kozlov, Yu. P., and Manukhina, E. B.,** Prevention of stress disturbances to heart contractile function in prolonged stress with prior adaptation to short stress exposures (in Russian), *Byull. Eksp. Biol. Med.,* 12, 25, 1983.
34. **Vorontsova, E. Ya., Pshennikova, M. G., and Meerson, F. Z.,** Effect of stress on extensibility, Starling mechanism, and resistance of myocardium to hypoxia (in Russian), *Kardiologiya,* 11, 68, 1982.
35. **Meerson, F. Z., Dolgikh, V. T., Smolentseva, V. N., and Batrachenko, E. R.,** Prevention of disturbances to metabolism and function of the cardiac muscle in immobilization stress with prior adaptation to short stress exposures (in Russian), *Vopr. Med. Khim.,* 3, 41, 1985.
36. **Fallen, E. T., Elliot, W., and Gorlin, R.,** Apparatus for study of ventricular function and metabolism is isolated perfused rat heart, *Fed. Proc., Fed. Am. Soc. Exp. Biol.,* 39, 1173, 1980.
37. **Polozhentsev, S. D. and Rudnev, D. A.,** Dynamics of some indices of lipid metabolism in young persons in the course of adaptation to prolonged physical and psychoemotional loads (in Russian), *Fiziol. Chel.,* 12, 151, 1986.
38. **Selye, H., Bajusz, E., Grasso, S., and Mendell, P.,** Simple technique for the surgical occlusion of coronary vessels in the rat, *Angiology,* 11, 398, 1960.
39. **Lowe, J. E., Reimer, K. A., and Jennings, R. B.,** Experimental infarct size as a function of the amount of myocardium at risk, *Am. J. Pathol.,* 90, 363, 1978.
40. **Reimer, K. A.,** Myocardial infarct size. Measurements and predictions, *Arch. Pathol. Lab. Med.,* 104, 225, 1980.
41. **Rasmussen, M. M., Reimer, K. A., Kloner, R. A., and Jennings, R. B.,** Infarct size reduction by propranolol before and after coronary ligation in dogs, *Circulation,* 56, 794, 1977.
42. **Reimer, K. A., Lowe, J. E., and Jennings, R. B.,** Effect of the calcium antagonist verapamil on necrosis following temporary coronary artery occlusion in dogs, *Circulation,* 55, 581, 1977.
43. **Meerson, F. Z.,** *Pathogenesis and Prevention of Stress and Ischemic Damages to the Heart* (in Russian), Meditsina, Moscow, 1984.
44. **Murry, C. E., Reimer, K. A., Long, G. B., and Jennings, R. B.,** Preconditioning with ischemia protects ischemic myocardium, *Circulation,* 72, pt II, 119, 1975.
45. **Nachlas, M. M. and Shnitka, T. K.,** Macroscopic identification of early myocardial infarcts by alterations in dehydrogenase activity, *Am. J. Pathol.,* 42, 379, 1963.
46. **Lie, J. T., Pairolero, P. C., and Holley, K. E.,** Macroscopic enzyme-mapping verification of large, homogeneous, experimental myocardial infarcts of predictable size and location in dogs, *J. Thorac. Cardiovasc. Surg.,* 69, 599, 1975.
47. **Kogan, A. Kh., Kudrin, A. N., and Mieégombyn, A.,** Method for determination of nonperfusible myocardial area in coronary-occlusive ischemia with Trypan Blue-stained microspheres (in Russian), *Farmakol. Toksikol.,* 6, 94, 1984.
48. **Lepran, I., Koltai, M. Siegmund, W., and Szekeres, L.,** Coronary artery ligation, early arrhythmias and determination of the ischemic area in conscious rats, *J. Pharmacol. Methods,* 9, 219, 1983.
49. **Lillie, R. D.,** *Histopathologic Technique and Practical Histochemistry,* McGraw-Hill, New York, 1965.
50. **Nepomnyashchikh, L. M.,** *Pathologic Anatomy and Ultrastructure of the Heart,* (in Russian), Nauka, Novosibirsk, 1981.
51. **Gang, E., Bigger J., and Livelli, F.,** A model of chronic ischemic arrhythmias: the relation between electrically inducible ventricular tachycardia, ventricular fibrillation threshold and myocardial infarct size, *Am. J. Cardiol.,* 50, 469, 1982.

52. **McGovern, B., Dimarco, J., Garan, H., and Ruskin, J.,** New concepts in the management of ventricular arrhythmias and sudden death, *Curr. Probl. Cardiol.*, 7, 1, 1983.
53. **El-Sherif, N., Mehra, R., Gough, W., and Zeiler, R.,** Ventricular activation patterns of spontaneous and induced ventricular rhythmus in canine one-day-old myocardial infarction, *Circ. Res.*, 51, 152, 1982.
54. **Sherlag, B., El-Sherif, N., Hope, R., and Lazzara, R.,** Characterization and localization of ventricular arrhythmias resulting from myocardial ischemia and infarction, *Circ. Res.*, 35, 372, 1974.
55. **Penkoske, P., Sobel, B., Corr, P., and Burton, E.,** Disparate electrophysiological alteration accompanying dysrhythmia due to coronary occlusion and reperfusion in the cat, *Circulation,* 58, 1023, 1978.
56. **Kaplinsky, E., Ogava, S., Michelson, E., and Dreifus, L.,** Instantaneous and delayed ventricular arrhythmias after reperfusion of acutely ischemic myocardium: evidence for multiple mechanisms, *Circulation,* 63, 333, 1981.
57. **Sumarokov, A. V.,** Impairment of cardiac excitability in delayed terms after experimental myocardial infarction in dogs (in Russian), *Patol. Fiziol. Eksp. Ter.*, 6, 26, 1959.
58. **Ablidskov, J.,** Recognition of cardiac states at high risk of ventricular arrhythmias by means of electrocardiographic waveform, *Jpn. Circ. J.*, 44, 691, 1980.
59. **Wilhelmsson, L., Wilhelmsson, C., Vedin, A., and Elmfeldt, D.,** Effects of infarct size, smoking, physical activity and some psychological factors on prognosis after myocardial infarction, *Adv. Cardiol.*, 29, 119, 1982.
60. **Jenkins, C., Zyzanski, S., and Rosenman, R.,** Risk of new myocardial infarction in middle-aged men with manifest coronary heart disease, *Circulation,* 53, 342, 1976.
61. **Meerson, F. Z., Radzievskii, S. A., Vorontsova, E. Ya., Golubeva, L. Yu., and Chuvil'skaya, L. M.,** Possibility of reflect activation of stress-limiting systems and prevention of cardiac rhythm disturbances with the use of electroacupuncture (in Russian), *Kardiologiya,* 1, 88, 1980.
62. **Krokhina, E. M.,** *Functional Morphology and Histochemistry of the Cardiac Vegetative Innervation* (in Russian), Nauka, Moscow, 1973.
63. **Manukhina, E. B., Vorontsova, E. Ya., Volina, E. V., and Meerson, F. Z.,** Study of the dynamics of norepinephrine content in the hepatic portal vein and the auricle of rats in stress (in Russian), *Byull. Eksp. Biol. Med.*, 12, 673, 1981.
64. **Skinner, J. E., Beder, S. D., and Entman, M. L.,** Psychological stress activates phosphorylase in the heart of conscious pig without increasing heart rate and blood pressure, *Proc. Natl. Acad. Sci. U.S.A.*, 80, 4513, 1983.
65. **Vasil'ev, Yu. N.,** Neuropharmacological analysis of acupunctural analgesia, in *Pharmacological Aspects of Anesthesia* (in Russian), Abstr. All-Union Conf., Leningrad, 1983, 19.
66. **Jing Xue, An-Zhing Zhang, Xi Aue, and Ding Cao,** Inhibitor effect of analogous electroacupuncture on experimental arrhythmias, *J. Acupuncture Electrother. Res. Int.*, 10, 13, 1985.
67. **Omura, J.,** Pathophysiology of acupuncture treatment: effect of acupuncture on cardiovascular and nervous systems, *J. Acupuncture Electrother. Res. Int.*, 1, 51, 1975.

Chapter 4

CENTRAL STRESS-LIMITING SYSTEMS AND CARDIOPROTECTIVE EFFECTS OF THEIR MEDIATORS AND ACTIVATORS

I. INTRODUCTION

Before considering the specialized modulatory stress-limiting systems of the organism, it should be noted that certain possibilities of self-restraint are inherent in the very mechanism of the stress reaction and its realization at the cell level. Table 1 reflects the results of our work[1] showing that upon 6-h emotional pain stress (EPS), besides the well-known shifts such as decreased content, synthesis, and neuronal uptake of norepinephrine, there is a considerable increase in the content of dopamine (almost threefold in the adrenal glands and 70% in the heart).

The fact that increased consumption and decreased content of norepinephrine and epinephrine in stress are consistently accompanied by dopamine accumulation in both organs can only be explained, within the present day concept of the catecholamine biosynthetic pathway, by the fact that in stress their formation is limited not in the first step (tyrosine hydroxylase which converts tyrosine to dopa), but at the dopamine β-hydroxylase step converting dopamine to norepinephrine. This would result in the events observed in our experiment: mobilization of the catecholamine reserve, combining with a significant elevation in dopamine in both the stress-effecting (adrenal glands) and the executive (heart) organs. In assessing the possible physiological role of dopamine accumulation in the response to a strong protracted exposure to stress, it should be borne in mind that dopamine, being a motor activator,[2] vasodilator, and natriuretic,[3] participates in the adaptive effect of stress and at the same time exerts a regulatory influence on the stress reaction itself. Thus, dopamine inhibits pituitary secretion of ACTH[4] and suppresses the ACTH-induced adrenal biosynthesis of corticosterone.[5] It acts, therefore, as a factor restricting the hypophysial-adrenal link in the stress reaction.

Basically similar self-restraint is observed for stress hormones acting at the cell membrane level. One of the mechanisms of self-controlled cell activation in response to an excessive stress signal is associated with release of arachidonic acid. As already mentioned in Chapter 1, hydrolysis of cell membrane phospholipids caused by agonists of Ca^{2+}-mobilizing receptors, besides diacylglycerol (DAG) and inositol triphosphate (IP_3), produces arachidonic acid; it gives rise to prostaglandins E_1, E_2, and I_2, which can effectively restrict cell activation by adrenergic stimuli through suppressing norepinephrine "discharge" from sympathetic terminals.[6]

Self-restraint mechanisms operate at the intracellular level as well; an example is stimulation of the cAMP phosphodiesterase by calmodulin,[7] which checks cAMP elevation and thereby cell activation by catecholamines and other hormones acting on the adenylate cyclase and the cAMP circuit.

Thus, into the design of the stress reaction the evolution has built such features as allow the developing reaction to restrict itself. However, this does not appear to completely solve the problem, and accordingly the stress reaction is modulated by specialized stress-limiting systems. We shall consider three important examples, namely the GABA-ergic system and the linked system of benzodiazepine receptors; the opioidergic system and linked serotinin mechanisms; and parasympathetic neural regulation of the heart, whose role in restricting the arrhythmogenic adrenergic effects is known, but turns out to need further study.

TABLE 1
Effect of a 6-h EPS on Neuronal Uptake of ^{3}H-Norepinephrine, ^{3}H-Catecholamine Synthesis (10^3 cpm/g tissue), and Catecholamine Content (μg/g) in the Rat Heart and Adrenal Glands

Indices	Heart		Adrenal glands	
	Control	EPS	Control	EPS
Neuronal uptake of ^{3}H-norepinephrine	70.7 ± 4.5	48.6 ± 3.5[a]	53.9 ± 2.7	41.2 ± 3.9[b]
Synthesis of ^{3}H-norepinephrine	7.4 ± 0.5	5.2 ± 0.6[b]	7.2 ± 0.6	5.3 ± 0.2[b]
Synthesis of ^{3}H-dopamine	1.9 ± 0.08	2.2 ± 0.26	4.3 ± 0.32	4.3 ± 0.54
Content of norepinephrine	0.99 ± 0.19	0.56 ± 0.10[c]	213 ± 26	149 ± 15[c]
Content of epinephrine	—	—	402 ± 39	209 ± 23[a]
Content of dopamine	0.1 ± 0.01	0.17 ± 0.01[c]	2.51 ± 0.3	7.10 ± 0.8[a]

[a] $P < 0.001$.
[b] $p < 0.01$.
[c] $p < 0.05$.

II. GABA-ERGIC SYSTEM AND BENZODIAZEPINE RECEPTORS*

At present the GABA system is regarded as the main regulatory checking system of mostly central action. On the other hand, in recent years it has been ascertained that besides the central nervous system (CNS, where the GABA system is represented by GABA-ergic neurons) GABA, enzymes of its synthesis and breakdown (respectively, glutamate decarboxylase [GDC] and GABA-transaminase [GABA-TA]), and its receptors are found in almost all organs and tissues[8,9] where GABA is involved as a modulator of their neurohumoral regulation.[9]

For us it is essential that the GABA-ergic system is well represented at all levels of cardiac regulation: in the frontal cortex[8,10] where there are neurons responsible for activation of sympathetic and parasympathetic cardiac regulation in stress;[11,12] in the hypothalamic vegetative centers[13,14] forming the common efferent "outlet" to the heart;[15] in the nuclei of the brain stem parasympathetic cardiovascular center;[16] in the cardiac afferentation center, i.e., nucleus tractus solitarius of the medulla oblongata;[17] in the cardiac sympathetic nuclei of the spinal cord;[18] and finally in the heart itself.[9] Such full representation of the GABA system in heart and its regulatory apparatus points to the indubitable importance of GABA in control of cardiac function. This has indeed been proved in the works of recent years that will be considered later.

The coupling of the GABA-ergic system with the stress-effecting system manifests itself first of all as GABA elevation in stress in various brain regions: frontal cortex, hypothalamus, striatum, thalamus,[10,19] increased glutamate formation and GABA content in brain hemispheres,[20] etc.; the excess of catecholamines[21] and corticosteroids[22] arising in the stress reaction depresses the activity of GABA-TA, the breakdown enzyme, entailing a rise in brain GABA content. In EPS, GABA increases in just those brain regions where GABA-TA declines.[10] The coupling between the GABA and the stress-effecting system also reveals itself in direct activation of the GABA neurons by catecholamines released in the brain adrenergic structures in the stress reaction. Direct evidence is available for activation of the GABA system in the cortex and hypothalamus by norepinephrine and electrostimulation of adrenergic neurons.[19,23]

Such activation of the GABA-ergic system can in its turn restrict the activity of the

* With M. G. Pshennikova.

stress-effecting systems and the stress reaction itself through negative feedback. This stress-limiting function of GABA appears to be performed by two basic mechanisms.

First, in the hypothalamus GABA has been found to restrict at the postsynaptic level the secretion of the ACTH-releasing factor and thereby the activation of the adrenal-hypophysial link of the stress reaction.[24,25] Further, GABA exerts a tonic inhibitory influence on the population of "command" neurons in the hypothalamus. This population, when activated, may generate an integrative multisystem response consistently found in emotional stress, i.e., enhanced vegetative organ function, behavioral reactions, etc., constituting the stress reaction (see Reference 13 for references). Thus, activation of the GABA system can restrict the stress reaction at the central level.

Second, at the presynaptic level GABA can attenuate norepinephrine release from sympathetic terminals that innervate organs and tissues, and thereby restrict adrenergic activation both in the brain and in the target organs.[6,26]

The above is schematically presented in Figure 1. In accordance with the abundance of the GABA system at all levels of cardiac regulation, in recent years it has been shown that the GABA-ergic neurons exert a tonic inhibitory influence on the brain centers regulating cardiac and vascular function, and cessation or weakening of this influence results in altered heart rate, hypertension, and cardiac rhythm disturbances. Thus, blocking the GABA receptors with bicuculline and picrotoxin or deficit of GABA induced with 3-mercaptopropionic acid lead to activation of the posterior hypothalamic centers of sympathetic control of the cardiovascular system[13,14] with ensuing tachycardia, hypertension, tachyarrhythmias, and extrasystole. Administration of a $GABA_A$-receptor agonist muscimol or a β-adrenoblocker propranolol prevents these events.[13,14,27] The GABA neurons also display such tonic inhibitory influence on the cardiac parasympathetic regulation centers of the nucleus ambiguus of the brain stem. Cessation of this influence entails bradycardia and bradyarrhythmias that can be abolished by dissection of the vagus nerve.[16,27]

GABA has also been recently shown to block the afferent flow of pain impulses including the one from ischemic myocardium,[28] which can prevent formation of an excitation focus in the large hemisphere cortex responsible for cardiac arrhythmias.[11]

Of special interest for us is the influence of the GABA system on the hypothalamic centers of cardiac sympathetic regulation, since it is these centers that are responsible for activation of the cardiac function in the stress reaction. In particular, it is in the posterior hypothalamus that the local blood flow is enhanced in response to emotional stress, indicating enhanced metabolic activity resulting from local neuronal excitation.[29] Destruction of this zone in baboons eliminates the cardiovascular response to acute emotional stress.[30]

Taken together with the data on the role of GABA in suppression of the hypophysial-adrenal link of the stress reaction, the available *facts give grounds for supposing that GABA deficiency caused by hereditary defects of mediator turnover, brain tissue injury, or other factors can impair the cardiac and vascular regulation and potentiate the stress reaction and its detrimental action on the cardiovascular system; conversely, augmented capacity of the GABA system can prevent such damage.*

Indeed, spontaneously hypertensive rats have been shown to display increased activity of the sympathetic nerves which is normalized upon administration of the $GABA_A$-receptor agonist muscimol into brain ventricles,[31] and to have congenital deficiency of GABA-ergic activity in the posterior hypothalamus,[32] i.e., in the zone where GABA exerts its tonic inhibition of the centers of sympathetic regulation of vascular tone. Thus, hypertension in these animals can be thought to result from enhanced activity of vascular sympathetic regulation because of the lack of GABA-ergic inhibition.[14,29]

On the other hand, adaptation to stress exposures, which restrict activation of stress-effecting systems and the detrimental effects of the stress reaction (see the preceding chapter), is accompanied with an increase in the functional capacity of the GABA-ergic system.[33,34]

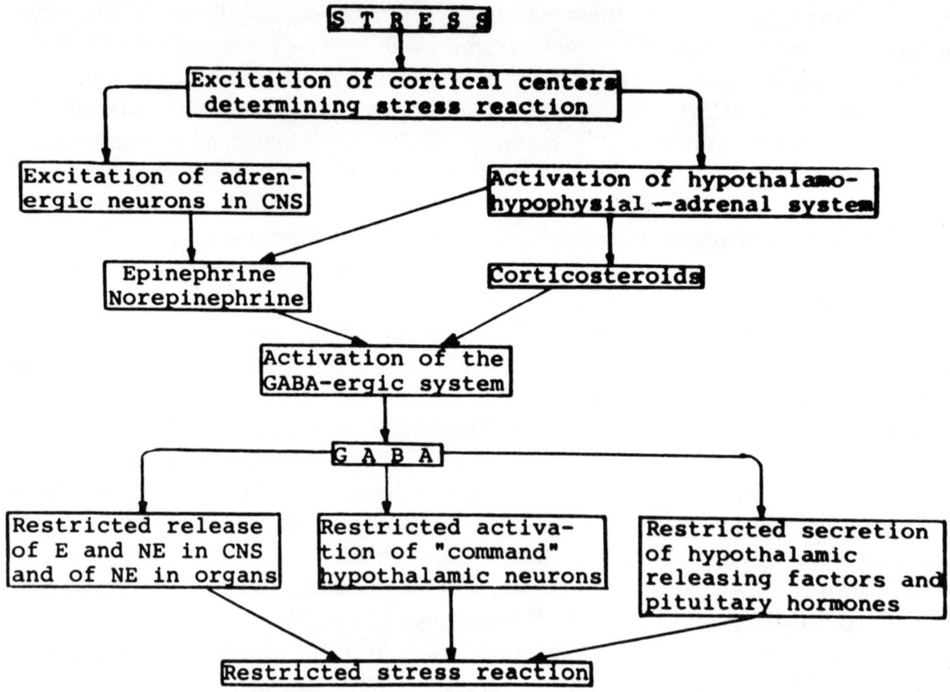

FIGURE 1. Coupling of the GABA-ergic system with the stress-effecting systems, and GABA-mediated restriction of the stress reaction. For explanations see text.

Thus, our studies show that in adaptation of rats to short immobilization stresses the activity of GDC in the large cerebral hemispheres increases while the GABA-TA activity remains the same, and accordingly the GABA content rises almost by 70%.[33]

This agrees with the recent data that adaptation of rats to repeated immobilization stress activates the GABA system in the frontal cortex as manifest by increased GDC activity and GABA turnover in this brain region.[34] The authors emphasize that activation of the GABA system in adapted animals combines with attenuated function of the peripheral sympathetic system which is controlled by GABA-inhibitable sympathetic centers.[34] All these data are also in line with the known facts that adaptation to repeated stress enhances animal resistance to the convulsive action of electric current and GABA antagonists,[35] and that administration of GABA or its active metabolite GHBA suppresses the stress reaction and prevents its detrimental effect.[36]

On the whole, the above gave grounds for using activators of the GABA system and its active metabolite GHBA to prevent cardiac stress damage as well as diseases in which the stress reaction is pathogenetically important, and first of all stress-induced and ischemic arrhythmias.

A previously published monograph[37] presented the data from our laboratory that GHBA can restrict the stress reaction as judged by blood corticosterone and simultaneously prevent such manifestations of stress damage as enzymemia, ulcerous lesions of the gastric mucosa, enhanced myocardial lipid peroxidation, and impaired cardiac contractile function. These data are in accord with clinical observations on the use of GHBA as an antiarrhythmic. Here we shall consider new material on the cardioprotective action of the GABA-ergic activator sodium valproate, which consistently raises the GABA content in the brain[38] and in the blood,[39] but has not heretofore been applied in cardiology.

At the first stage of this work[40] we studied the effect of sodium valproate on arrhythmias attending acute cardiac ischemia produced in conscious animals according to Lepran et al.[41]

TABLE 2
Effect of Sodium Valproate on Cardiac Rhythm Disturbances in Acutely Ischemic Conscious Rats

	Control (n = 20)	Valproate (n = 20)
Extrasystole		
Number of animals	12	6
Total duration in group	211	83
Mean duration per animal	10.6 ± 9.6	4.2 ± 5.8
Ventricular tachycardia		
Number of animals	13	6
Total duration in group	394	122
Mean duration per animal	19.7 ± 17.3	6.1 ± 6.4
Ventricular fibrillation		
Number of animals	12	2
Total duration in group	562	56
Mean duration per animal	28.1 ± 23.7	2.8 ± 5.0
All arrhythmias		
Number of animals	15	6
Total duration in group	1107	261
Mean duration per animal	55.4 ± 36.4	13.1 ± 15.2
Deaths	7	0

The study was carried out on 40 male Wistar rats weighing 230 to 280 g; half of the animals received 200 mg valproate per kilogram *per os* 90 min before acute ischemia, and the other 20 served as controls. Table 2 shows that acute ischemia was attended with grave arrhythmias in most of the controls: 13 animals (65%) developed ventricular tachycardia, and 12 animals (60%) ventricular fibrillation with a lethal outcome in 7 cases. In the group that had received sodium valproate the incidence of all types of arrhythmia, extrasystole, and ventricular tachycardia decreased by a factor of 2 to 2.5. The incidence of fibrillation fell sixfold and, most importantly, deaths were completely averted. It should also be noted that the overall duration of all types of arrhythmia decreased more than fourfold (ventricular fibrillation tenfold).

Thus, we can see that the antiarrhythmic effect of adaptation in acute myocardial ischemia in conscious animals can be efficiently mimicked by activating one of the main stress-limiting systems of the organism, the GABA-ergic one.

Next, experiments were run on anesthetized rats to assess the effect of sodium valproate on the drop of ventricular fibrillation threshold in acute ischemia and on the extent of ischemic arrhythmias. Before acute ischemia, the fibrillation thresholds were about the same in both groups: 10.8 ± 1.1 mA in the control and 11.7 ± 0.8 mA with valproate. Acute ischemia drastically decreased the fibrillation threshold in the control group: the drop was thirteenfold ($p < 0.01$), whereas after valproate administration the decrease was less so that the ischemic threshold (2.5 mA) was still three times higher than in the control ($p < 0.01$). It is also noteworthy that acute ischemia resulted in a substantial lengthening of the QT interval ($p < 0.01$), which reflects the onset of the vulnerable period.[42] This can probably be explained by depression of the rest potential (RP) of cardiac cells in acute ischemia,[43] which results in decreased cell excitability and longer refractory state.[44] Sodium valproate not only lessened the drop of the fibrillation threshold, but also substantially prevented the changes in QT, i.e., most likely restricted the depression of the RP and associated alterations in cell excitability.

Thus, prior administration of the GABA-ergic activator sodium valproate significantly decreased the probability of fibrillation in acute myocardial ischemia.

Next, the effect of sodium valproate was studied on arrhythmias developing in acute ischemia imposed with left coronary artery ligation in anesthetized animals. These experiments confirmed the well-known fact that anesthesia substantially restricts the stress reaction and thereby decreases the overall extent of arrhythmia in cardiac ischemia as compared to conscious animals. Nevertheless, even under such conditions the antiarrhythmic effect of sodium valproate proved definite enough. Thus, in the control all animals had extrasystoles and ventricular tachycardia, and eight out of ten developed cardiac fibrillation which, however, was reversible. Prior administration of sodium valproate appreciably diminished the incidence of fibrillation and decreased the total duration of all types of arrhythmia threefold ($p < 0.01$), decreased the duration of extrasystole by about 25%, ventricular tachycardia by 30%, and fibrillation sevenfold. There was also a tendency to a decrease in the mean duration of different types of arrhythmia. *So, the antiarrhythmic effect of valproate in acutely ischemic anesthetized rats was similar to the one in conscious animals.*

The second stage of our work was aimed at assessing the influence of sodium valproate on cardiac electric stability in experimental myocardial infarction. The studies were carried out with rats 48 h after coronary artery occlusion according to Selye. The acute tests were performed under anesthesia. The cardiac fibrillation threshold and ectopic activity were determined as described in Chapter 2. Sodium valproate did not appreciably change the heart rate (Table 3), but largely prevented the drop of the fibrillation threshold in infarction and practically eliminated the extrasystoles commonly observed with vagal stimulation in infarction.

Thus, the GABA-ergic activator prevents profound impairment of cardiac electric stability typical of myocardial infarction.

Since many antiarrhythmics are known to depress cardiac contractile function, it was important to find out the "costs" of this effect. Table 4 shows that *valproate did not additionally depress the parameters of cardiac contractile function in experimental myocardial infarction. In essence, the above experiments were aimed at prevention of cardiac arrhythmias in ischemic damage, i.e., represented experimental prophylaxis.*

At the third and final stage, we tried to use sodium valproate for experimental therapy of cardiac electric stability disorders in postinfarction cardiosclerosis, 2 months after experimental myocardial infarction. These experiments were carried out with larger rats (350 to 400 g) who therefore had a lower heart rate under anesthesia. The results are presented in Table 5 and are quite similar to those obtained in infarction.

In the aggregate, the beneficial antiarrhythmic effects of sodium valproate in acute ischemia in both conscious and anesthetized animals, in myocardial infarction, and in postinfarction cardiosclerosis make most topical a study of the antiarrhythmic action of such GABA-ergic activators in clinical cardiology.

It is now known that the GABA system is regulated, besides other mechanisms, by benzodiazepine receptors localized in the synaptic structures of the CNS and allosterically coupled with the postsynaptic $GABA_A$ receptors.[8,45] The main function of the classical ligands of benzodiazepine receptors — 1,4-benzodiazepines — is potentiation of the GABA relay at all CNS levels, actualized in the form of anticonvulsive, anxiolytic, and hypnotic efforts.[45,46] Antagonists and inversive agonists of these receptors, on the contrary, weaken the inhibitory action of GABA and accordingly aggravate convulsions, fear, excitement, etc.[45] Benzodiazepines act allosterically on the GABA receptor to potentiate the GABA-induced opening of the chloride channel and chloride entry into the neuron.[45,46] It can thus be supposed that benzodiazepines enhance the above mentioned GABA-ergic tonic inhibition of the hypothalamic and brain stem neurons realizing the sympathetic influence on the heart, vessels, and other organs,[13,14,29] and can thereby restrict activation of these neurons in stress. In particular, a benzodiazepine diazepam (Valium®) has been shown effective in preventing stress-induced hypertension.[47] Benzodiazepines probably also augment the checking effect of GABA in the cortex, which is rich in benzodiazepine receptors.[8]

At present there is no doubt that activation of the benzodiazepine receptors relieves emotional tension and excessive psychomotor reactivity in stress. Basing on this, we used

TABLE 3
Effect of Sodium Valproate on the Cardiac Fibrillation Threshold and Ectopic Activity in Myocardial Infarction

Series	Heart rate (min^{-1})	Fibrillation threshold (mA)	Total number of extrasystoles in vagal bradycardia
Control (n = 8)	400 ± 19	6.4 ± 0.37	0
Infarction (n = 8)	438 ± 18	2.6 ± 0.51[a]	103
Valproate (n = 8)	412 ± 13	6.8 ± 0.42	0
Infarction plus valproate (n = 8)	422 ± 17	5.5 ± 0.71[b]	2

[a] $p_{1\text{-}2} < 0.01$.
[b] $p_{4\text{-}2} < 0.01$.

TABLE 4
Effect of Sodium Valproate on the Left Ventricular Contractile Function 48 h After Myocardial Infarction

Series	Heart rate (min^{-1})	Developed pressure (mmHg)	IFS
Control (n = 10)	448 ± 4	118 ± 4.4	87.2 ± 4.7
Infarction (n = 10)	407 ± 18	87 ± 3.9[a]	66.7 ± 4.1[a]
Valproate (n = 11)	441 ± 6	119 ± 2.8	93.1 ± 4.4
Infarction plus valproate (n = 9)	381 ± 16	79 ± 2.2[b]	62.0 ± 4.2[b]

[a] $p_{1\text{-}2} < 0.01$.
[b] $p_{3\text{-}4} < 0.01$.

TABLE 5
Normalization of Cardiac Electric Stability in Postinfarction Cardiosclerosis With Sodium Valproate

Series	Heart rate (min^{-1})	Fibrillation threshold (mA)	Total number of extrasystoles in vagal bradycardia
Control (n = 11)	389 ± 11	6.8 ± 0.7	19
Cardiosclerosis (n = 11)	379 ± 8	2.3 ± 0.3[a]	401
Control plus valproate (n = 11)	380 ± 13	6.4 ± 0.7	0
Cardiosclerosis plus valproate (n = 11)	380 ± 12	6.3 ± 0.3	40

[a] $p < 0.01$.

a known benzodiazepine receptor agonist, phenazepam, to restrict ischemic and reperfusion arrythmias and disturbances to cardiac electric stability in infarction and postinfarction cardiosclerosis.

Phenazepam is well known as a psychotropic and anticonvulsive drug. Therefore, we first studied the antiarrhythmic action of phenazepam in the above conditions and then briefly collated the antiarrhythmic and the anticonvulsive properties of this benzodiazepine receptor agonist.

Table 6 demonstrates the effect of phenazepam (1 mg/kg intraperitoneally, 1 h before ischemia) in acute ischemia and subsequent reperfusion. The total duration of all types of cardiac rhythm disorders was much less than in controls; the mean duration of all arrhythmias per animal decreased more than twofold in ischemia and almost fivefold in reperfusion. It is noteworthy that both the incidence and the mean duration of a grave form of arrhythmia

TABLE 6
Effect of Phenazepam on Cardiac Rhythm Disorders in Acute Ischemia and Reperfusion in the Whole Organism

Indices	Ischemia Control (n = 12)	Ischemia Phenazepam (n = 12)	Reperfusion Control (n = 12)	Reperfusion Phenazepam (n = 12)
Extrasystole				
Number of animals	12	12	12	10
Total duration	395	287	76	49
Mean duration	33 ± 4	24 ± 3	6 ± 2	4 ± 2
Ventricular tachycardia				
Number of animals	12	10	12	11
Total duration	509	162	572	139
Mean duration	43 ± 9	14 ± 3[a]	48 ± 9	12 ± 4[a]
Ventricular fibrillation				
Number of animals	8	5	7	2
Total duration	203	18	272	6
Mean duration	17 ± 7	1.5 ± 2[a]	23 ± 15	0.5 ± 1[a]
All arrhythmias				
Total duration	1107	467	920	194
Mean duration	92 ± 19	39 ± 6[a]	77 ± 15	16 ± 6[a]

[a] Difference from respective controls significant at $p < 0.01$.

TABLE 7
Effect of Phenazepam on Cardiac Fibrillation Threshold and Vagally Elicited Ectopic Activity in Acute Myocardial Infarction

Series (n = 10 each)	Initial heart rate	Total no. of extrasystoles	Mean no. of extrasystoles	Fibrillation threshold (mA)
Control	393 ± 12	2	0.2	6.3 ± 0.5
Phenazepam	402 ± 9	0	0	6.9 ± 0.2
Infarction	403 ± 16	325	32.5 ± 12	1.5 ± 0.2
Infarction plus Phenazepam	398 ± 18	59	5.9 ± 5	4.0 ± 0.5
$p_{3\text{-}4}$			<0.05	<0.001

— ventricular fibrillation — were markedly lower in both conditions after phenazepam administration. Thus, it has been proved that in the whole organism phenazepam has a pronounced antiarrhythmic effect in acute ischemia and reperfusion of the heart. Notably, this drug was ineffective in analogous experiments with isolated heart; i.e., unlike sodium valproate, it acted exclusively at the neural regulation.

The data in Table 7 reflect the results of phenazepam injection in acute myocardial infarction. The drug (1 mg/kg) was injected twice: before coronary occlusion and 1 h before testing the electric stability.

The disturbances of cardiac electric stability in unprotected animals were typical of acute myocardial infarction: enhanced suppression of the sinus node automatism upon vagal stimulation, numerous extrasystoles evolving at this background, and a fourfold drop of the electric fibrillation threshold. Phenazepam itself did not appreciably affect these parameters in normal animals, but largely attenuated the above disturbances in myocardial infarction (see Table 7).

To appreciate the real significance of this protective effect of phenazepam, one should consider the data on mortality from myocardial infarction in our experiments. In total, to

TABLE 8
Effect of Phenazepam on Cardiac Fibrillation Threshold and Vagally Elicited Ectopic Activity in Postinfarction Cardiosclerosis

Series (n = 9 each)	Initial heart rate	Total no. of extrasystoles	Mean no. of extrasystoles	Fibrillation threshold
Control	367 ± 11	5	0.5	5.5 ± 0.3
Phenazepam	347 ± 10	0	0	6.4 ± 0.2
Cardiosclerosis	352 ± 10	249	28 ± 14	2.0 ± 0.2
Cardiosclerosis plus phenazepam	338 ± 10	15	2 ± 2	4.0 ± 0.3
$p_{3\text{-}4}$			<0.01	<0.001

produce acute infarction and postinfarction cardiosclerosis, coronary occlusion was performed in 70 rats without any protection; the first-day mortality was 47%. In 20 animials coronary occlusion was performed after single administration of phenazepam in the above dosage; only one animal died within the first day. Thus, in our hands phenazepam, by improving the cardiac electric stability in the acute period of experimental myocardial infarction, markedly decreased mortality.

Table 8 shows the results of experimental therapy of the disturbances of cardiac electric stability in postinfarction cardiosclerosis with phenazepam injected at 1 mg/kg intraperitoneally three times in 2 d prior to testing, the last injection 1 h before assaying the electric stability. As follows from Table 8, postinfarction cardiosclerosis was attended with pronounced ectopic activity of the heart; in vagal bradycardia there were numerous ventricular extrasystoles. The electric fibrillation threshold was lowered threefold. These data are in accord with the clinical observations of the high probability of arrhythmias and fibrillation in patients with postinfarction cardiosclerosis. Phenazepam practially completely abolished ventricular extrasystoles in vagal bradycardia (i.e., suppressed the ectopic activity of the heart) and doubled the fibrillation threshold (i.e., diminished the probability of fibrillation).

It is quite essential that the antiarrhythmic effect in acute myocardial infarction and postinfarction cardiosclerosis was achieved with doses or phenazepam that did not adversely affect arterial pressure. Indeed, Table 9 shows that in the absence of stress (in control and in postinfarction cardiosclerosis) the drug had no effect at all on the pressure in the carotid artery; in acute myocardial infarction the pressure in phenazepam-treated animals proved higher than in unprotected ones. This agrees nicely with prevention of mortality in experimental infarction shown above.

In the aggregate, *the experimental results testify that the benzodiazepine receptor agonist phenazepam to a large extent abolishes the disturbances of cardiac electric stability both in acute experimental myocardial infarction and in chronic postinfarction cardiosclerosis, diminishing in both cases the probability of ventricular arrhythmias and cardiac fibrillation.*

These facts are in accord with the results of another work[45] demonstrating a direct antiarrhythmic effect of this drug in acute ischemia and reperfusion, which takes place in the whole organism, but not in isolated heart and is therefore central.

In interpreting the antiarrhythmic action of phenazepam, it should be remembered that benzodiazepine receptors widely represented in the synaptic structures of the cortex[8] and other brain regions are important for potentiation of the GABA effects at all CNS levels;[45,46] on the other hand, activation of the central adrenergic mechanisms is decisive in impairment of cardiac electric stability in acute ischemia, and accordingly ischemic arrhythmias can be prevented with intracisternal administration of a β-blocker[48] as well as removal of the stellate ganglion.[49] Therefore, diazepines including phenazepam can be thought to boost the GABA-ergic tonic inhibition of the neurons exerting the adrenergic influence on the heart. As a result, excessive activation of these neurons usual in response to acute cardiac ischemia is checked upon administration of phenazepam, producing at the central level the above-shown antiarrhythmic effect.

TABLE 9
Effect of Phenazepam on Blood Pressure In the Carotid Artery in Acute Myocardial Infarction and Postinfarction Cardiosclerosis

Series	Blood pressure (mmHg)	
	Systolic	Diastolic
Control (n = 10)	132 ± 4	108 ± 3
Phenazepam (n = 10)	128 ± 12	97 ± 12
Infarction (n = 10)	84 ± 5	71 ± 6
Infarction plus phenazepam (n = 10)	104 ± 3[a]	86 ± 6
Cardiosclerosis (n = 9)	107 ± 5	97 ± 4
Cardiosclerosis plus phenazepam (n = 9)	106 ± 5	94 ± 5

[a] $p_{3\text{-}4} < 0.01$.

Thus, the data obtained point out that benzodiazepine receptor agonists, as well as other GABA activators, in addition to their conventional psychotropic action display pronounced antiarrhythmic activity and deserve thorough clinical study.

By and large, it can be stated that *the concept of the GABA-ergic system is quite important for cardiology, since deficiency of this or the benzodiazepine receptor system can be involved not only in epilepsy, but in arrhythmias as well,* and pharmocological activation of the GABA-ergic system, either direct or through benzodiazepine receptors, is a promising approach to treating arrhythmias.

III. OPIOIDERGIC SYSTEM*

The opioid peptides (OPs) were initially regarded as endogenous analgetic factors; it was just this action, similar to that of morphine preparations, that gave them their name (i.e., morphine-like). Now, however, there is no doubt that OPs are in fact regulators of numerous processes while their analgetic effect is only one manifestation of their modulatory function. The OPs and their receptors, i.e., both components of the opioidergic system, have been found in the cells of different brain and spinal cord regions,[50,51] peripheral divisions of the nervous system,[50,52] as well as in adrenal glands[53] and other organs, including the heart.[6]

The coupling between the opioidergic and the stress-effecting systems is well studied, and it is known that the opioidergic system can directly participate in the stress reaction as a regulator of sensitivity to pain and as a modulator of emotional, behavioral, and other components of the reaction. This is based on two groups of experimental data. First, during the stress reaction production and liberation of OPs is stimulated in various brain regions, and their blood level rises. This is accompanied with such defensive reactions as elevation of the pain threshold and analgesia,[54] altered behavior,[55] hyperthermia,[56], etc., these reactions being prevented by opiate receptor blockers like naloxone or by opiate synthesis inhibitors. It must be mentioned that in electro- and acupuncture (which can be regarded as brief noninjurious stresses), the analgesia is also accompanied with OP elevation in the blood and in the cerebrospinal fluid, and inhibited with naloxone.[57] Second, administration of OPs or their synthetic analogs produces a dose-dependent analgetic effect and other defensive reactions observed in stress.

The coupling of the opioidergic system to the stress-effecting one, which determines its activation in stress, can be ensured by genetic programming as well as by feedback. An

* With M. G. Pshennikova.

example of genetic coupling is the equimolar release at ACTH and beta-endorphin from the anterior pituitary body,[58,59] which is due to ACTH and beta-endorphin being produced from the common polypeptide precursor pro-opiomelanocortin by the Leu-Phe peptidase.[59,60] Analogously, coupled release of catecholamines and enkephalins from the adrenal glands[62] is due to their common localization in the chromaffin vesicles.[53] A manifestation of feedback is the suppression of both ACTH and beta-endorphin production in the anterior pituitary body through inhibition of the Leu-Phe endopeptidase glucocorticoids released in response to ACTH.[60] The coupling between opioidergic and the stress-effecting systems appears to be manifold, and is reflected, in particular, in that the systems are intimately associated topologically and functionally both in the CNS and in the periphery.[52,63,64]

With regard to the problem of cardiac neural regulation and cardiac arrhythmias, it is noteworthy that the thoracic segments of the spinal cord harbor cholinergic neurons whose axons innervate the sympathetic ganglia, being preganglionic, and the adrenal medulla, ending there on the chromaffin cells. At least a substantial portion of these neurons have been found to contain in their axonic vesicles both acetylcholine and enkephalins.[52] Therefore, when these spinal neurons are activated their axons, besides acetylcholine (stimulating the sympathetic cells of the ganglia and release of adrenal catecholamines), also liberate enkephalins which can inhibit the release of acetylcholine and thereby restrict the neurotransmission in the sympathetic ganglia.[65]

For understanding the direct stress-limiting effect of OPs, it is important that they are secreted substances accumulating biosynthetically in secretory granules or vesicles in the nerve endings or secretory cells. Their release is not constitutive, but is triggered by certain physiological conditions and signals, such as acute changes in the activity of the neurohormonal system, which is definitive for their modulatory function. Thus it has been found that, being localized in the nerve terminals together with norepinephrine, OPs are not released during moderate impulse activity of the nerve, i.e., during moderate liberation of the mediator; only in high and prolonged neural impulsation typical of stress reaction, they are released to inhibit further liberation of the mediator and to prevent its excessive activity.[63]

Thus, *the coupling between the opioidergic and the stress-effecting systems evolved in such a way that opioids are released timely and economically, only in a great or excessive adrenergic stress reaction.*

This means that in the course of adaptation to stress the increasing power of the opioidergic system should reveal itself as direct accumulation of OPs in the corresponding brain and adrenal structures. Only this would allow the adapted animals to check the excitation evoked by adrenergic and cholinergic agents in the brain structures such as the frontal cortex, which has been pointed out as the probable site of formation of an arrhythmogenic excitation focus in acute cardiac ischemia.[11]

Our studies have shown that OPs are indeed accumulated during adaptation to stress, and the catecholamine- or acetylcholine-induced excitation of the frontocortical neurons is indeed suppressed. Thus, using a radioimmunoassay technique we have been able to demonstrate[66] that adaptation to short stress exposures increases the concentrations of enkephalins and beta-endorphin in all brain structures examined and in the adrenal glands (Table 10). Clearly, a result of such adaptation would be that in stress or just upon a strong enough stimulation of the brain neurons the coupled release of OPs (and maybe mediators of other stress-limiting systems) would be enhanced and consequently the adrenoresponsiveness or cholinoresponsiveness of the neurons could be attenuated. To assess the reality of such attenuation at the brain-cortical level, we studied the effect of adaptation to short stresses on the chemoreactive properties of the neurons of the sensomotor cortex, namely on their sensitivity to acetylcholine and norepinephrine.[67] To this end, animals were paralyzed with alpha-tubocurarine, and with the use of a micromanipulator fastened to the cranium a three-bore microelectrode was submerged to the level of the IV-V layer of the cerebral

TABLE 10
Opioid Peptide Content in Brain Structures and Adrenal Glands in Adaptation to Short Stress Exposures

	Peptide content (pmol/mg tissue)		
	Met-enkephalin	**Leu-enkephalin**	**β-Endorphin**
Control (n = 7)			
Cerebellum	22.3 ± 7.8	20.2 ± 3.8	
Hypothalamus	226.7 ± 9.2	123.3 ± 22.9	10.2 ± 0.8
Striatum	263.2 ± 8.9	186.0 ± 17.5	
Cortex	60.5 ± 7.5	49.1 ± 5.7	
Adrenal glands	53.7 ± 1.7	71.8 ± 8.4	
Adaptation (n = 7)			
Cerebellum	40.9 ± 7.1[a]	37.2 ± 6.8[a]	
Hypothalamus	422.3 ± 45.4[b]	271.9 ± 41.2[b]	17.8 ± 1.5[a]
Striatum	468.8 ± 44.0[b]	538.9 ± 40.5[c]	
Cortex	65.8 ± 5.1	56.5 ± 5.0	
Adrenal glands	134.0 ± 29.3[b]	156.7 ± 42.4[a]	

Difference from respective controls significant at:
[a] $p < 0.05$.
[b] $p < 0.01$.
[c] $p < 0.001$.

sensomotor cortex. The bores were filled with 3 *M* NaCl (recording electrode), 2 *M* acetylcholine, and 0.2 *M* norepinephrine bitartrate. The neuromediators were administered to the neurons with an electrophoretic current of 30 to 40 nA for 30 s, and 60-s recordings of the impulse activity before and after administration of the compounds were compared; the criterion of neuronal reaction was at least a 20% change in the pulsation rate. In total, 111 neurons have been thus registered in control and 48 in adapted animals. In the relative numbers of activated, unresponsive, and inhibited neurons upon acetylcholine and norepinephrine administration, the adapted animals differed markedly from the controls. The portion of unresponsive neurons in adapted animals increased 2 to 2.7-fold, while that of responsive neurons fell by 39 to 56% with the number of inhibited neurons declining to a greater extent. A more detailed study showed that the average reaction of neurons to acetylcholine and norepinephrine was much less pronounced in adapted animals. Thus with activated neurons the effect of norepinephrine was twofold in control, but only 34% in adapted animals; with inhibited neurons norepinephrine decreased their activity by 77% in control and by 34% in adapted animals. The responses to acetylcholine were also attenuated, albeit to a much smaller extent.

As shown in recent years, OPs can restrict the adrenergic regulation and other links of the stress reaction by several concrete mechanisms. First, at the presynaptic level the norepinephrine release from sympathetic terminals in the CNS and in the periphery can be suppressed by the action of OPs on the opiate receptors on the terminals.[6,68,69] Second, OPs can also inhibit the adrenergic neurons themselves in the CNS and in the peripheral sympathetic ganglia,[63,70] and block liberation of catecholamines from the adrenal glands and their action on the effector organs, which takes place through the postsynaptic opiate receptors.[63,70] Third, besides restricting the activity and the effects of the adrenergic system, OPs can modulate the release of hormones. Beta-endorphin produced in the pituitary body has been shown to locally inhibit there the liberation of a stress hormone vasopressin.[71] OPs inhibit the biosynthesis and liberation of corticosteroids, including glucocorticoids.[72] On the other hand, OPs can activate the secretion of insulin,[73] usually depressed in stress, and secretion of thyrocalcitonin and somatotropin[74] participating in the adaptive effects of stress reaction (see Chapter 1).

In other words, OPs check the mobilizing effect of stress, preventing its transition to a detrimental one (Chapter 1). This was the basis for introducing OPs and their analogs to suppress the stress reaction and its injurious effects, in particular to prevent or attenuate the stress-induced and ischemic damage to the heart.

In stress caused in rats by 18-h hanging by the cervical fold, prior administration of a leu-enkephalin analog (0.1 mg/kg) substantially alleviated the complex of nonspecific stress damage (gastric ulceration, eosinopenia, and atrophy of the thymus) and checked the glucocorticoid elevation in blood.[75] Again, in stress caused by acute myocardial ischemia some leu-enkephalin analogs attenuated the stress-induced elevation of blood cortisol and prevented the rise in aldosterone,[76,77] as well as attenuated twofold to threefold the stress increase in catecholamine excretion with urine.[78] Concurrently, OP administration before such stress prevented the stress decline in insulin secretion and the phenomenon of "stress diabetes".[78] Finally, prior administration of OPs efficiently prevented the rise in blood vasopressin in stress from acute myocardial ischemia or trauma.[76]

It must be accentuated that restriction of the stress reaction with OPs is associated with prevention or alleviation of the stress damage and functional disturbances to the heart. Thus, we have shown that prior administration of beta-endorphin is effective against the stress-induced impairment of the contractile function of nonischemic myocardial regions in rats with acute experimental myocardial infarction.[79] Similarly, a leu-enkephalin analog dalargin substantially restricted myocardial damage caused by a 6-h EPS.[80] In this work, the damage was assessed by accumulation of labeled technetium pyrophospate in the myocardium and by the creatine phosphokinase level in the serum, i.e., by the generally accepted criteria of cardiomyocyte membrane damage. Introduction of dalargin decreased more than by half the label accumulation at the peak of injury (12 h after stress) and reliably attenuated the stress elevation of the enzyme in blood. In the mechanism of protective action of OPs against cardiac stress injury, which is largely adrenergic in nature (see Chapter 1), an important place besides checking the catecholamine "discharge" is occupied by suppression of catecholamine action on the heart owing to adenylate cyclase inhibition through opiate receptors on the cardiac cells. Indeed, the adrenergic novodrin injury, displaying features of stress and ischemic damage and attended with release of cardiomyocyte markers into the blood, is associated with a rise in myocardial cAMP; prior administration of dalargin completely prevents this activation of adenylate cyclase,[76] i.e., virtually blocks the intracellular effects of adrenomimetics. Thus, *the protective effect of OPs against cardiac stress damage appears to involve their inhibitory influence on the centers of cardiac adrenergic regulation and also the influence on the heart proper where they inhibit norepinephrine release from sympathetic terminals and its action on the adenylate cyclase system.*

On this basis, we have recently for the first time used dalargin to prevent ischemic and reperfusion arrhythmias.[81] Table 11 demonstrates that in intact animals pretreatment with dalargin decreases more than by half the overall duration of all types of arrhythmia both in ischemia and in reperfusion, including the grave forms such as ventricular fibrillation, the mean duration of which in reperfusion is four times less in dalargin-treated animals. It is quite essential that dalargin markedly diminishes the incidence of fibrillation and prevents death from fibrillation (Table 11). Thus, *in the whole organism dalargin exhibits a protective antiarrhythmic action in acute ischemia and reperfusion.* With isolated hearts, no such effect of this OP could be observed.

Attention should be paid to the fact that the opioidergic system is topologically and functionally linked not only with the stress-effecting, but also with other regulatory systems that now can be referred to as stress-limiting ones. In particular, it is most tightly connected with the serotoninergic system, as shown by two lines of evidence. First, opiates and OPs markedly increase formation and liberation of serotonin from serotonergic neurons.[82-84] Second, the analgetic action of OP is in large measure realized with the help of the sero-

TABLE 11
Effect of Dalargin on Cardiac Rhythm Disorders in Acute Ischemia and Reperfusion in the Whole Organism

	Ischemia (10 min)		Reperfusion (10 min)	
Indices	Control (n = 11)	Dalargin (n = 11)	Control (n = 10)	Dalargin (n = 10)
Extrasystole				
Number of animals	10	11	9	9
Total duration	259	243	66	92
Mean duration	24 ± 4	22 ± 7	7 ± 4	9 ± 4
Ventricular tachycardia				
Number of animals	11	9	10	9
Total duration	895	240	1364	467
Mean duration	81 ± 19	22 ± 8[a]	136 ± 29	47 ± 13[a]
Ventricular fibrillation				
Number of animals	8	2	5	2
Total duration	386	252	502	120
Mean duration	35 ± 17	23 ± 28	50 ± 36	12 ± 18[a]
All arrhythmias				
Total duration	1540	735	1924	679
Mean duration	140 ± 22	67 ± 25	192 ± 43	68 ± 24[a]
Deaths	1	1	5	0

[a] Difference from respective controls significant at $p < 0.01$.

toninergic system and dependent on serotonin metabolism. In rats the antinociceptive activity of OP introduced into the cerebral ventricles is potentiated by serotonin and weakened by prior reserpinization and depletion of the serotonin depot;[85] suppression of serotonin reuptake enhances,[85] while blocking the serotonergic receptors weakens the OP effect.[86] These data and the results of direct electrophysiological studies on the effect of OPs on interneuronal transmission at different levels on the CNS give grounds for supposing that OP can inhibit the interneuronal transmission of excitation, which in the spinal marrow takes place through activation of the serotoninergic system by the opiate receptors of corresponding neurons.

In the words, *the emerging notion is that the stress-effecting system is coupled, through the opioidergic one or in a more direct way to the serotoninergic system, whereby the latter acquires a stress-limiting function.*

Indeed, already in 15 to 30 min after the onset of immobilization stress in rats there is an elevation of serotonin in the hypothalamus and of its metabolite 5-hydroxyindole acetic acid in the hypothalamus, tonsil, hippocampus, and medulla oblongata.[87,88] Serotonin, on the one hand, is involved in stimulating the hypothalamic production of the ACTH-releasing factor and ensuing secretion of ACTH and endophins by the pituitary gland,[89] and on the other hand the OP-induced activation of the serotoninergic system has been shown above to produce a stress-limiting effect itself. It is quite instructive that even when these notions were only emerging, Rabinowtiz and Lown,[90] on the basis of the first data on the ability of serotonin to check the excitation of the brain adrenergic centers, undertook a successful attempt to achieve an antiarrhythmic effect by augmenting the serotonin concentration in the brain. This was done by combined administration of three substances: (1) the serotonin precursor tryptophan, (2) a decarboxylase inhibitor to interrupt tryptophan conversion to serotonin in all tissues except the brain, and (3) a monoamine oxidase inhibitor to prevent serotonin breakdown in the brain. The resulting elevation of the brain serotonin content produced a stable increase in the cardiac threshold for stimuli causing extrasystole.

We have recently undertaken a study[91] of the effect of adaptation to stress on the serotonin content in the midbrain where in the region of the raphe there is a large congregation of serotonergic neurons. The fluorimetric assay showed that the serotonin content increased by about 60%. Since such adaptation has a pronounced antiarrhythmic effect, at the next stage of our work we tried to prevent arrhythmias caused in conscious rats according to Lepran et al.[41] with a synthetic serotonin analog 4-nitro-5-methoxytryptamine hydrochloride synthesized by Petrunin of the D. I. Mendeleev Chemical-Technical Institute, Moscow. Prior administration of this serotonin analog decreased threefold the total duration of all types of arrhythmia and fivefold the incidence of cardiac fibrillation in conscious acutely ischemic animals; mortality was completely abolished.

In the aggregate the above signifies that the opioidergic and linked serotoninergic systems can restrict the stress reaction, and accordingly their mediators or synthetic analogs thereof have stress-limiting and specifically cardioprotective and antiarrhythmic effects. This is summarized in Figure 2.

Among other things, the proposed concept implies that genetic or acquired deficiency of the opioidergic system can augment the vulnerability of the organism to stress, whereas enchanced power of this system, conversely, can increase the organismic resistance to such influences. Indeed, in four lines of mice with differing innate density of opiate receptors in the brain this feature clearly correlated with the extent of analgesia in stress.[92] Spontaneously hypertensive rats with enhanced activity of the sympathetic system[93] display a congenitally low OP content in tissues.[94] Furthermore, in myocardial infarction patients the severity of the stress component, pain syndrome, and enzymemia is the greater the lower is the beta-endorphin content in the blood.[95] This is the reason for adaptational or pharmacological activation of the opioidergic system, or "pharmacoprosthetics" with its mediators or their synthetic analogs.

IV. PARASYMPATHETIC SYSTEM, ITS CARDIOPROTECTIVE EFFECTS, AND ANTIARRHYTHMIC ACTION OF AN ACETYLCHOLINE ANALOG

Increasing vagal tone or vagal stimulation under certain conditions are known to raise the cardiac fibrillation threshold and even to stop the developing arrhythmias.[96] This is commonly thought to result from restriction of the excessive adrenergic influence on the heart in stress and ischemia.[11,12] The adrenergic action is limited because acetylcholine acts as an agonist of muscarinic receptors to suppress norepinephrine release from sympathetic terminals[97,98] and also restricts the response to norepinephrine at the receptor level.[98] Further, it should be borne in mind that in the heart the muscarinic receptors are coupled through guanine nucleotide-binding proteins with K^+ efflux channels, and with the β-receptor-linked adenylate cyclase. Acetylcholine acting on the muscarinic receptors activates the K^+ channels to enhance K^+ efflux from the cell, but inhibits the adenylate cyclase to restrict the cAMP-dependent Ca^{2+} entry. This results in hyperpolarization and decreasing excitability of the cardiocyte membrane.[99,100] Increasing concentrations of acetylcholine have also been shown to attenuate the potential-dependent entry of Na^+ and Ca^{2+}, which also favors hyperpolarization.[100,101]

On the whole, the cardiac cholinergic apparatus restricts the excessive adrenergic stress effects on the heart, favors maintenance of a high enough RP of the myocardial cells, and thus acts as a stress-limiting antiarrhythmic factor.[101]

Obviously, through this mechanism, increasing tonicity of the cardiac parasympathetic regulation can play an important part in the protective, antiarrhythmic effect of adaptation to stress.

To test this suggestion, together with Kuznetsov we carried out experiments in which the mobility of rats was largely restrained by placing the animals in small boxes; this created a relatively mild immobilization stress which the animals experienced for 5 d and thus

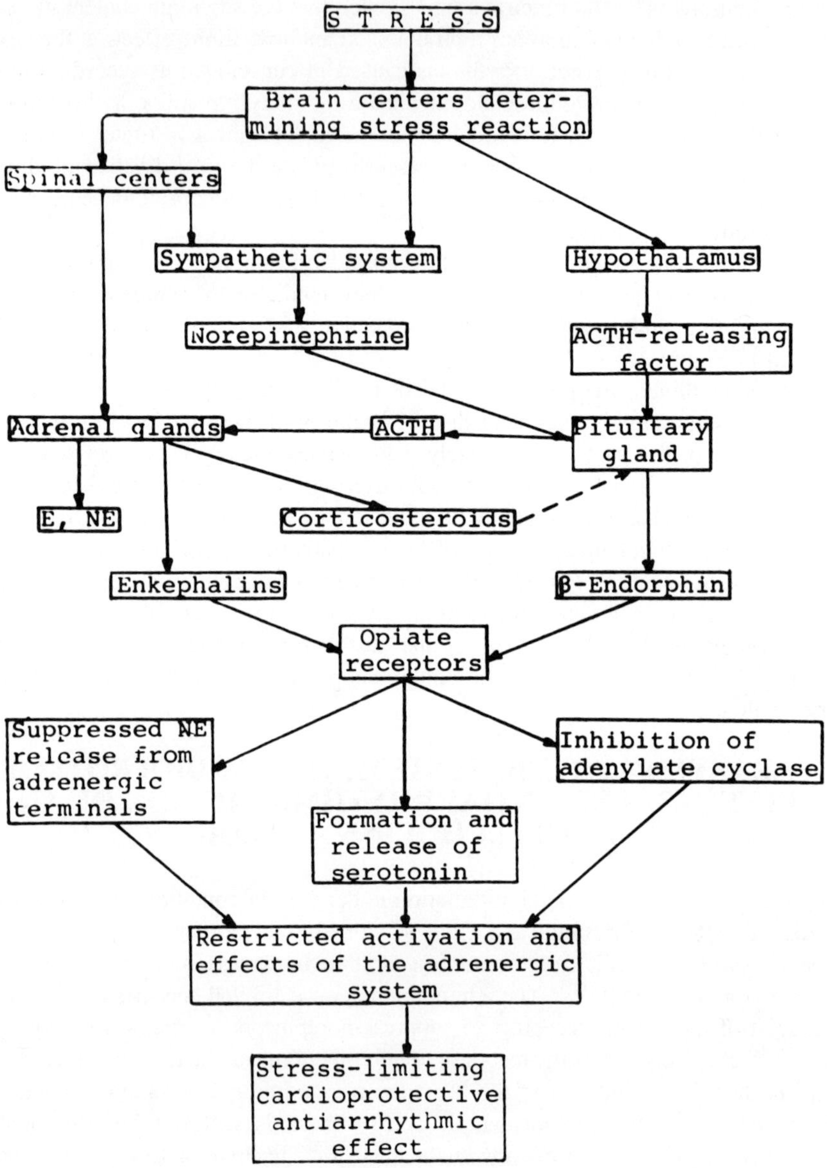

FIGURE 2. Coupling of the opioidergic system with the stress-effecting and the serotoninergic system; the stress-limiting cardioprotective effect of the opioidergic system. The broken arrow denotes the inhibitory influence of corticosteroids on ACTH and OP formation in the pituitary gland. For explanations see text.

adapted to this moderate stress. The results presented in Table 12 show that after 1 d of stress there was no appreciable change in the heart rate, whereas the ventricular fibrillation threshold decreased by half. By the fifth day bradycardia grew definite, while the fibrillation threshold was restored to normal. Administration of atropine at this time normalized the heart rate, but again decreased the fibrillation threshold. Thus, a 5-d adaptation to relatively mild stress resulted in increasing tonic negatively chronotropic vagal influence on the heart with concomitant restitution of the initially lowered cardiac fibrillation threshold.

Next, the animals were subjected to a 10-min ischemia followed by reperfusion as described earlier (see Chapter 3) to register the developing arrhythmias. Table 13 shows

TABLE 12
Rat Heart Rate and Fibrillation Threshold in Adaptation to Continuous 5-d Stress and Blockade of the Cholinergic Innervation

Series	Heart rate (min^{-1})	Fibrillation threshold (mA)
Control (n = 10)	441 ± 8	7.84 ± 0.24
1-d stress (n = 10)	413 ± 20	4.10 ± 0.57
5-d stress (n = 7)	354 ± 11	7.64 ± 0.58
5-d stress plus atropine (n = 8)	492 ± 13	5.07 ± 0.62
$p_{1\text{-}2}$		<0.001
$p_{1\text{-}3}$	<0.001	
$p_{3\text{-}4}$	<0.001	<0.01

that adaptation decreased the overall duration of grave arrhythmias (ventricular tachycardia and fibrillation) more than sevenfold in ischemia and about threefold in reperfusion. In both cases this protective effect was abolished by atropine (10 mg/kg).

Thus, in the course of adaptation to continuous stress there is a gradual increase in the tonic vagal influence on the heart manifesting itself as bradycardia, normalization of the fibrillation threshold, and markedly enhanced resistance of the heart to the arrhythmogenic action of ischemia and reperfusion.

The gradually increasing tonic influence of the parasympathetic system on the heart in adaptation to continuous stress can serve as a natural stress-limiting antiarrhythmic factor. It is noteworthy that in this case resistance to such potent arrhythmogens as ischemia and reperfusion is enhanced not at the expense of heavy episodic exposures of the heart to negatively chronotropic influences, which can well be dangerous, but owing to a steadily enforced cholinergic regulation of the heart.

Basing on the principle of ''imitating'' the natural stress-limiting systems of the organism, we arrived at an idea that the new data on the role of parasympathetic regulation in antiarrhythmic mechanism of adaptation make topical a search for new cardioprotectors which would in full measure possess the adrenolytic and hyperpolarizing properties of acetylcholine, but would be free of its excessive negatively chronotropic effect, thus making optimal antiarrhythmics. It stands to reason that, first of all, attention should be paid to natural and synthetic compounds structurally close to acetylcholine. A family of this kind is formed by γ-butyrobetaine derivatives constantly produced in the brain and the heart.[102,103]

An analogous compound, which was synthesized by Kalvins and co-workers in the Institute of Organic Synthesis, Latvian Academy of Sciences, and which we had an opportunity to test, is ethyl-3(2-ethyl-2,2-dimethylhydrazinium) propionate (EDIHYP).

Figure 3 shows the chemical structure of acetylcholine and EDIHYP; there is obvious similarity, yet certain differences in properties and activity could be expected, taking account of the fact that acetylcholine esterase does not hydrolyze γ-butyrobetaine esters.[104,105]

Our studies with Abdikaliev were aimed at evaluating the antiarrhythmic properties of EDIHYP in clinically pertinent experimental models and elucidating the mechanism of its action.

The antiarrhythmic effects of EDIHYP were assessed in acute aschemia and reperfusion in anesthetized rats, in acute myocardial infarction, and in postinfarction cardiosclerosis. In all cases the drug was administered at 25 mg/kg *per os* 2 h before the tests. The main issues from the experiments were as follows:

1. In ischemia caused by a 10-min clamping on the left coronary artery, EDIHYP does not appreciably alter the number of extrasystoles, but decreases by half the mean

TABLE 13
Effect of Adaptation to Moderate Stress on Cardiac Rhythm Disorders in Ischemia and Reperfusion with Intact and Blocked Cholinergic Innervation

	Ischemia				Reperfusion			
Indices	**Control (n = 11)**	**Atropine (n = 11)**	**Adaptation (n = 8)**	**Adaptation + atropine (n = 9)**	**Control (n = 11)**	**Atropine (n = 11)**	**Adaptation (n = 8)**	**Adaptation + atropine (n = 9)**
Extrasystole								
Number of animals	11	11	8	9	10	11	8	8
Total number of extrasystoles	324	421	178	737	219	305	70	204
Ventricular tachycardia								
Number of animals	6	6	2	5	10	10	6	7
Total duration	29	63	4	55	202	148	64	118
Mean duration	2.7 ± 2.5	5.7 ± 5.3	0.5 ± 0.7[a]	6.1 ± 5.5[b]	18.4 ± 5.2	13.4 ± 4.2	7.6 ± 4.4[a]	13.1 ± 5.2
Ventricular fibrillation								
Number of animals	2	2	0	2	3	3	0	2
Total duration	11	13	0	7	45	78	0	18
Mean duration of grave arrhythmias	3.7 ± 4.0	6.9 ± 6.4	0.5 ± 0.7[a]	6.9 ± 6.5[b]	22.5 ± 9.3	20.4 ± 10.3	7.6 ± 4.4[a]	15.1 ± 9.1

Difference with respective (a) ''control'' or (b) ''adaptation'' significant at $p < 0.05$.

1 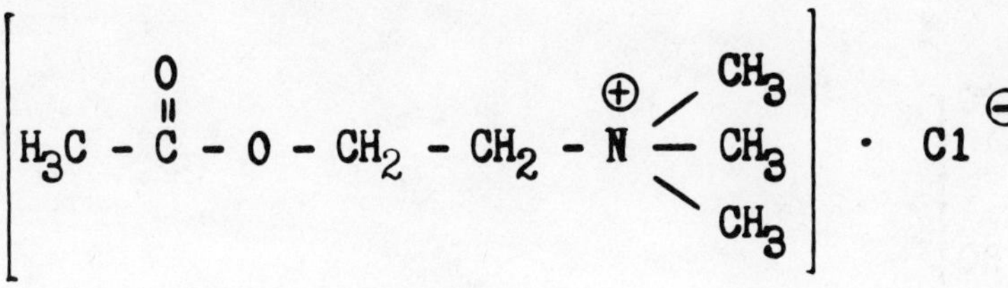

ACETYLCHOLINE

2 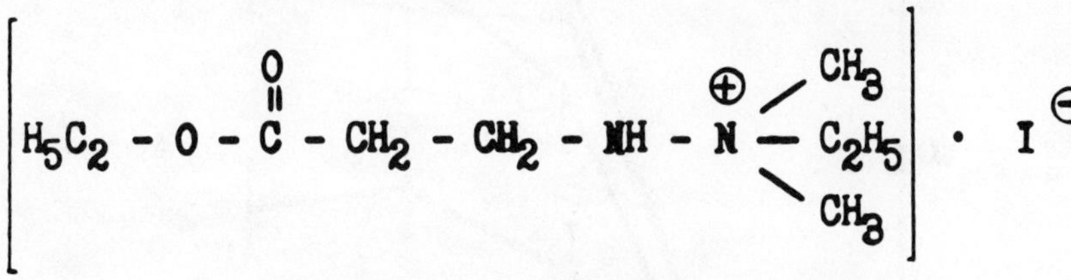

ETHYL-3-(2,2-DIMETHYL-2-ETHYLHYDRAZINIUM) PROPIONATE (EDIHYP)

FIGURE 3. Structural formulas of (1) acetylcholine and (2) EDIHYP.

duration per animal of ventricular tachycardia, and diminishes 5-fold the incidence of fibrillation in acute ischemia (accordingly, the mean duration per animal of such arrhythmias falls 90-fold). In reperfusion the number of extrasystoles is decreased 2.5-fold, and mean durations of ventricular tachycardia and ventricular fibrillation decreased 5-fold and 3-fold, respectively. Thus, the antiarrhythmic effect of EDIHYP is greater in ischemic than in reperfusion arrhythmias.

2. In acute myocardial infarction and postinfarction cardiosclerosis, experimental therapy with EDIHYP abolishes the drop in ventricular fibrillation threshold commonly observed in these conditions, and decreases 7-fold to 8-fold the number of extrasystoles elicited in vagal bradycardia. Thus, *EDIHYP suppresses the ectopic activity of the heart in acute myocardial infarction and postinfarction cardiosclerosis.*

In studying the mechanism of this pronounced antiarrhythmic effect, we took account of the fact that the conditions of our model are rather close to the clinical ones, and on the other hand the most potent clinical antiarrhythmics are found among blockers of β-adrenoreceptors and of slow Ca^{2+} channels. This is explained by the fact that such compounds restrict or abolish the cardiotoxic action of high catecholamine and calcium concentrations, i.e., eliminate the two major pathogenetic links of arrhythmias. In this context we studied the adrenolytic and Ca-protective effects of EDIHYP. In all experiments with whole animals and isolated hearts we used atropine to check the extent to which the protective effect of EDIHYP as an acetylcholine analog is due to its binding with muscarinic receptors.

To assess the effect of EDIHYP on the cardiac damage by toxic epinephrine concentrations, four series of experiments were performed with isolated isotonically contracting hearts perfused according to Langendorf: (1) 15 min of perfusion with $5 \cdot 10^{-5}$ *M* epinephrine; (2) addition of 10^{-5} *M* EDIHYP before epinephrine; (3) 10^{-7} *M* atropine before epinephrine; and (4) EDIHYP, atropine, and epinephrine. In these experiments two issues have been established:

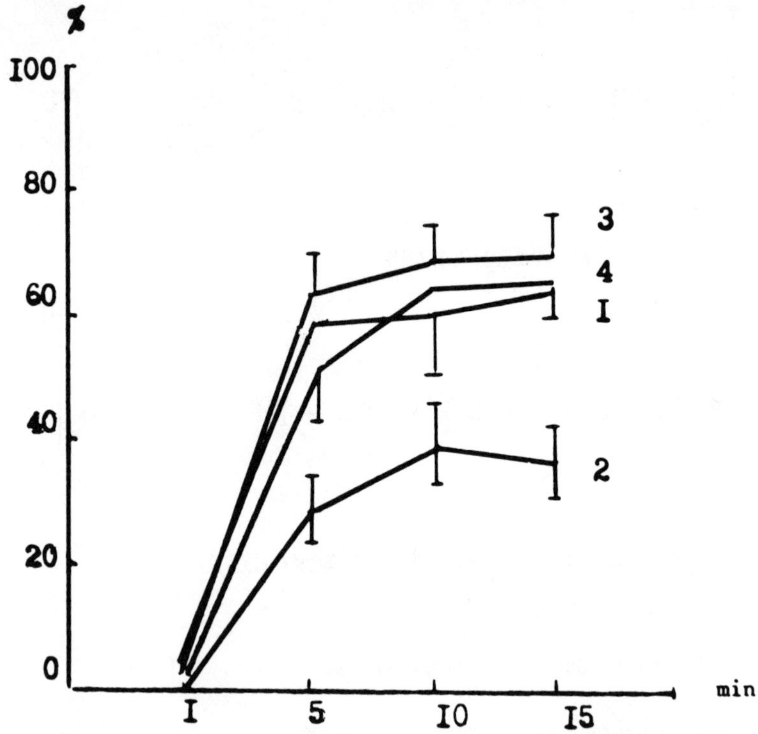

FIGURE 4. Effect of EDIHYP on the contracture caused with cardiotoxic doses of epinephrine. (1) Epinephrine; (2) EDIHYP plus epinephrine; (3) EDIHYP plus atropine plus epinephrine; (4) atropine plus epinephrine. The abscissa is time after administration, in minutes; the ordinate is extent of contracture, percent of the initial contraction amplitude.

1. Epinephrine at this concentration causes contracture of isolated hearts and decreases approximately threefold the main parameters of their contractile function: amplitude and velocity of contraction and velocity of relaxation. Figure 4 shows that EDIHYP reliably attenuates the adrenotoxic contracture, and by virtue of this checks the depression of the contraction amplitude. It can further be seen that atropine abolishes this anticontractural effect of EDIHYP which can therefore be supposed to take place through the muscarinic receptors, though, under these conditions it is not attended with a negatively chronotropic effect (no bradycardia is observable).
2. Moderate extrasystole (mean 77 extrasystoles per heart) develops by the tenth minute of exposure to epinephrine, which is reduced threefold ($p < 0.05$) with EDIHYP. Atropine by itself does not affect the extent of adrenotoxic arrhythmia, and in combination with EDIHYP does not change its antiarrhythmic effect. Hence, *the antiarrhythmic action of EDIHYP in adrenotoxic damage to the isolated heart does not involve the muscarinic receptors.*

In further studies, to assess the role of the antiadrenergic component in the protective effect of EDIHYP, we made use of a rather arbitrary model which is nevertheless accepted in modern pharmocology of arrhythmias, namely the arrhythmias evoked with intravenous administration of toxic doses (200 mg/kg) of calcium chloride; they are often regarded as the result of activation of adrenergic centers and enhanced discharge of catecholamines.[106] No matter how true is this opinion, the ability of some nontoxic substance to prevent at single administration the lethal arrhythmias caused by calcium chloride is obviously a reliable indication of its high antiarrhythmic activity.

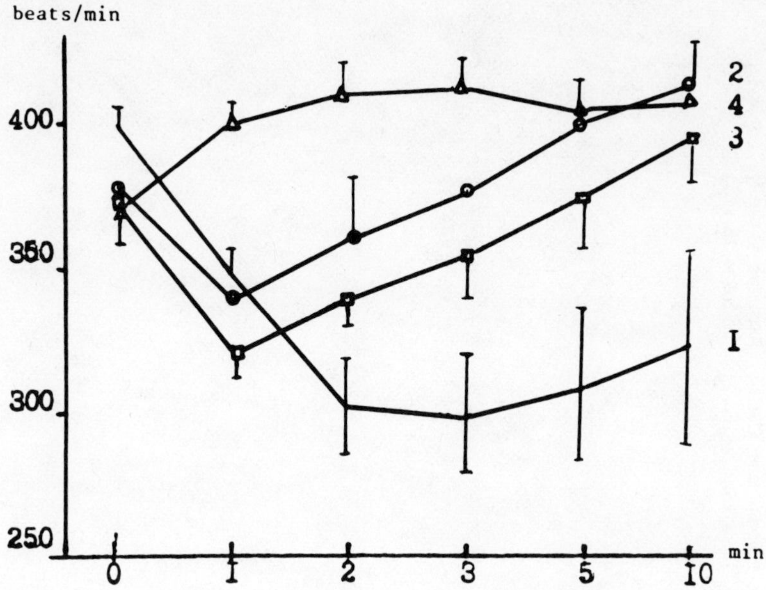

FIGURE 5. Effect of EDIHYP on the heart rate in $CaCl_2$-induced arrhythmia. (1) $CaCl_2$; (2) EDIHYP plus $CaCl_2$; (3) atropine plus $CaCl_2$; (4) atropine plus EDIHYP plus $CaCl_2$. The abscissa is time in minutes; the ordinate is heart rate in beats per minute.

In these experiments EDIHYP was administered at 5 mg/kg intravenously, 5 min before calcium chloride. The results are presented in Table 14 and Figure 5 and yield three main points.

1. EDIHYP administered before calcium chloride exhibits a pronounced antiarrhythmic effect. Indeed, in the control series 9 animals out of 15 died of fibrillation and ensuing cardiac arrest that occurred within 10 min following calcium chloride injection. The animals pretreated with EDIHYP developed no ventricular tachycardia or fibrillation and none of them died within the whole observation period. The mere comparison of mortality (60% in controls vs. none in protected animals) leaves no doubt about the powerful protection provided by EDIHYP against lethal $CaCl_2$-induced arrhythmias.
2. The antiarrhythmic action of EDIHYP does not appear to involve a cholinergic component. Indeed, the ''cholinergic'' side effects — salivation and lacrimation — observed in the first minute after EDIHYP injection are completely abolished with a low dose of atropine (0.1 mg/kg, i.e., one tenth that used to block the muscarinic receptors) which does not at all attenuate the radical antiarrhythmic effect of EDIHYP.
3. The effect of EDIHYP and low doses of atropine in $CaCl_2$ arrhythmias is peculiarly synergistic. Atropine by itself at low doses does not appreciably change the number of extrasystoles or mortality, and even shortens by half the time from $CaCl_2$ injection to cardiac arrest (Table 14, $p < 0.001$), which is in line with the present day notion of the stabilizing action of the parasympathetic system on cardiac rhythm.[107] However, when introduced with EDIHYP, atropine not only does not interfere with its antiarrhythmic action, but even further diminishes the number of extrasystoles (Table 14). Moreover, Figure 5 shows that bradycardia observed in the first 10 min after $CaCl_2$ injection is only shortened, yet still manifest with either drug alone, but completely abolished with the combination of EDIHYP and low atropine.

TABLE 14
Effect of EDIHYP on the $CaCl_2$-Induced Arrhythmias

Indices	Control + $CaCl_2$ (n = 15)	EDIHYP + $CaCl_2$ (n = 15)	EDIHYP + atropine + $CaCl_2$ (n = 15)	Atropine + $CaCl_2$ (n = 15)
Estrasystole				
Number of animals	13	6	2	9
Total number of extrasystoles	245	22	5	270
Ventricular tachycardia				
Number of animals	9	0	0	8
Total duration	236	0	0	135
Ventricular fibrillation				
Number of animals	10	0	0	6
Total duration	365	0	0	163
Mean time from $CaCl_2$ to cardiac arrest	6.6 ± 2.0			3.2 ± 0.4
Deaths within 10 min from $CaCl_2$	9	0	0	7

In the aggregate, the data obtained unequivocally testify to the pronounced protective action of EDIHYP against arrhythmias caused with toxic doses of calcium chloride. Thus, we are dealing with a promising antiarrhythmic.

Next, we assessed the ability of EDIHYP to check the contractural and arrhythmogenic action of high calcium concentrations on the isolated heart. Experiments were run with isotonically contracting hearts obtained from control animals and from those subjected to a 2-h immobilization stress. When the Ca^{2+} concentration in the perfusing solution was raised from 1.36 to 10 m*M*, pronounced contracture developed in the control hearts; it was still two to three times greater in the poststress hearts, more than half of which (6 of 11) went into fibrillation in 2 to 4 min of exposure to high calcium. The main result was that virtually no contracture or fibrillation was observed in the hearts of animals that received EDIHYP (25 mg/kg *per os* immediately before stress or 2 h before taking the hearts). *Hence, a single peroral administration of a relatively small nontoxic dose of this acetycholine analog, without causing bradycardia, not only protects the heart from stress-induced impairment of its contractile function, but markedly enhances myocardial resistance to the cardiotoxic action of high calcium concentrations — calcium contracture and cardiac fibrillation. Since excess* Ca^{2+} *is a common central link of the pathogenesis of most various kinds of cardiac damage (viz. adrenergic, ischemic, reperfusion, hereditary cardiomyopathic), the discovered cardioprotective effect appears quite important.*

The pronounced antiarrhythmic and anticontractual effects of EDIHYP raised a question whether or not this acetylcholine analog can act on the muscarinic receptors *in vitro* when there is no competition from acetylcholine. A typical experiment presented in Figure 6 shows that introduction by a high EDIHYP concentration (10^{-4} *M*) into the perfusing solution of the isolated heart decreases the contraction rate by 100 beats per minute (cf. lanes a and b); addition of 10^{-7} *M* atropine almost completely abolishes this effect (lane c), although by itself atropine does not change the contraction rate (lane d). Thus, at a high concentration and without competition from acetycholine existing in the whole organism, EDIHYP can act on the muscarinic receptors to cause bradycardia. The next question arising in this connection is whether or not this action is anyhow involved in the antiarrhythmic effect of EDIHYP or whether or not it can take place under complete blockade of the muscarinic receptors.

The answer comes from Table 15, showing the effect of 10^{-4} *M* EDIHYP, 10^{-7} *M* atropine, and their combination on ischemic and reperfusion arrhythmias produced in the isolated heart. We can see that either agent produces hardly any effect by itself, but together they prove highly protective in both conditions. The ischemic arrhythmias are known to be largely neurogenic in origin.[11,12] and only weakly pronounced in the isolated heart; yet EDIHYP plus atropine decreases threefold to fivefold the number of hearts with extrasystole and the total number of extrasystoles as compared with other series. Their combined effect is still more striking in reperfusion; the mean duration of fibrillation is diminished by more than an order of magnitude, and all hearts keep contracting by the fifth minute of reperfusion when most of them have stopped in other series.

Summing up, though *in principle EDIHYP may produce a negative chronotropic effect via the muscarinic receptors, this has nothing to do with its antiarrhythmic action, which in the whole organism (in acute ischemia and reperfusion, myocardial infarction, or postinfarction cardiosclerosis, see above) is never attended with bradycardia or other cholinergic effects, and in the isolated heart is effectual just under blockade of the muscarinic receptors and absence of bradycardia.*

Of course, the exact mechanism of EDIHYP action is to be elucidated with the techniques of molecular pharmacology. At present it can only be supposed that this acetylcholine analog has a lower affinity for the muscarinic receptors than their natural agonist acetylcholine. Therefore, in the organism EDIHYP can usually add nothing to the tonic influence of the

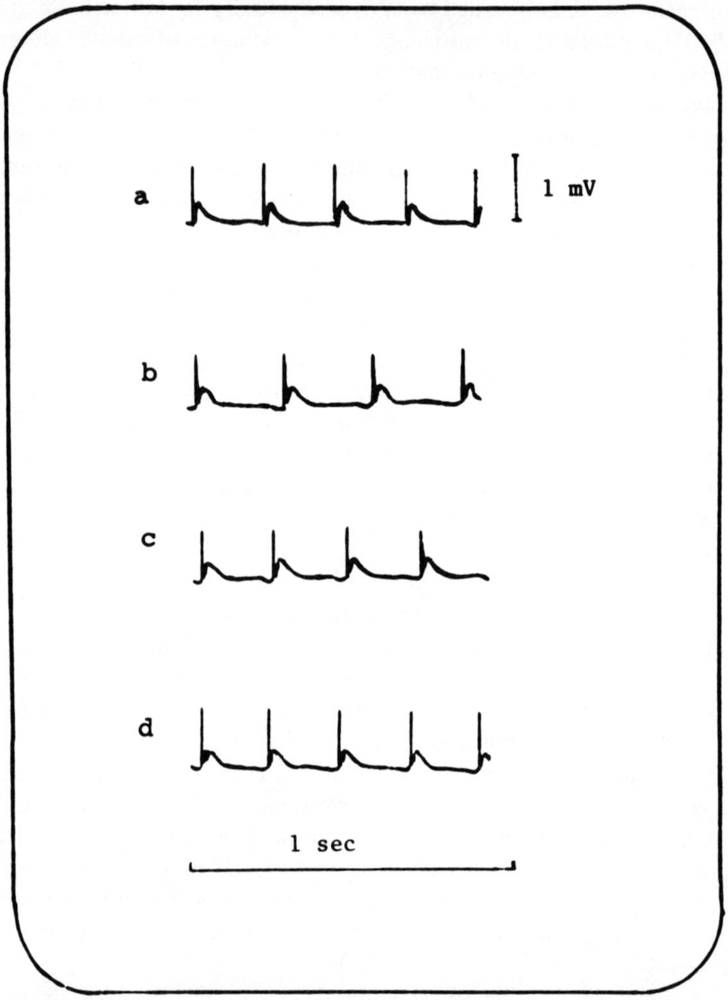

FIGURE 6. Effects of EDIHYP, atropine, and their combination on isolated heart contraction (electrograms). (a) Control; (b) 10^{-4} *M* EDIHYP; (c) 10^{-4} *M* EDIHYP plus 10^{-7} *M* atropine; (d) 10^{-7} *M* atropine.

parasympathetic cholinergic system on the heart and causes no bradycardia. It is obvious, on the other hand, that the powerful cardioprotective and specifically antiarrhythmic action of EDIHYP must involve some other regulatory mechanisms of the cell. To mention a couple of yet speculative possibilities, EDIHYP may act directly on the K^+ channels linked to the receptors via the regulatory G-protein,[99,108] but unlike tetraethylammonium[100] does not block, but activates them, producing an acetylcholine-like hyperpolarization and enhancing thereby the myocardial resistance to arrhythmogenic factors. Again, EDIHYP may act like the pertussoid toxin[108] via the G-protein α-subunit to inhibit the adenylate cyclase and to limit thereby the cAMP-dependent Ca^{2+} entry into the cells; this would hinder membrane depolarizaton in ischemia, reperfusion, or excess of catecholamines, contributing thus to the antiarrhythmic effect of EDIHYP.

This question, however, awaits further detailed and first of all biochemical studies with the use of labeled ligands and EDIHYP. In the context of this book, *it is noteworthy how the ''principle of imitation'' applied even to the most studied stress-limiting system such as the parasympathetic one can somewhat unexpectedly yield novel potent cardioprotective drugs.*

TABLE 15
Effects of EDIHYP, Atropine, and Their Combination on Rhythm Disturbances in Ischemia and Reperfusion of the Isolated Heart (in Each Series n = 10)

Indices	Ischemia				Reperfusion			
	Control	EDIHYP	EDIHYP + atropine	Atropine	Control	EDIHYP	EDIHYP + atropine	Atropine
Extrasystole								
Number of animals	7	8	2	3	8	8	10	9
Total number of extrasystoles	400	435	90	310	310	375	825	315
Ventricular tachycardia								
Number of animals	1	0	0	3	10	9	9	10
Total duration	28	0	0	26	535	412	133	325
Mean duration					54 ± 22	41 ± 12	13 ± 5	33 ± 8
Ventricular fibrillation								
Number of animals	0	0	0	0	8	7	5	8
Total duration					1516	978	82	1987
Mean duration					152 ± 29	98 ± 22	8 ± 8[a]	199 ± 28
Grave arrhythmias (VT + VF)								
Mean duration					205 ± 34	139 ± 25[a]	22 ± 13[a]	231 ± 34
Hearts working in 5 min of reperfusion					3	5	10	2

[a] Difference with control significant at $p < 0.01$.

REFERENCES

1. **Meerson, F. Z., Malyshev, V. V., Petrova, V. A., and Lifant'ev, V.I.,** Prevention of activation of the hypophysial-adrenal system and cardiac damage in stress with the antioxidant ionol (in Russian), *Kardiologiya,* 9, 85, 1982.
2. **Pycock, C. J., Horton, R. W., and Carter, C. J.,** Interaction of hydroxytryptamine and γ-aminobutyric acid with dopamine, *Adv. Biochem. Pharmacol.,* 19, 323, 1978.
3. **Schwartz, J.,** The dopaminergic system in the periphery, *J. Pharmacol.,* 15, 401, 1984.
4. **Beaulieu, S., DiPaolo, T., and Barden, N.,** Roles of the noradrenergic, dopaminergic and serotoninergic systems in the modulation of the ACTH response to stress by the amygdaloid central nucleus, *Can. J. Neurol. Sci.,* 12, 214, 1985.
5. **Matsuki, M., Nishida, S., and Kashiwa, Y.,** Effect of dopamine on ACTH-induced glucocorticoid secretion in rat adrenal suspended cells, *Horm. Metal. Res.,* 17, 429, 1985.
6. **Fuder, H.,** Selected aspects of presynaptic modulation of noradrenaline release from heart, *J. Cardiovasc. Pharmacol.,* 7, (Suppl. 5), 2, 1985.
7. **Vorontsova, E. Ya., Pshennikova, M. G., and Meerson, F. Z.,** Effect of stress on myocardial extensibility, Starling mechanism, and resistance to hypoxia (in Russian), *Kardiologiya,* 11, 68, 1982.
8. **Sergeev, V. P. and Shimanovskii, N. A.,** *Receptors of Physiologically Active Substances* (in Russian), Meditsina, Moscow, 1987.
9. **Erdö, S. L.,** Peripheral GABA-ergic mechanisms, *Trends Pharmacol. Sci.,* 6, 205, 1985.
10. **Andreev, B. V., Galust'yan, G. É., Ignatov, Yu. D., Nikitina, Z. S., and Sytinskii, I. A.,** Effect of emotional pain stress on the gamma-aminobutyric acid system (in Russian), *Ukr. Biokhim. Zh.,* 55, 652, 1983.
11. **Skinner, J. E.,** Psychosocial stress and sudden cardiac death: brain mechanisms, in *Stress Heart Disease,* Beamish, R. E., Singal, P. K., and Dhalla, N. S., Eds., Martinus Nijhoff, Boston, 1985, 44.
12. **Lown, B., Desilava, R. A., Reich, P., and Murawski, B. J.,** Psychophysiologic factors in sudden cardiac death, *Am. J. Psychiatry,* 137, 1325, 1980.
13. **Di Micco, J. A., Abshire, V. M., Hankins, K. D., Sample, R. H., and Wible, J. H.,** Microinjection of GABA antagonists into posterior hypothalamus elevates heart rate in anesthetized rats, *Neuropharmacology,* 25, 1063, 1986.

14. **Wible, J. H., Luft, F. C., and Di Micco, J. A.,** Hypothalamic GABA suppresses sympathetic outflow to the cardiovascular system, *Am. J. Physiol.*, 254, 680, 1988.
15. **Natalson, B. H.,** Neurocardiology, an interdisciplinary area for the 80s, *Arch. Neurology,* 42, 178, 1985.
16. **Di Micco, J. A., Gale, K., Hamilton, B., and Gillis, R. A.,** GABA-receptor control of parasympathetic outflow to heart: characterization and brain stem localization, *Science,* 204, 4397, 1106, 1979.
17. **Hwang, B. H. and Gang-Yen Wu.,** Ultrastructural studies on catecholaminergic terminals and GABA-ergic neurons in nucleus tractus solitarius of the rat medulla oblongata, *Brain Res.*, 302, 57, 1984.
18. **Gordon, F. J.,** Spinal GABA receptors and central cardiovascular control, *Brain Res.*, 328, 165, 1985.
19. **Yoneda, Y., Kanmori, K., Ida, S., and Kuriyama, K.,** Stress-induced alterations in metabolism of γ-aminobutyric acid in rat brain, *J. Neurochem.*, 40, 350, 1983.
20. **Meerson, F. Z.,** *Adaptation, Stress, and Prophylaxis* (in Russian), Nauka, Moscow, 1981.
21. **Ebadi, M. and Govitrapong, P.,** Biogenic amine-mediated alteration of pyridoxal phosphate formation in rat brain, *J. Neurochem.*, 32, 845, 1979.
22. **Banay-Schwarts, M., Zanchin, G., Guzman, F. De, and Lajtha, A.,** The effect of corticosteroids on amino acid content of brain tissue preparations, *Psychoneuroendocrinology,* 4, 207, 1979.
23. **Moroni, F., Bianchi, C., and Moneti, G.,** Release of GABA from guinea pig neocortex induced by electrical stimulation of the locus coeruleus or by norepinephrine, *Brain Res.*, 232, 216, 1982.
24. **Hökfelt, T., Everitt, B., Meister, B., Melander, T., Schalling, M., and Johansson, O.,** Neurons with multiple messengers with special reference to neuroendocrine systems, *Recent Prog. Horm. Res.*, 42, 1, 1986.
25. **Andreev, B. V., Ignatov, Yu. A., Nikitina, Z. S., and Sytinskii, I. A.,** The antistress role of the brain GABA-ergic system (in Russian), *Zh. Vyssh. Nervn. Deyat. im. I. P. Pavlova,* 32, 511, 1982.
26. **Bowery, N. G., Hill, D. R., and Hudson, A. L.,** Heterogeneity of mammalian GABA receptors, in *Actions and Interactions of GABA and Benzodiazepines,* Bowery, N. G., Ed., Raven Press, New York, 1984, 81.
27. **Di Micco, J. A. and Gillis, R. A.,** Neuro-cardiovascular effects produced by bicuculline in the cat, *J. Pharmacol. Exp. Ther.*, 210, 1, 1979.
28. **Frolov, V. A., Bilibin, D. P., Shevelev, S. A., and Khodorovich, N. A.,** Cardiac afferentation in some myocardial pathologies (in Russian), *Byull. Eksp. Biol. Med.*, 1, 22, 1987.
29. **Di Micco, J. A. and Abshire, V.,** Evidence for GABA-ergic inhibition of a hypothalamic sympathoexcitatory mechanism in anesthetized rats, *Brain Res.*, 402, 1, 1987.
30. **Smith, D. A., Astley, C. A., De Vito, J. L., Stein, J. M., and Walsh, K. E.,** Functional analysis of hypothalamic control of the cardiovascular responses accompanying emotional behavior, *Fed. Proc., Fed. Am. Soc. Exp. Biol.*, 39, 2487, 1980.
31. **Under, T., Becker, H., and Dietz, R.,** Antihypertensive effect of the GABA receptor agonist muscimol in spontaneously hypertensive rats, *Circ. Res.*, 54, 30, 1984.
32. **Hambley, J. W., Jonston, G. A. R., and Shaw, J.,** Alterations in a hypothalamic GABA system in the spontaneously hypertensive rat, *Neurochem. Int.*, 6, 813, 1984.
33. **Meerson, F. Z., Pshennikova, M. G., Shabunina, E. V., Sazontova, T. G., and Belkina, L. M.,** Stress-limiting systems of the organism and prevention of cardiac fibrillation (in Russian), *Vestn. Akad. Med. Nauk SSSR,* 6, 47, 1987.
34. **Otero Losada, M. E.,** Changes in central GABA-ergic function following acute and repeated stress, *Br. J. Pharmacol.*, 93, 483, 1988.
35. **Wielosz, M., Stelmasiac, M., Ossowska, G., and Kleinrok, Z.,** Effects of electroconvulsive shock on central GABA-ergic mechanism, *Pharmacol. Pharm.*, 37, 113, 1985.
36. **Meerson, F. Z., Malyshev, V. V., Popova, N. K., and Markovskaya, G. I.,** Decreased stress reaction and gastric ulceration under the influence of GHBA (in Russian), *Byull. Eksp. Biol. Med.*, 12, 659, 1979.
37. **Meerson, F. Z.,** *Adaptation, Stress and Prophylaxis,* Springer-Verlag, Berlin, 1984.
38. **Löescher, W. and Vetter, M.,** Drug-induced changes in GABA content of nerve endings in 11 rat brain regions, correlation to pharmacological effects, *Neurosci. Lett.*, 47, 325, 1984.
39. **Löescher, W. and Schmidt, D.,** Increase of human plasma GABA by sodium valproate, *Epilepsia,* 21, 611, 1980.
40. **Meerson, F. Z., Shabunina, E. V., Belkina, L. M., and Pshennikova, M. G.,** Prevention of arrhythmias and cardiac fibrillation with a factor causing GABA accumulation in the brain (in Russian), *Kardiologiya,* 5, 87, 1987.
41. **Lepran, L., Kolbai, M., Siegmund, W., and Scekeres, L.,** Coronary artery ligation, early arrhythmias and determination of the ischemic area in conscious rats, *J. Pharmacol. Methods,* 9, 219, 1983.
42. **Han, J.,** Electrophysiologic mechanisms of ventricular fibrillation, in *Cardiology: Proc. 8th World Congr.*, Tokyo, 1979, 903.
43. **Clusin, W. T., Blake, K., Smith, N. A., and Buchbinder, M.,** Mechanism of cellular depolarization in the acutely ischemic heart, in *Membranes and Muscle: Proc. Int. Symp.*, Cape Town, 1985, 291.

44. **Hiraoka, M.,** Role of fast and slow inward current in the genesis of arrhythmias, in *Cardiology: Proc. 8th World Congr.,* Tokyo, 1979, 898.
45. **Martin, I. L.,** The benzodiazepines and their receptors: 25 years of progress, *Neuropharmacology,* 26, 957, 1987.
46. **Haefely, W., Polc, P., Pieri, L., Schaffner, R., and Laurent, J. P.,** Neuropharmacology of benzodiazepines: synaptic metchanisms and neural basis of action, in *The Benzodiazepines: From Molecular Biology to Clinical Practice,* Kosta, E., Ed., Raven Press, New York, 1983, 21.
47. **Segel, M.,** Effect of diazepam (valium) on chronic stress-induced hypertension in the rat, *Experientia,* 37, 298, 1981.
48. **Skinner, J. E. and Reed, J. C.,** Blockade of a frontocortical-brain-stem pathway prevents ventricular fibrillation of the ischemic heart in pigs, *Am. J. Physiol.,* 24, H156, 1981.
49. **Cox, W. and Robertson, H. F.,** Effects of stellate ganglionectomy on the cardiac function of intact dogs and its effects on the extent of myocardial infarction and on the cardiac function following coronary occlusion, *Am. Heart J.,* 12, 285, 1936.
50. **Miller, R. J.,** Peptides as neurotransmitters: focus on the enkephalins and endorphins, *Pharmacol. Ther.,* 12, 73, 1981.
51. **Pert, C. B., Kuhar, M. J., and Snyder, S. H.,** Opiate receptors: autoradiographic localization in rat brain, *Proc. Natl. Acad. Sci. U.S.A.,* 73, 3729, 1976.
52. **Kondo, H., Kuramoto, H., Wainer, B. H., and Yanaihara, N.,** Evidence for the coexistence of acetylcholine and enkephalin in the sympathetic preganglionic neurons of rats, *Brain Res.,* 335, 309, 1985.
53. **Lewis, J. W., Tordoff, M. G., Sherman, J. E., and Libski, J. C.,** Adrenal medullary enkephaline-like peptides may mediate opioid stress analgesia, *Science,* 217, 557, 1982.
54. **Carnody, J. and Cooper, K.,** Swim stress reduces chronic pain in mice through an opioid mechanism, *Neurosci. Lett.,* 74, 358, 1987.
55. **Amir, S. and Amit, Z.,** Opiate ligands may mediate stress-induced changes in the affective properties of pain-related behaviour in rats, *Life Sci.,* 18, 1143, 1978.
56. **Millan, M. J., Przewlocki, R., Jerlicz, M., Gramsch, Ch., Höllt, V., and Herz, A.,** Stress-induced release of brain and pituitary β-endorphin: major role of endorphins in generation of hyperthermia, *Brain Res.,* 208, 325, 1981.
57. **Clement-Jones, V., Tomlin, S., and Rees, L.,** Increased beta-endorphin but not met-enkephalin levels in human cerebrospinal fluid after acupuncture for recurrent pain, *Lancet,* 8201, 946, 1980.
58. **Fraioloi, F., Moretti, C., Paolucci, D., Aliciccio, E., Crescenzi, F., and Fortunio, G.,** Physical exercise stimulates marked concomitant release of beta-endorphin and ACTH in peripheral blood in man, *Experientia,* 36, 987, 1980.
59. **Guillemin, K., Vargo, Th., Rossier, J., Minick, S., Ling, N., Rivier, C., Vale, W., and Blooms, F. E.,** β-Endorphin and adrenocorticotropin are secreted concomitantly by the pituitary gland, *Science,* 197, 1367, 1977.
60. **Lebouille, J. L. M., Burbach, J. P., De Kloet, E. R., Wilgant, V. M., Sweep, C. G., and Wied, D. D.,** Leu-Phe-cleaving endopeptidase activity, γ-endorphin, and β-endorphin in the rat pituitary gland and brain, *Neuroendocrinology,* 47, 7, 1988.
61. **Berkenbosch, F., Tilders, F. J., and Vermes, I.,** β-Adrenoreceptor activation mediates stress-induced secretion of α-endorphin-related peptides from intermediate but not anterior pituitary, *Nature,* 305, 237, 1983.
62. **Tigranyan, R. A. and Vakulina, O. P.,** Opioid peptide content in rat tissues in prolonged restraint of motile activity (in Russian), *Kosm. Biol. Aviakosmicheskaya Med.,* 18, 83, 1984.
63. **Hökfelt, T., Everitt, B., Meister, B., Melander, T., Schalling, M., and Johansson, O.,** Neurons with multiple messengers with special reference to neuroendocrine systems, *Recent Progr. Horm. Res.,* 42, 1, 1986.
64. **Izquierdo, I.,** Opioid-catecholamine and opioid-cholinergic interactions in memory regulation, *Trends Pharm. Sci.,* 6, 192, 1985.
65. **Konishi, S., Tsunoo, H., and Otsuka, M.,** Enkephalin as a transmitter for presynaptic inhibitor in sympathetic ganglia, *Nature,* 294, 80, 1981.
66. **Meerson, F. Z., Dmitriev, A. D., Zayats, V. M., Rozhitskaya, I. I., and Kizim, E. A.,** Effects of stress, infarction, and adaptation to short stress exposures on the opioid peptide content in the brain (in Russian), *Vopr. Med. Khim.,* 5, 32, 1985.
67. **Markarova, M. Yu., Koshtoyants, O. Kh., Kruglikov, R. I., and Meerson, F. Z.,** Effect of adaptation to short stress exposures on the chemoreactivity of the sensomotor cortical neurons (in Russian), *Vopr. Med. Khim.,* 6, 1174, 1987.
68. **Amir, S. and Amit, Z.,** Endogenous opiate ligands may mediate stress-induced changes in the affective properties of pain-related behaviour in rats, *Life Sci.,* 18, 1143, 1978.
69. **Starke, K., Schoffel, E., and Illes, P.,** The sympathetic axons innervating the sinus node of rabbit possess presynaptic opioid κ- but not μ- or σ-receptor, *Naunyn-Schmiedeberg's Arch. Pharmacol.,* 329, 206, 1985.

70. **Berridge, M. J.,** Inositol triphosphate and diacylglycerol as second messengers, *Biochem. J.*, 220, 345, 1984.
71. **Knepel, W., Nutto, D., and Herting, G.,** Evidence for inhibition by β-endorphin of vasopressin release during foot shock-induced stress in the rat, *Neuroendocrinology*, 34, 353, 1982.
72. **Taylor, T., Dluhy, R., and Williams, G.,** Beta-endorphin suppressed adrenocorticotropin and cortisol levels in 9 normal human subjects, *J. Clin. Endocrinol. Metab.*, 57, 592, 1983.
73. **Green, I., Ray, K., and Perrin, D.,** Opioid peptide effects on insulin release and cAMP in islets of Langerhans, *Horm. Metab. Res.*, 15, 124, 1983.
74. **Penalva, A., Villanueva, L., and Casanueva, F.,** Cholinergic and hostaminergic involvement in the growth hormone releasing effect of an enkephalin analog FK-33814 in man, *Psychopharmacol.*, 80, 120, 1983.
75. **Lishmanov, Yu. B., Amosov, E. N., Slepushkin, V. D., and Yaremenko, K. V.,** A study of the antistress effect of D-Ala^2-Leu^5-enkephalin(in Russian), *Byull. Eksp. Biol. Med.*, 8, 199, 1984.
76. **Slepushkin, V. D., Lishmanov, Yu. B., Zoloev, G. K., and Prum, I. A.,** Present-day concepts of some unconventional neuroendocrine mechanisms of stress (in Russian), *Usp. Fiziol. Nauk*, 4, 106, 1985.
77. **Lishmanov, Yu. B., Slepushkin, V. D., and Prum, I. A.,** Effect of enkephalins on activity of several stress hormones in acute myocardial ischemia (in Russian), *Patol. Fiziol. Eksp. Ter.*, 3, 22, 1985.
78. **Lishmanov, Yu. B., Lasukova, T. V., and Alekminskaya, L. A.,** Enkephalins and hormonal-metabolic reactions in experimental stress of varying severity (in Russian), *Byull. Eksp. Biol. Med.*, 3, 269, 1985.
79. **Meerson, F. Z., Zayats, V. I., and Pshennikova, M. G.,** Prevention of impairment of the contractile function of nonischemic heart regions in experimental infarction with beta-endorphin (in Russian), *Kardiologiya*, 7, 102, 1985.
80. **Lishmanov, Yu. B.,** Use of enkephalins to prevent cardiac stress damage in the experiment (in Russian), *Byull. Eksp. Biol. Med.*, 9, 271, 1986.
81. **Meerson, F. Z., Pshennikova, M. G., Belkina, L. M., Abdikaliev, N. A., and Malishev, I. J.,** Prevention of ischemic arrhythmias by activation of stress-limiting systems of the organism, *CV World Res.*, in press.
82. **Pshennikova, M. G.,** Role of opioid peptides in organismic reaction to stress (in Russian), *Patol. Fiziol. Eksp. Ter.*, 3, 85, 1987.
83. **Yaksh, T. L.,** Direct evidence that spinal serotonin and noradrenaline terminals mediate the spinal antinociceptive effects of morphine in the periaqueductal gray, *Brain Res.*, 160, 180, 1979.
84. **Garcia-Sevilla, J. A., Magnusson, T., and Carlsson, A.,** Effects of enkephalins and two enzyme-resistant analogues on monoamine synthesis and metabolism in rat brain, *Naunyn-Schmiedeberg's Arch. Pharmacol.*, 310, 211, 1980.
85. **Lee, R. L., Sewell, R., and Spencer, P. S.,** Antinociceptive activity of D-Ala^2-D-Leu^5-enkephalin (BW 180C) in the rat after modification to central 5-hydroxytryptamine function, *Neuropharmacology*, 18, 711, 1979.
86. **Kharkevich, D. A. and Titov, M. I.,** Peptides with analgetic activity (in Russian), *Vestn. Akad. Med. Nauk SSSR*, 5, 54, 1982.
87. **Culman, J., Kvetnansky, R., Torda, T., and Murgas, K.,** Serotonin concentration in individual hypothalamic nuclei of rats exposed to acute immobilization, *Neuroscience*, 5, 1503, 1980.
88. **Tanaka, M., Kohno, Y., Nakagawa, R., Matsuo, K., and Nagasaki, N.,** Changes of serotonin and 5-hydroxyindolacetic acid in rats by immobilization, *Jpn. J. Pharmacol.*, 28, (Suppl. 54P), 1978.
89. **Buckingham, J. C. and Hodges, J. R.,** Hypothalamic receptors influencing the secretion of corticotrophin releasing hormone in the rat, *J. Physiol.*, 290, 421, 1979.
90. **Rabinowitz, S. H. and Lown, B.,** Central neurochemical factors related to serotonin metabolism and cardiac ventricular vulnerability for repetitive electrical activity, *Am. J. Cardiol.*, 41, 516, 1978.
91. **Shabunina, E. V., Petrunin, I. A., Vinograd, L. Kh., Manukhina, E. B., and Meerson, F. Z.,** Prevention of arrhythmias during acute ischemia in conscious animals with a serotonin analog (in Russian), *Byull. Eksp. Biol. Med.*, 10, 410, 1988.
92. **Marek, P., Yirmiya, R., and Liebeskind, J. C.,** Strain differences in the magnitude of swimming-induced analgesia in mice correlate with brain opiate receptor concentration, *Brain Res.*, 447, 188, 1988.
93. **Westfall, T. C. and Meldrum, M. J.,** Alternations in the release of norepinephrine at the vascular neuroeffector junction in hypertension, *Annu. Rev. Pharmacol. Toxicol.*, 25, 621, 1985.
94. **Di Giulio, A., Yang, H., and Fratta, W.,** Decreased content of immunoreactive enkephalin-like peptide in peripheral tissues of spontaneously hypertensive rats, *Nature*, 278, 646, 1979.
95. **Stoupel, E., Pinchas, A., Gilad, I., Laren, Z., and Agmon, J.,** Beta-endorphins in acute myocardial infarction, *Clin. Cardiol.*, 9, 409, 1986.
96. **Kent, K. M., Smith, E. R., Redwood, D. K., and Epstein, S. E.,** Electrical stability of acutely ischemic myocardium. Influences of heart rate and vagal stimulation, *Circulation*, 47, 291, 1973.
97. **Levy, M. N. and Blattberg, B.,** Effect of vagal stimulation on the overflow of norepinephrine into the coronary sinus during cardiac sympathetic nerve stimulation in the dog, *Circ. Res.*, 38, 81, 1976.

98. **Verrier, R. L.,** Mechanisms of behaviorally induced arrhythmias, *Circulation,* 76, 1, 1987.
99. **Breitwieser, G. E. and Szabo, G.,** Uncoupling of cardiac muscarinic and β-adrenergic receptors from ion channels by a guanine nucleotide and analogue, *Nature,* 317, 538, 1985.
100. **Löffelholz, K. and Pappano, A. J.,** The parasympathetic neuroeffector junction of the heart, *Physiol. Rev.,* 37, 1, 1985.
101. **Baly, J. C., Kovacs, R. J., and Rardon, D. P.,** Anatomical, biochemical and electrophysiologic evidence for parasympathetic innervation of the ventricle, in *Mechanisms and Treatment of Cardiac Arrhythmias: Relevance of Basic Studies to Clinical Management,* Reiser, H. J. and Horowitz, L. N., Eds., Baltimore, 1985, 370.
102. **Hosein, E. A., Kato, A., Vine, E., and Hile, A. M.,** Identification of acetyl(-)carnitylcholine in rat brain extracts and the comparison of its cholinomimetic properties with acetylcholine, *Can. J. Physiol. Pharmacol.,* 48, 709, 1970.
103. **Hosein, E. A. and Koh, T. Y.,** Influence of deep narcosis on the content of substance with acetylcholine-like activity in heart of rat, *Rev. Can. Biol.,* 25, 25, 1966.
104. **Burgen, A. S. V. and Hobbiga, F.,** Pharmacology of the Me and benzyl ester of γ-crotonic betaine, *Br. J. Pharmacol.,* 4, 229, 1949.
105. **Thomitzec, W.-D., Strack, E., and Lorenz, F.,** Über den Einfluss ein Derivate aliphatis den Trimethylbetaine auf die Acetylcholinesterase und über die Hydrolyse von Betainestern, *Acta Biol. Med. Ger.,* 11, 353, 1963.
106. **Golburn, R. W., Goodwing, F. K., Bunney, E., and Davis, J. M.,** Effect of lithium on the uptake of noradrenaline by synaptosomes, *Nature,* 215, 1395, 1967.
107. **Verrier, R. L. and Hageston, E. L.,** Naural mechanism of cardiac arrhythmias, in *Mechanisms and Treatment of Cardiac Arrhythmias: Relevance of Basic Studies to Clinical Management,* Reiser, H. J. and Horowitz, L. N., Eds., Baltimore, 1985, 76.
108. **Nier, E. J. and Clapham, D. E.,** Roles of G-protein subunits in transmembrane signalling, *Nature,* 333, 129, 1988.

Chapter 5

LOCAL STRESS-LIMITING SYSTEMS AND THEIR CARDIOPROTECTIVE EFFECTS

I. INTRODUCTION

Operation of the stress-limiting systems exclusively by blocking or restricting the stress reaction at the central level can hardly be considered an optimal solution of the problem of modulating this reaction in the course of adaptation. Indeed, during adaptation to the changing set of environmental factors, in some working organs the strong effect of the stress hormones and mediators is absolutely indispensable, while in others it is quite needless. At the same time the stress reaction is known to be a generalized link of adaptation. Hence the most nearly perfect adaptation can in all probability be achieved owing to the participation of the local modulatory systems that either restrict or, conversely, potentiate the action of stress hormones and mediators in the organs and cells. Since the very concept of the stress-limiting systems is rather recent,[1,2] the important question of the relations of the central and the local stress-limiting systems in general, and in the cardioprotective effect of adaptation specifically, has not been discussed heretofore.

As the reader will be able to see, the materials presented in Chapter 6 provide unequivocal evidence that all the protective effects of adaptation to repeated stress (enhanced resistance to toxic levels of catecholamines or calcium, etc.) are in full measure found in the isolated hearts of adapted animals. This issue, which will be the subject of special consideration, implies that besides the central neurohumoral regulatory systems an important part in the adaptational protection of the heart is played by local mechanisms forming in the course of adaptation in the organ. *A priori,* it can be envisaged that such local protection is provided by the antioxidant system, the adaptive changes in the calcium membrane transport, the adenosinergic and the prostaglandin systems, etc. Accordingly, we shall further deal with the data available to date on the changes in these systems in adaptation to stress and on the cardioprotective and first of all antiarrhythmic significance of such changes.

II. ANTIOXIDANT HEART PROTECTION FROM ISCHEMIC, REOXYGENATIVE, AND STRESS DAMAGES

Disturbances of the free-radical homeostasis, their role in cardiac injury, and methods of their correction constitute a rapidly developing trend of modern cardiology. Its origin can be traced back to two main sources from apparently remote fields of science. One is the fundamental studies of Bakh,[4] Demenov,[5] and Fridovich[6] into the theory of free-radical oxidation. The other is the works in vitaminology[7,8] demonstrating that the lack of α-tocopherol and other vitamins inhibiting free-radical oxidation may result in rapid injury to the cardiac muscle.

Further development of the notions of the role of free-radical reactions in cardiac pathology has gone through several stages.

Thus, when in 1969 superoxide dismutase (SOD) was discovered by McCord and Fridovich[9] and proved to be highly active in the cardiac muscle, it became clear that cardiomyocytes had evolutionarily acquired a specific enzyme system for scavenging free radicals, and hence free-radical oxidation proceeds constantly in the myocardium.

In 1973, Hearse et al.[3] described the oxygen paradox as cardiac muscle injury upon resumed supply of oxygen after a long enough period of anoxia. Owing to further studies by their laboratory and to the works of Guarniery et al.[10] on the antioxidant action of

TABLE 1
Activity of Antioxidant Enzymes and Content of LPO Products in Heart Ventricles

Indices	Right ventricle (n = 10)	Left ventricle (n = 10)
Superoxide dismutase (arb. U/min·mg)	218 ± 21	333 ± 25[a]
Catalase (nmol H_2O_2/min·mg)	256 ± 16	475 ± 25[a]
Schiff bases (arb. fluorescence units)	1.64 ± 0.12	1.00 ± 0.15[a]
Lipid hydroperoxides ($OD^{0.1\%}_{1\ cm}$)	1.49 ± 0.20	1.03 ± 0.13[a]

[a] $p < 0.05$.

α-tocopherol and reduced glutathione, this important phenomenon got an explanation in terms of the free-radical oxidation theory. Finally, in 1976 Kogan et al.[11] obtained direct evidence for the involvement of free-radical oxidation in the pathogenesis of myocardial infarction, having demonstrated enhanced chemiluminescence in the ischemic zone and having attributed it to activation of free-radical processes. Simultaneously, our laboratory showed that activation of free-radical oxidation is a major element of the generalized stress damage to the organism (see Chapter 1). Emotional pain (EPS) and immobilization stress proved to cause accumulation of the lipid peroxidation (LPO) products in liver, lungs, heart, aorta, brain, and eye retina; antioxidants protected these organs from stress injuries. These data lay into the foundation of the concept of the role of LPO activation in the primary noncoronarogenic stress-induced damage to the heart.[12,13] The mentioned studies reinforced the idea of the real significance of LPO activation in cardiac pathology, and now permit us to point out three basic mechanisms of LPO activation in the heart.

1. Primary excessive generation of active oxygen forms and lipid hydroperoxides in hyperbaric oxygenation, stress-induced excess of catecholamines, excess of variable-valency metals in hemolytic anemia, etc.
2. Primary decline in the power of the antioxidant systems in vitamin E deficiency, acatalasia, intoxication with enzyme poisons, etc.
3. Combination of primary LPO activation and deterioration of the antioxidant systems in hypoxia-reoxygenation, ischemia-reperfusion.

This concept predetermined the order of presentation in this section. We shall consecutively consider the mechanisms of LPO activation and the possibilities of the antioxidant protection of the heart in ischemia-reperfusion; LPO activation and antioxidant protection in cardiac stress injury; the role of LPO in arrhythmias and the experimental and clinical effects of antioxidants; and finally, some prospects for further studies.

In assessing the mechanism of enhancement of free-radical oxidation in ischemia and reperfusion, it should be borne in mind that in mitochondria, as electrons are transferred to cytochrome oxidase, under normal conditions there can occur a single-electron "side-drop" to dioxygen, giving rise to the active oxygen forms which react with the endogenous substrates in the cell structures, first and foremost with phospholipids. This free-radical lipid oxidation yields peroxide compounds and accordingly the whole process has been termed lipid peroxidation. Our data in Table 1 show that the LPO products are always present and hence the process is always operative in the normal ventricular myocardium. It can also be seen that the intensity of LPO is inversely correlated with the activity of the natural antioxidant agents.

LPO is enhanced in ischemia and reperfusion. Panel 1 in Figure 1 shows that normal four-electron reduction of oxygen on cytochrome oxidase proceeds in uninterrupted and

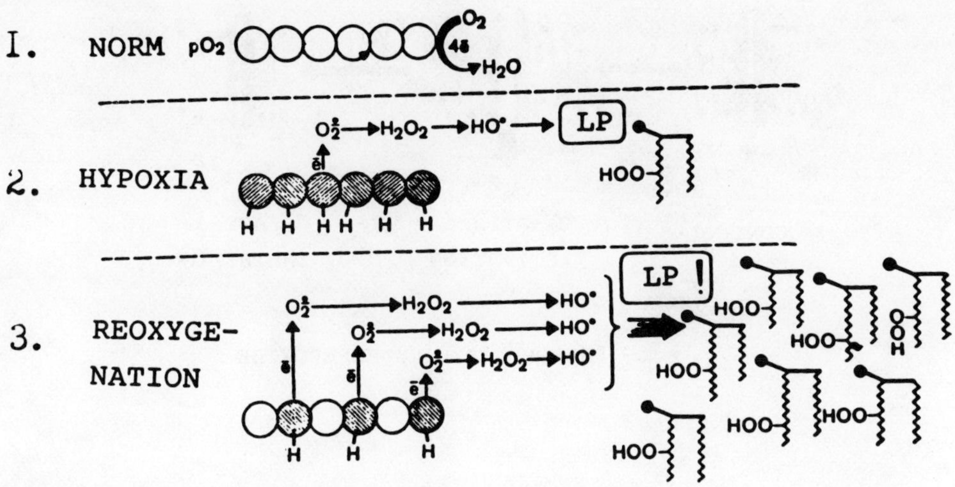

FIGURE 1. Activation of lipid peroxidation in hypoxia and reoxygenation. For explanations see text.

coordinated operation of the respiratory chain, i.e., at normal oxygen tension. Panel 2 shows that when the respiratory chain is blocked in its terminal link, as in ischemic hypoxia, the reduction of the preceding carriers causes the oxygen dissolved in the membrane lipid milieu to be reduced; however, this is not the four-electron reduction to water, but partial reduction producing active oxygen forms. Of course, with the lack of oxygen, accumulation of its active forms and LPO is only limited and slow. Panel 3 shows that much greater amounts of active oxygen and LPO products are formed when the reduced state of the respiratory-chain carriers (electron donors) combines with a high enough oxygen tension. This happens in reoxygenation following hypoxia and ischemia, i.e., after each coronary attack in recirculation through ischemic myocardial regions, and upon restoration of oxygen transport to the anoxic heart.

Initially, the active oxygen combines with unsaturated fatty acyl residues in phospholipids to produce unstable hydroperoxides. Their accumulation entails several rather important modifying effects studied *in vitro* by Arkhipenko et al.[14]

Figure 2A exemplifies, with the Ca ATPase of the sarcoplasmic reticulum (SR), one of the effects of this kind when hydroperoxides are accumulated and the amount of unsaturated lipids decreases in the lipid milieu of the integral proteins, which are the chief functional proteins of the membrane. Moderate LPO increases the mobility of the phospholipid chains, which as a rule is accompanied with enhanced catalytic activity of the enzymes. In pronounced LPO activation greater significance is acquired by the decreasing content of unsaturated phospholipids, which results in the integral proteins turning out to "freeze into" the more rigid milieu, with restricted conformational mobility of their polypeptide chains.

Figure 2B attempts to correlate these changes with the response of the isolated auricle to such an LPO inducer as hydrogen peroxide. It can be seen that initially H_2O_2 affects the atrial contractile function like catecholamines: the contraction amplitude increases and there is even a decrease in the tension at rest. Then the second stage develops, with pronounced bradyarrhythmia ending in cardiac arrest.

The second modifying effect is that of oxidized phospholipids accumulating as the result of LPO from ordered groups known as peroxide clusters. Figure 3 shows the process of their formation. Owing to the lateral diffusion of whole associations of oxidized phospholipids in each membrane layer, they come to be located opposite each other to form permeability channels allowing, in particular, passage of Ca^{2+}. Appearance of such clusters upon LPO activation caused by ischemia and especially reperfusion can be thought to play an importaant part in accumulation of excess calcium and its cardiotoxic effect.

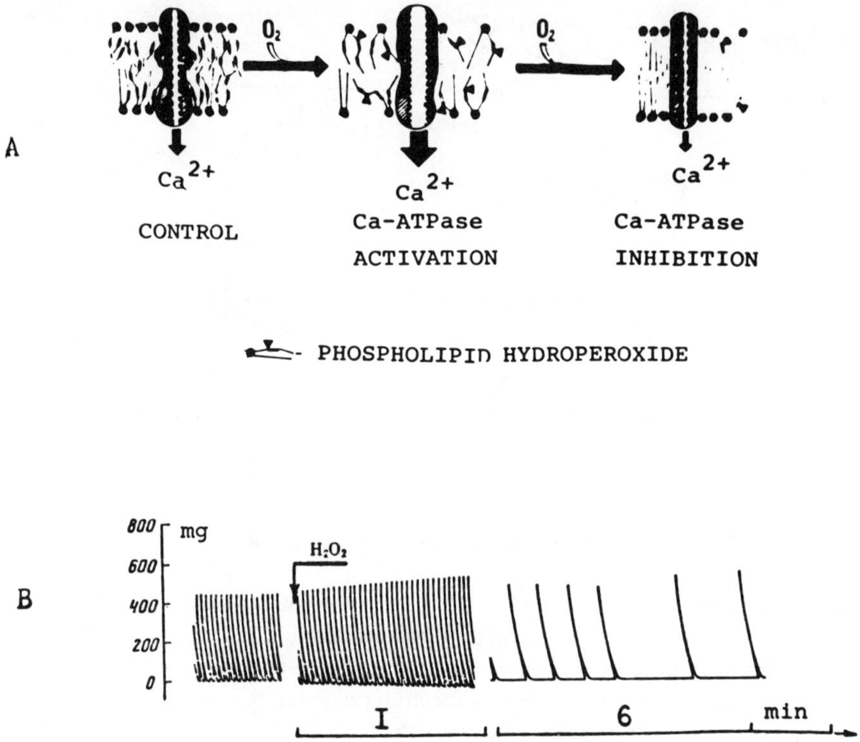

FIGURE 2. (A) Changes in the activity of the Ca ATPase of the SR as LPO proceeds in its lipid milieu, and (B) progressive disturbance to contraction of the isolated right auricle in exposure to H_2O_2.

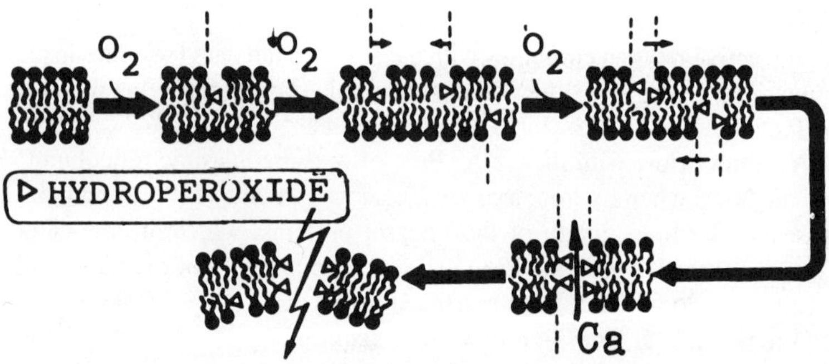

FIGURE 3. Formation of "peroxide clusters" and membrane fragmentation in LPO. The empty triangles denote peroxide groups. For explanations see text.

The above effects of LPO are essentially reversible. On the contrary, two other, namely protein intermolecular linking and inactivation of sulfhydryl groups, appear irreversible.

Figure 4 shows one of these irreversible effects. The hydroperoxide produced in the reaction between phospholipid and activated molecular oxygen splits into a lysophospholipid-like compound with an abbreviated fatty chain and a short aliphatic dialdehyde which can interact with the amino groups of two protein molecules as a bifunctional linking agent.

Through these detrimental effects, LPO can cause more or less pronounced inactivation of the three important types of membrane proteins: cation pumps, ion channels, and signal-transmitting receptor systems. This impairs the electric stability and contractile function of

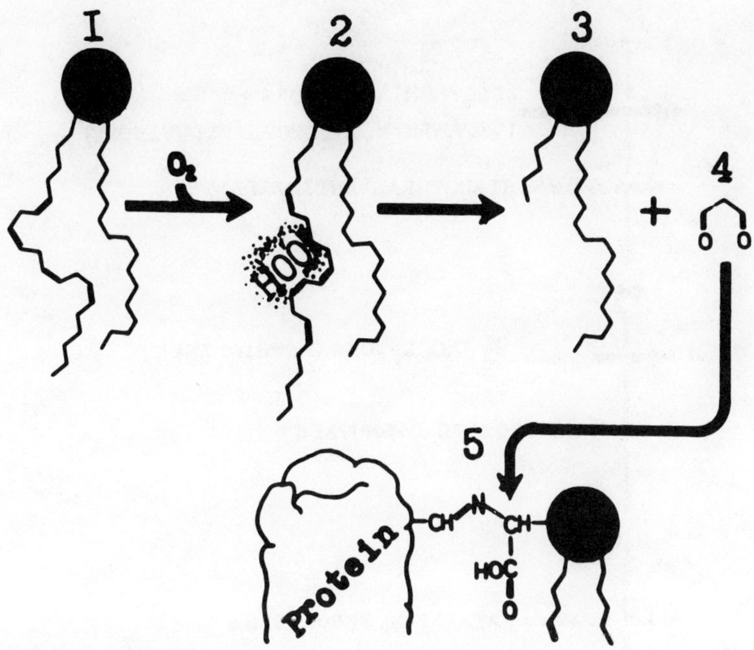

FIGURE 4. Formation of links and inactivation of membrane enzymic proteins in LPO. For explanations see text.

TABLE 2
Main Mechanisms Activating Free-Radical Oxidation in the Myocardium in Ischemia and Reperfusion

1. Activation of free-radical lipid oxidation by electron carriers (see text)
2. Activation of free-radical lipid oxidation by the xanthine oxidase system[15,16]
3. pH-dependent activation of free-radical lipid oxidation[17]
4. Generation of free radicals by leukocytes[18,19]
5. Deterioration of the antioxidant system in cardiomyocytes[20-22]

the heart as a whole. Hence the problem of antioxidant protection acquires much clinical importance.

To evaluate the possibilities of antioxidant protection it is expedient to consider first the main mechanisms augmenting free-radical oxidation in the myocardium in ischemia and reperfusion; these are listed in Table 2.

The first one — formation of free radicals through partial reduction of oxygen by the respiratory chain — has already been discussed above. Other mechanisms of LPO activation are well known from recent works. Here it is reasonable to dwell on the last one listed, namely deterioration of the antioxidant system in the cardiomyocytes; indeed, were the myocardial antioxidant capacity unlimited, none of these factors could have caused LPO activation.

The scheme in Figure 5 shows that the cellular antioxidant mechanism operates as a cascade of specialized steps. Thus formation of the superoxide radical can be prevented by competing electron acceptors like vitamins E or K_3; conversion of the superoxide radical to hydrogen peroxide is blocked by anion-radical acceptors such as the sulfur-containing amino acids methionine and cysteine. Further, coordinated action of two enzymes — SOD and catalase — suppresses formation of hydroxyl radicals; since the latter readily interact with polyenic lipids, this enzyme system is central to regulation of LPO at the initiation stage.

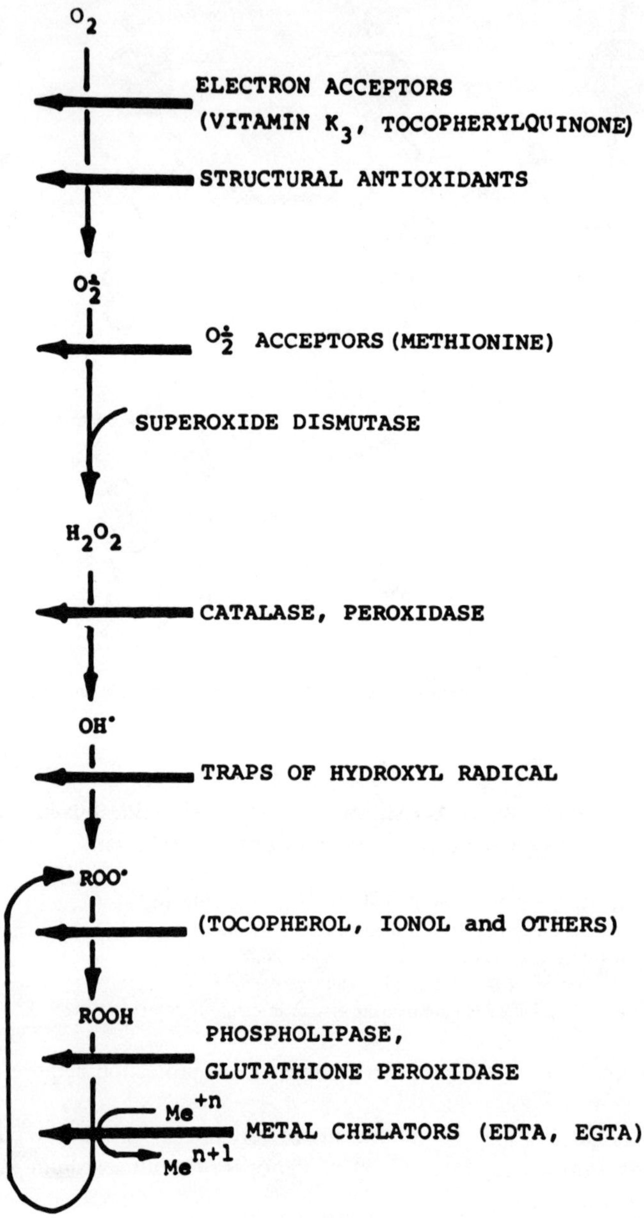

FIGURE 5. The antioxidant system of the cell.

The works of recent years in our laboratory have shown that the reliability of this antioxidant protection system is determined not only by its biological design, but also by its remarkable ability to increase its power upon repeated exposure of the organism to factors inducing LPO activation. This, in particular, is what happens in adaptation to repetitive stress.

Augmentation of the antioxidant system in the course of this process has recently been demonstrated with the use of a simple technique of inducing LPO by adding hydrogen peroxide or organic peroxides into the solution perfusing the contracting cardiac muscle.[23] When H_2O_2 was added to the oxygenated solution bathing the isolated auricles of control and stress-adapted rats, LPO was activated as manifest in accumulation of malonic dialdehyde

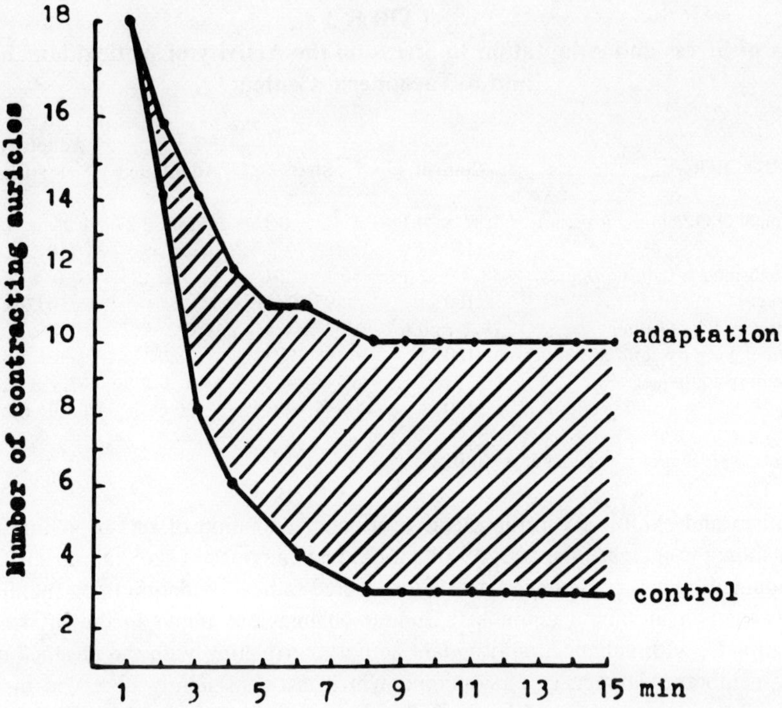

FIGURE 6. Effect of adaptation to short stress exposures on the resistance of isolated auricles to H_2O_2-induced LPO. The abscissa is time after addition of H_2O_2, min; the ordinate is the number of contracting auricles.

(MDA), and there were typical triphasic alterations in the atrial function ending in brady-arrhythmia and cardiac arrest.[24]

Figure 6 compares the response of 18 control and 18 ''adapted'' auricles to an equal amount of H_2O_2. One can see that within 10 min after adding the peroxide, 10 adapted, but only 3 control preparations continued to function, i.e., the auricles of adapted animals were appreciably more resistant to the LPO inducer. In accord with this, special experiments showed that upon LPO induction with the Fe/ascorbate system in the ventricular homogenates from adapted animals, MDA accumulated three times more slowly than in the control.[25] Thus, we observed actually increased resistance of the myocardium of adapted animals to factors inducing LPO.

The data in Table 3 shed some light on this phenomenon. As can be seen, after a single 6-h EPS the catalase activity in the myocardium declines by 20% while the activity of other antioxidant enzymes — SOD and glutathione peroxidase (GPO) — and the α-tocopherol content do not change appreciably. Upon adaptation to repeated stress catalase increases almost by half and SOD by 15%, while GPO and α-tocopherol remain the same. It should be recalled that catalase in the cells is essential to elimination of hydrogen peroxide which inhibits SOD; accordingly, their activities under optimal conditions change in synchrony,[31,32] as observed in our case: in animals adapted to repeated stress and exposed to a single prolonged EPS the activities of antioxidant enzymes do not drop below control levels.

This activation of the antioxidant enzymes appears to be one of the factors of the cytoprotective action of adaptation to stress which, as we could have seen, does not at all decrease the ischemic zone in coronary artery ligation, but decreases the necrotic zone in infarction by over 40% (see Chapter 3) and checks the reperfusion arrhythmias (see above).

It is essential that not only adaptation to stress can augment the antioxidant capacity of

TABLE 3
Effects of Stress and Adaptation to Stress on the Activity of Antioxidant Enzymes and α-Tocopherol Content

Indices	Control	Stress	Adaptation	Adaptation + stress	Assay (Ref.)
Catalase (nmol H_2O_2/min per g tissue)	1.82 ± 0.11 (100%)	1.47 ± 0.18[a] (80.7%)	2.52 ± 0.27[a] (138.5%)	1.96 ± 0.21 (107.8%)	26
Superoxide dismutase (arb. un./min per g tissue)	58.7 ± 2.1 (100%)	56.1 ± 2.1 (95.3%)	67.9 ± 2.5[a] (115.7%)	64.0 ± 2.5 (109.3%)	27
Glutathione peroxidase (μmol NADPH/min per g tissue)	19.2 ± 0.6 (100%)	18.7 ± 0.4 (95.8%)	19.0 ± 0.7 (98.9%)	19.4 ± 0.2 (101.2%)	28,29
α-Tocopherol (μg/g tissue)	66.7 ± 2.1 (100%)	63.4 ± 4.3 (95.1%)	64.5 ± 2.9 (96.6%)	67.8 ± 2.6 (101.6%)	30

[a] Difference with control significant at $p < 0.05$.

the organism and exhibit a cardioprotective effect. Adaptation of rats to swimming loads has been shown to increase the activity of antioxidant enzymes in skeletal muscle,[2,33] which is accompained by less pronounced activation of free-radical oxidation upon maximal physical loads than in untrained animals.[34] Similar changes are found in the myocardium of trained animals, with enhanced antioxidant activity correlating with the absence of cardiomyocyte membrane damage or enzymemia, which are consistently observed in untrained animals under maximal physical loads.[35] There are full grounds for believing that the enhanced activity of the antioxidant systems is one of the elements determining the widely known cardioprotective effect of training and specifically the attenuation of the IHD risk factors (a comprehensive review of this problem can be found in a recent monograph).[2]

Of course, this cytoprotective effect also involves other regulatory and first of all stress-limiting systems of the organism. In essence, the data on activation of the antioxidant systems in adaptation to stress or physical load mean that in using natural or synthetic antioxidants we, as in many other cases, follow the principle of mimicking the natural organismic defense mechanisms.

It might seem that the efficient and adaptively reinforcible antioxidant system should safeguard the cell against excessive LPO and membrane damage. However, in point of fact this system is rapidly deteriorated in ischemia and reperfusion as shown by Gutkin and Petrovich.[20] According to their data depicted in Figure 7, 30 min after coronary artery ligation the leakage of SOD into the perfusate from the isolated heart increases to roughly the same extent as that of the marker enzyme lactate dehydrogenase. These authors observed no release of such important antioxidant enzymes as GPO and catalase, which was in line with the earlier data of Guarniery et al.[36]

However, further studies have shown that these two enzymes are inactivated in the ischemic myocardium. As is evident in Figure 8, GPO activity falls more than eightfold within 60 min (and most likely irreversibly) and SOD activity falls by half; these changes prove dramatic for the myocardial cells.

The scheme in Figure 9 depicts that familiar chain of events: the superoxide anion derived from several sources dismutates in the SOD reaction to a less dangerous compound, hydrogen peroxide, which is then disposed of by GPO and catalase. It is easily conceivable that the near-complete inactivation of GPO shown above would lead to accumulation of hydrogen peroxide. In the presence of substantial amounts of variable-valency metals, and first of all iron, this would inevitably result in immense activation of the Haber-Weiss reaction and intense generation of the rather toxic hydroxyl radical. This detrimental situation becomes self-sustaining, since the superoxide anion under conditions of acidosis can inhibit catalase, and hydrogen peroxide inhibits SOD. The combined action of the three active

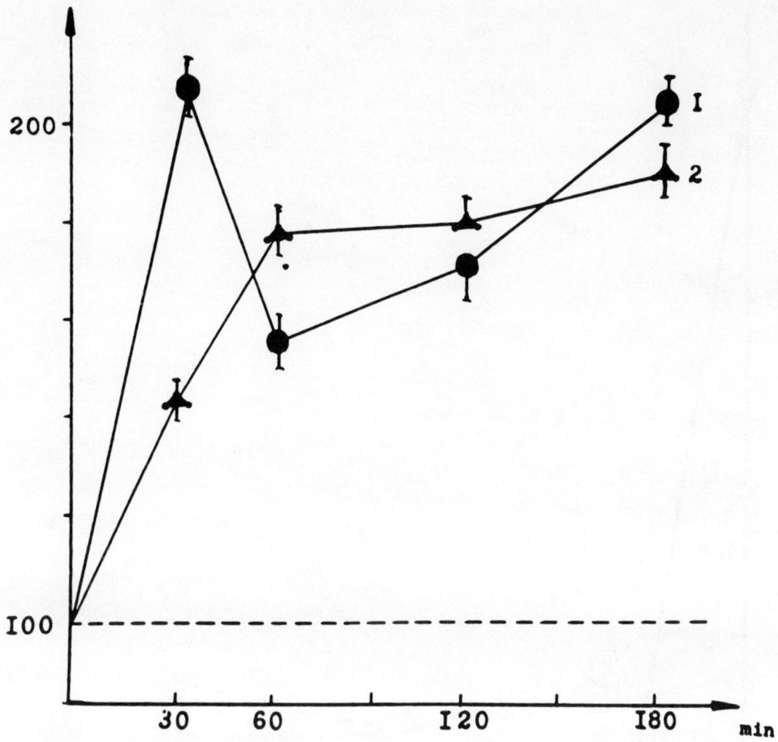

FIGURE 7. Leakage of lactate dehydrogenase (1) and superoxide dismutase (2) from the myocardium of the isolated heart into the perfusate upon coronary artery occlusion. The abscissa is time after occlusion in minutes; the ordinate is relative enzyme content in the perfusate, percent of that prior to occlusion.

oxygen forms results in profound damage to cell structures, increasing calcium concentration and its cardiotoxic effect, actuating or potentiating the whole pathogenetic chain of ischemic damage.

The phenomenon of ischemic breakdown of the myocardial antioxidant enzyme system at present raises no doubt, and in this case LPO is activated under conditions of a great lack of oxygen. This naturally raises the question, what is primary in ischemia: breakdown of the antioxidant system or enhanced free radical generation? Regardless of the answer, which is yet to found, it can be stated that all the modern antioxidant protection in ischemia and reperfusion is based on compensating for the deficiency of the myocardial own system. Just this is the aim of administering α-tocopherol, ubiquinones, SOD, catalase, mannitol, glutathione, methionine, sodium selenite, or ionol, hydroxypyridines, and others.

The protective effects of these antioxidants observed by different authors are far from being similar. Table 4 presents the results from several laboratories that have tried to restrict the size of necrosis in ischemia and reperfusion using a number of antioxidants. The first three works listed demonstrate that 1 d after coronary artery occlusion the necrotic area is decreased by a nonspecific inhibitor of xanthine oxidase, allopurinol. However, in one of these works the effect was totally lacking when assessed after 2 d of ischemia.

Next is a group of important works where a short or rather long ischemia was followed by reperfusion of various duration. It turned out that in all cases antioxidants exhibit a protective effect even after 6 h of ischemia, but in subsequent reperfusion it is reliably observed only for a limited time, which usually does not reach 2 d. This has led the researchers

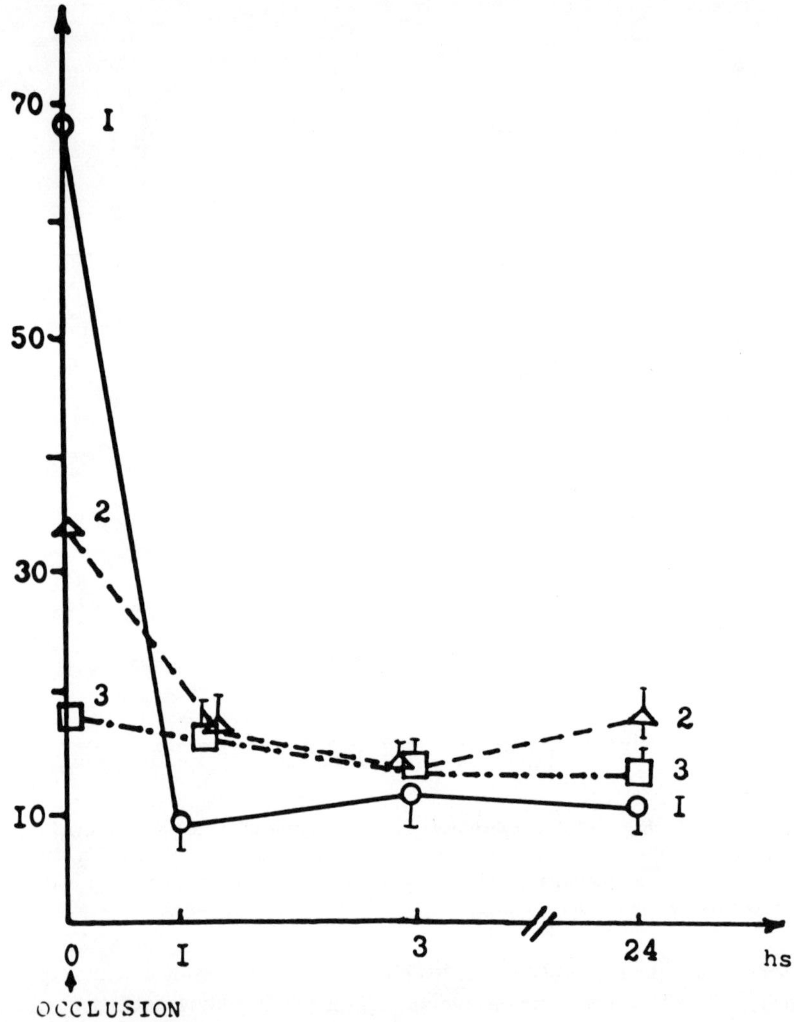

FIGURE 8. Changes in the activity of antioxidant enzymes in the zone of myocardial ischemia upon coronary occlusion. (1) Glutathione peroxidase, (2) superoxide dismutase, (3) catalase. The abscissa is time after occlusion, hr; the ordinate is enzyme activity: GPO, nmol/min; SOD, arb. units (inhibition of a O_2-dependent reaction); catalase, μmol/min.

to the common conclusion that the antioxidants only slow down the development of necrosis, but do not affect its final size.

We have studied the possibility of restricting the volume of necrotic tissue in experimental infarction with the synthetic antioxidant ionol (butylated hydroxytoluene) which, for half a century, has been used as a food additive.

In these studies[47] ionol was administered at 50 mg/kg in vegetable oil daily for 3 d before creating the infarction and for 2 d after. Myocardial infarction in rats was produced by left coronary artery ligation according to Selye.

The left part of Table 5 shows that 2 d after the infarction in the ischemic zone the content of LPO intermediates, dienic conjugates, is enhanced threefold and that of final LPO products, Schiff bases, fourfold. Administration of ionol has no effect whatsoever on these indices and hence on LPO activation. The right part shows that LPO activation in the ischemic zone is accompanied with a more than twofold decrease in GPO and catalase

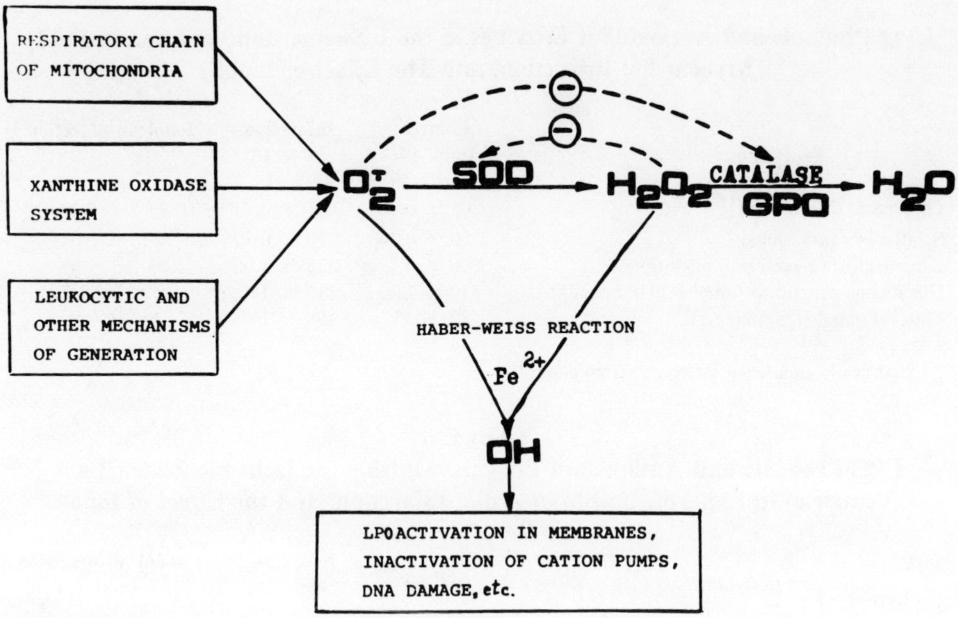

FIGURE 9. LPO activation and its detrimental effect in myocardial ischemia. For explanations see text.

TABLE 4
Effects of Antioxidant Agents on the Size of Ischemic Necroses

Agent	Object	Duration of Ischemia	Duration of Reperfusion	Necrotic size reduction (% of control)	Ref.
Allopurinol	Dog	24 h	—	68	37
	Dog	24 h	—	63	38
	Dog	24 h	—	18	39
	Dog	48 h	—	0	39
	Dog	40 min	4 d	0	40
	Dog	60 min	4 h	50	16
SOD plus catalase	Rabbit	45 min	4 h	32	39
	Rabbit	45 min	3 d	0	39
	Dog	90 min	24 h	52	41
	Dog	6 h	—	45	42
	Dog	6 h	30—48 h	0	42
Antiserum to neutrophils	Dog	90 min	6 h	45	43
	Dog	90 min	24 h	37	44
	Dog	4 h	6 h	0	44
Ibuprofen	Dog	90 min	2—3 d	30	45
	Dog	3 h	3 d	0	46

activities and a somewhat lesser decrease in SOD. Neither of these changes is affected by ionol. This is the situation in the ischemic zone — in the left ventricle; it is different beyond, as shown in Table 6.

One can see that outside the ischemic region — in the right ventricle — LPO is also enhanced and the antioxidant enzymes are also partly inactivated. However, ionol practically abolishes these alterations. This difference may be attributed to greater activation of LPO and destruction of the local antioxidant system in the ischemic region, and inaccessibility of the ischemic zone for ionol

At the same time it should be borne in mind that LPO activation outside the infarct

TABLE 5
LPO Products and Antioxidant Enzymes in the Ischemic Zone in Experimental Myocardial Infarction, and The Effect of Ionol

Indices	Control (n = 18)	Infarction (n = 18)	Ionol + infarction (n = 17)
Conjugated dienes ($OD^{0.1\%}_{1\ cm}$)	1.03 ± 0.08	2.91 ± 0.24[a]	2.79 ± 0.24[a]
Schiff bases (arb. units)	1.00 ± 0.14	4.30 ± 0.19[a]	4.18 ± 0.14[a]
Superoxide dismutase (un./min·mg)	29.6 ± 2.1	16.8 ± 1.08[a]	18.2 ± 1.4[a]
Glutathione peroxidase (nmol NADP/min·mg)	280 ± 11	115 ± 11[a]	129 ± 17[a]
Catalase (nmol H_2O_2/min·mg)	432 ± 30	198 ± 16[a]	219 ± 23[a]

[a] Statistically significant difference from control.

TABLE 6
LPO Products and Antioxidant Enzymes Outside the Ischemic Zone (Right Ventricle) in Experimental Myocardial Infarction, and the Effect of Ionol

Indices	Control (n = 18)	Infarction (n = 18)	Ionol + infarction (n = 17)
Conjugated dienes ($OD^{0.1\%}_{1\ cm}$)	1.36 ± 0.15	2.43 ± 0.29[a]	1.53 ± 0.16
Schiff bases (arb. units)	1.37 ± 0.11	2.46 ± 0.22[a]	1.41 ± 0.31
Superoxide dismutase (U/min·mg)	24.8 ± 0.9	21.4 ± 1.4	23.2 ± 1.6
Glutathione peroxidase (nmol NADP/min·mg)	241 ± 14	158 ± 14[a]	222 ± 11
Catalase (nmol H_2O_2/min·mg)	356 ± 23	247 ± 17[a]	298 ± 18[a]

[a] Statistically significant difference from control.

TABLE 7
Effect of Ionol on the Volume of Necrotic Tissue as Assessed by Visual and Computer Morphometry

	Necrotic volume (% of cardiac muscle)	
	Visual point count	Computer image analysis
Myocardial infarction	38.5 ± 2.9 (n = 9)	48.1 ± 2.8 (n = 8)
Myocardial infarction plus ionol	28.8 ± 1.4	36.6 ± 1.7

Note: $p < 0.05$.

results not from ischemia or reperfusion, but from the stress adrenergic attack which attends any myocardial infarction; it is consistently observed in EPS and prevented with β-blockers as well as with various antioxidants. In this connection we have estimated the influence of ionol on the size of necrosis in experimental infarction.[48] Table 7 shows the volume of necrotic tissue (percent of left ventricular myocardium) determined in sections stained for succinate dehydrogenase: the necrotic portion reaching 48% in unprotected animals is decreased by one fourth in ionol-treated ones.

This positive result might reasonably be explained by the cytoprotective effect of ionol in the periphery of the ischemic zone to which it had some access; however, the very fact of restriction of the necrotic area remains debatable.

It is known that ischemia and reperfusion are attended with catecholamine- and calcium-induced activation of phospholipases, detergent action of lysophospholipids and acylcarnitine, lysosome labilization, and release of lysosomal enzymes. Simultaneously, the lack of energy incapacitates the cation pumps, which in its turn leads to calcium myofibrillar contracture, cardiomyocyte swelling, etc. Thus, LPO activation is just one of the links of the pathogenetic chain of ischemic damage (see Chapter 2). This particularly appears to account for the limited extent and instability of the antinecrotic action of antioxidants in myocardial infarction. Notwithstanding, this gives no grounds for being pessimistic in considering the problem of heart protection with antioxidants. The matter is that LPO is activated in nonischemic regions of the heart under the influence of ischemic stress, throughout the heart in EPS as well as in reoxygenation following transient ischemia; it plays an important part in the pathogenesis of arrhythmias and in cardiac injury in hemolytic anemia;[12,49] it is also consistently elicited in response to large physical loads and decreases physical endurance in animals and humans.[50] In all these cases there is reversible but potentially dangerous injury to the cell membrane structures. Hence there is a need for efficient and differentiated antioxidant protection, and the problem is no less important than that of attenuating the myocardial necrosis in infarction. Accordingly, we shall further consider (with ionol and some other antioxidants) the possibilities of antioxidant protection in myocardial infarction, cardiac stress damage, arrhythmias, and physical loads.

Figure 10 presents the dynamics of left-ventricular developed pressure and contraction velocity at relative rest and under maximal load imposed by clamping the aorta for 25 s. One can see that both indices are substantially decreased in animals with experimental myocardial infarction, the depression being greatest by the 25th second of clamping as the remaining myocardial regions grow tired. Prior administration of ionol prevents such depression to a large extent.[51] This beneficial effect can in great measure be attributed to ionol protecting the nonischemic myocardial regions against the stress damage attending infarction. Indeed, Figure 11 shows that the marked decrease in the right atrial contraction force is largely abolished with the antioxidant.[52]

It is quite plausible that similar protection took place in the nonischemic regions of the ventricle, providing for its higher contractile function as shown in Figure 10.

Notably, administration of the antioxidant restricts not only the depression of contractile function, but also the disturbances of cardiac electric stability in infarction.[53]

Table 8 demonstrates the influence of prior administration of ionol on the fibrillation threshold and the ectopic activity of the heart, which are affected in myocardial infarction. The fibrillation threshold is more than threefold lower 2 d after infarction, and in vagally induced bradycardia numerous extrasystoles are observed. Ionol given for 3 d before and after infarction completely prevents the drop in the fibrillation threshold and diminishes six times the number of vagally elicited ventricular extrasystoles.

These data do not at all mean that ionol specifically should be used in human myocardial infarction, but point to the basic possibility of substantial antioxidant protection against disturbances of cardiac electric stability and contractile function in infarction. We are inclined to regard such protection as the result of restriction of the detrimental action of stress inevitably attending myocardial infarction.

The main mechanism by which stress damages the myocardium, and in particular the nonischemic heart regions in infarction, has been considered in detail in Chapter 1; the primary stress-induced noncoronarogenic damage is an independent phenomenon not linked to ischemia. Indeed, the works of Verrier and other researchers (see Chapter 1) have proved that in the heaviest behavioral stresses conscious animals display not constriction, but, contrariwise, adrenergic dilatation of the coronary vessels and enhancement of the coronary blood flow which, however, is accompanied by a significant drop in the cardiac fibrillation threshold. At the same time, our laboratory has shown that severe exogenous stress gives rise to a peculiar complex of damage which fits well into the concept of the ''primary stress heart''. In this case we are dealing with the β-adrenergic damage that closely resembles the

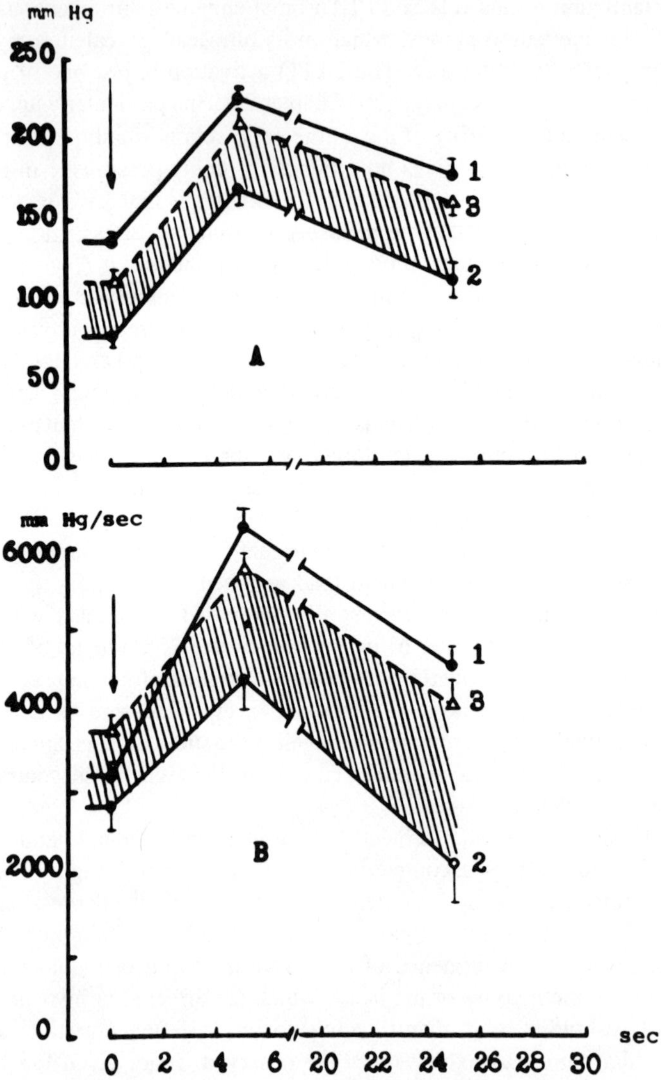

FIGURE 10. Attenuation of the depression of left-ventricular contractility in experimental myocardial infarction with the antioxidant ionol. (A) Developed pressure and (B) pressure buildup rate at relative physiological rest and under maximal cardiac load imposed by complete clamping of the aorta. (1) control, (2) infarction, (3) ionol plus infarction. The shaded zone reflects the protective effect of ionol. The arrow denotes the moment of aortic clamping.

isoproterenol-induced lesions first described by Rona et al.[54] in 1959. Nowadays there is much to make one believe that this complex is not just a lab finding, but an important pathophysiological and clinical syndrome — the primary stress damage to the heart extensively considered in Chapters 1 and 2.

In the present context, the main point of interest is that the chief constituents of cardiac primary stress damage are in great measure induced by LPO activation and can therefore be prevented with timely administration of antioxidants.

A 6-h EPS has been shown to cause accumulation of dienic conjugates and Schiff bases in the myocardium, which can be attenuated by pretreatment with ionol (Chapter 1).

Figure 12A shows that upon EPS the activity of the sarcolemmal Na,K ATPase is

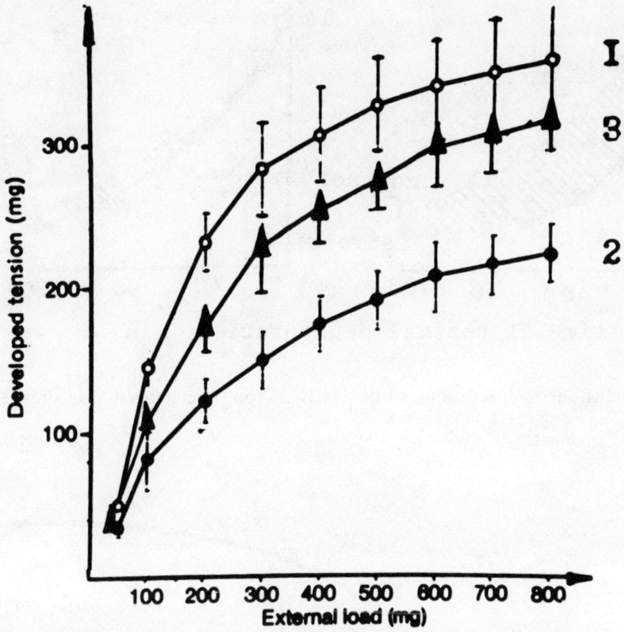

FIGURE 11. Effect of prior administration of ionol on the depression of right-atrial developed tension in experimental left-ventricular infarction. The abscissa is the stretching load, milligrams; the ordinate is developed tension, milligrams. (1) Control, (2) infarction, (3) ionol plus infarction.

TABLE 8
Effect of Ionol on Cardiac Electric Stability in Myocardial Infarction

Series	Heart rate (beats/min)	Fibrillation threshold (mA)	Number of extrasystoles in vagal bradycardia per group
Control (n = 10)	404 ± 13	7.0 ± 0.4	0
Myocardial infarction (n = 10)	394 ± 17	2.1 ± 0.2[a]	167
Ionol (n = 10)	409 ± 12	6.5 ± 0.3	0
Ionol plus infarction (n = 10)	386 ± 16	7.3 ± 0.3	27

[a] $p < 0.001$.

lowered and its thermal inactivation accelerated. Ionol (Figure 12B) prevents this: the shaded zone reflecting the effect of stress almost completely disappears.

As can be seen in Figure 13, the uptake of Ca^{2+} is impaired in SR vesicles isolated from the stress heart; the shaded zone here reflects the protective effect of the antioxidant.

The antioxidant protection against stress can prevent all disturbances to cardiac contractile function, metabolism, and, what is most important, to its electric stability as demonstrated in Figure 14, where prior administration of ionol virtually abolishes the stress-induced decline in the fibrillation threshold (A) and aggravation of vagal bradycardia (B).

These facts provide unequivocal evidence for the feasibility of preventing stress damage with antioxidants; they are important because pronounced LPO activation has now been proved for humans under stress (see Chapter 1) and because we could see that stress damages persist even after a single exposure to stress.

In real life, man, like animals, goes through countless stressful episodes, whose consequences may add up to evolve into noncoronarogenic, nonischemic cardiosclerosis that

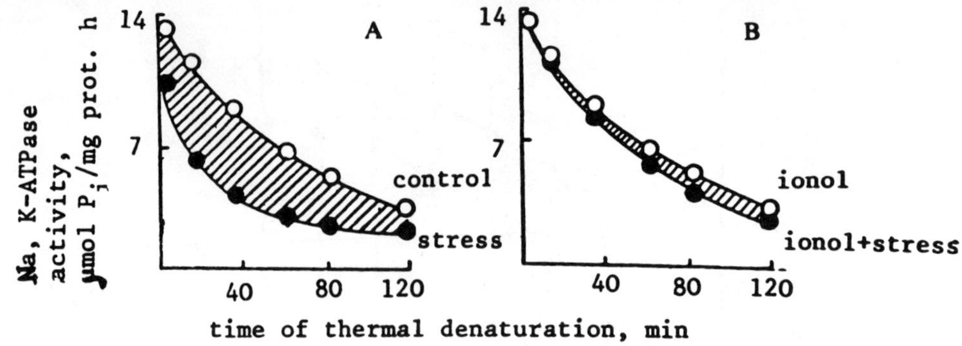

FIGURE 12. Accelerated thermoinactivation of the Na,K ATPase in emotional pain stress (A) and prevention of this with ionol (B).

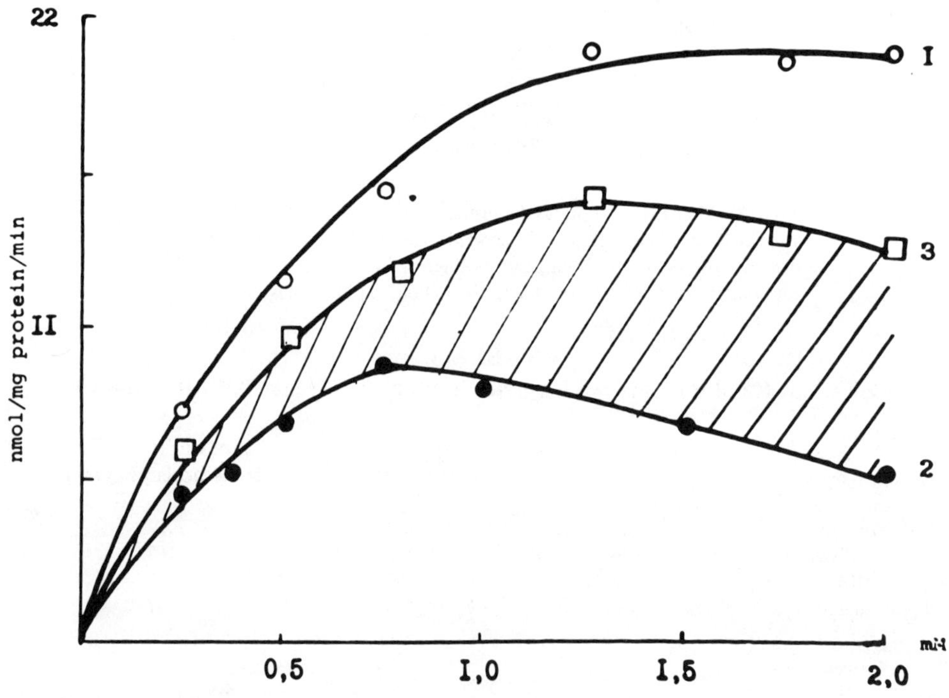

FIGURE 13. Attenuation of the stress-induced impairment of Ca^{2+} uptake by cardiac SR vesicles with ionol. The abscissa is Ca^{2+} concentration in the medium, m*M*; the ordinate is the rate of Ca^{2+} uptake, nmol/min per milligram protein. (1) Control, (2) stress, (3) ionol plus stress.

is, in our opinion, involved in heart diseases. This first of all applies to a large number of patients who have no ischemic disease, but suffer from stubborn, so-called idiopathic arrhythmias and blocks in various divisions of the conduction system, and sometimes from idiopathic cardiopathies leading to heart failure in patients without previous circulatory disorders. In many cases the idiopathic arrhythmias and cardiopathies are probably of stress origin. Therefore, a high content of natural antioxidants in food and special antioxidant protection in stress may attenuate the number of such often serious patients.

Of special significance is the antiarrhythmic action of antioxidants, since the combination of ischemia and stress is the main cause of grave arrhythmias, fibrillation, cardiac arrest, and sudden cardiac death. This situation can be most unambiguously reproduced with acute

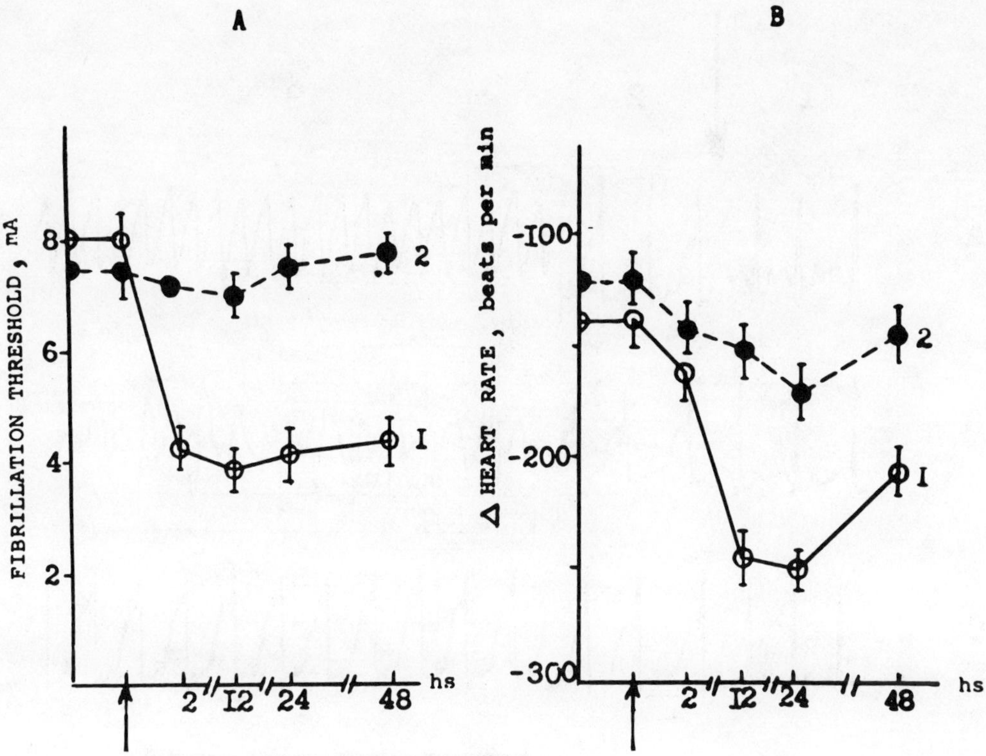

FIGURE 14. Effect of prior administration of ionol on (A) cardiac electric stability and (B) extent of vagal bradycardia in rats that have undergone stress. (1) Untreated animals; (2) ionol-treated animals. Arrows indicate stress. The abscissa is time after stress in hours; the ordinates are (A) fibrillation threshold, milliamperes; (B) drop in the heart rate upon vagal stimulation, beats per minute.

coronary artery occlusion in conscious animals; therefore, we thought it expedient to assess the potentialities of antioxidant protection in just these conditions.

The ECGs in Figure 15 reflect the results obtained with left coronary artery occlusion in conscious rats according to Lepran et al.[55] Ionol, though not abolishing the pronounced ischemic ECG alterations typical of coronary occlusion, nevertheless prevents ventricular tachycardia and fibrillation. Moreover, mortality within 20 min of occlusion was close to 60% (12/21) in the control unprotected group and four times less (3/21) in the ionol-pretreated group.

It is noteworthy that the antiarrhythmic action of antioxidants, unlike their antinecrotic action, has been unequivocally proved in many authoritative laboratories worldwide. Table 9 reviews the antiarrhythmic effects of a broad spectrum of antioxidants in reperfusion (i.e., the most severe) arrhythmias. One can see that antioxidants with quite different mechanisms of action — from xanthine oxidase inhibitors to iron-binding agents — are capable of reducing arrhythmias.

There is also a considerable body of testimony to the antiarrhythmic action of antioxidants in ischemia and adrenergic attack (see review).[63] All this means that antioxidants ought to have an important enough place in the panoply of modern antiarrhythmics.

By and large, collating the marked antiarrhythmic, antistress action of many antioxidants and their debatable effectiveness in restricting the size of ischemic necrosis, one cannot help concluding that the prospects for their use lie mostly in protection against stress and cardiac arrhythmias rather than against irreversible ischemia and necrosis.

Since neurogenic mechanisms are pathogenetically important in arrhythmias, the use of

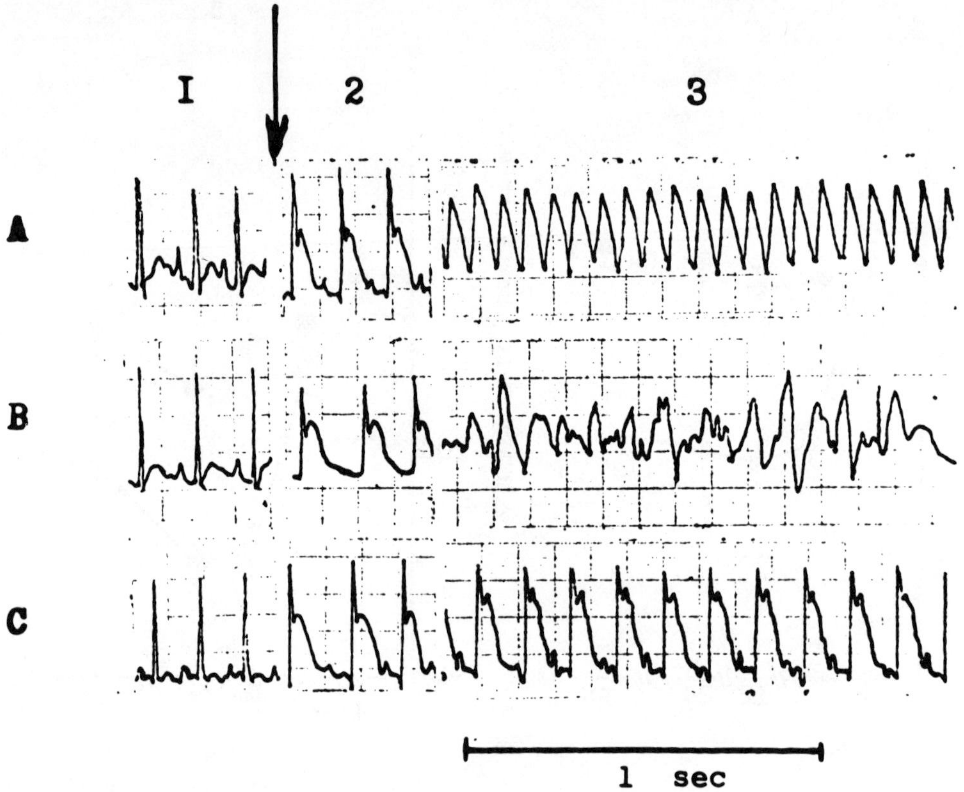

FIGURE 15. Effect of prior administration of ionol on cardiac rhythm disorders elicited by acute coronary occlusion in conscious animals. ECG (I indirect lead): (1) before, (2) 30 s, and (3) 5 min after occlusion. The arrow indicates the moment of occlusion. (A,B) Control, (C) ionol. Explanations in text.

TABLE 9
Effects of Antioxidants on the Incidence of Reperfusion Arrhythmias

Agent	Object	Conditions	Effect[a]	Ref.
Allopurinol	Rat	Anesthesia	D	56
	Dog	Anesthesia	N	57
SOD	Rat	Isolated heart	D	58,59
	Rat	Anesthesia	N	60
Catalase	Rat	Isolated heart	D	59
	Rat	Anesthesia	N	60
Glutathione	Rat	Isolated heart	D	58,59
Mannitol	Rat	Isolated heart	D	58,59
Vitamin E	Rat	Anesthesia	D	60
Vitamin C	Rat	Isolated heart	D	58
Coenzyme Q_{10}	Dog	Anesthesia	D	61
Folic acid	Rat	Anesthesia	D	62
Amflutisol	Rat	Anesthesia	D	62
Desferrioxamine	Rat	Isolated heart	D	59
L-Methionine	Rat	Isolated heart	D	59

[a] D, decrease; N, no effect.

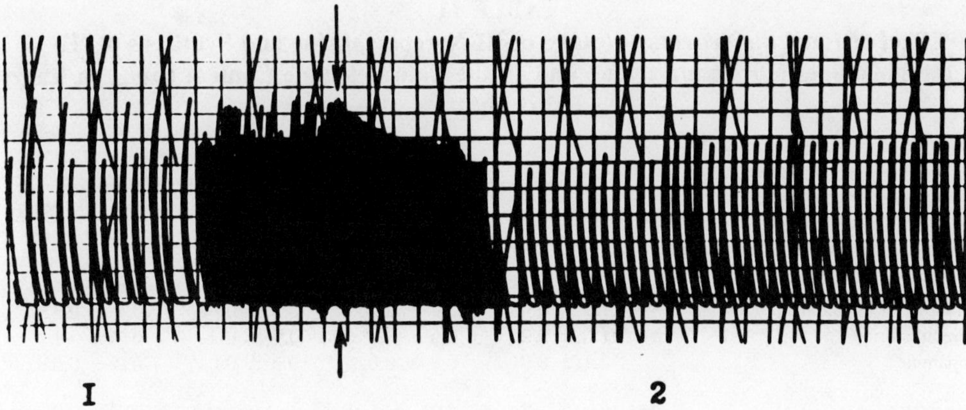

FIGURE 16. A hydroxypyridine antioxidant abolishes spontaneous arrhythmia in the isolated auricle. (1) Spontaneous bigeminy; (2) normalized rhythm. The arrow denotes addition of the antioxidant. Explanations in text.

TABLE 10

Effect of Ionol on Neuronal Uptake of ^{3}H-Norepinephrine and Synthesis of ^{3}H-Catecholamines (10^3 cpm/g Tissue) and on the Catecholamine Content (μg/g) in Rat Adrenal Glands in Stress

	Series (n = 12 each)			
Indices	**Control**	**Stress**	**Ionol**	**Ionol + stress**
Neuronal uptake of ^{3}H-norepinephrine	53.9 ± 2.7	41.2 ± 3.9[a]	56.3 ± 4.3	82.2 ± 3.0[a]
Synthesis of ^{3}H-norepinephrine	7.2 ± 0.6	5.3 ± 0.2[a]	7.2 ± 1.0	21.3 ± 1.6[b]
Synthesis of ^{3}H-dopamine	4.3 ± 0.3	4.3 ± 0.5	4.3 ± 1.1	17.8 ± 1.8[b]
Epinephrine	402 ± 39	209 ± 23[b]	410 ± 53	326 ± 26
Norepinephrine	213 ± 26	149 ± 15[c]	195 ± 19	185 ± 24
Dopamine	2.5 ± 0.3	7.1 ± 0.8[b]	2.1 ± 0.4	4.9 ± 0.7[c]

Difference with control:
[a] $p < 0.01$.
[b] $p < 0.001$.
[c] $p < 0.05$.

antioxidants as antiarrhythmics calls for a clearer notion of whether they only act directly on the heart or may have central action as well.

The direct cardiac action has now been demonstrated in numerous experiments. To give an example (Figure 16), a water-soluble hydroxypyridine antioxidant (2-ethyl-6-methyl-3-hydroxy-pyridine) added to the perfusing solution eliminates the spontaneous stable bigeminy of the isolated auricle. A large number of similar works available leave no doubt of the local cardioprotective ability of antioxidants. Their central action, however, has for a long time been much more questionable.

To elucidate this, we have studied the effect of ionol on the content and the synthesis of catecholamines and corticosterone in the stress reaction. The results proved somewhat unexpected. Table 10 presents the data on catecholamine metabolism in the adrenal glands. Besides the known fact that stress causes a discharge of epinephrine and norepinephrine whereby their content decreases in the adrenal medulla, ionol in stress rather surprisingly enhances severalfold the synthesis of dopamine and norepinephrine, preventing thus the decline in norepinephrine content in the adrenal glands; interestingly, despite greater synthesis with ionol, the dopamine content increases in a considerably smaller degree than without it. It appears that under the influence of ionol the adrenal glands become a source of dopamine.

TABLE 11
Effect of Ionol on Neuronal Uptake of ^{3}H-Norepinephrine and Synthesis of ^{3}H-Catecholamines (10^3 cpm/g tissue) and on the Catecholemine Content (μg/g) in Rat Heart in Stress

	Series (n = 12 each)			
Indices	**Control**	**Stress**	**Ionol**	**Ionol + stress**
Neuronal uptake of ^{3}H-norepinephrine	70.7 ± 4.5	48.6 ± 3.5[a]	74.6 ± 4.1	130.0 ± 11.3[a]
Synthesis of ^{3}H-norepinephrine	7.4 ± 0.5	5.2 ± 0.6[b]	9.3 ± 1.4	34.3 ± 0.4[a]
Synthesis of dopamine	1.9 ± 0.08	2.2 ± 0.26	6.3 ± 0.94[b]	23.1 ± 0.32[a]
Norepinephrine	1.0 ± 0.2	0.6 ± 0.1[b]	0.9 ± 0.2	0.7 ± 0.1
Dopamine	0.1 ± 0.01	0.2 ± 0.02[c]	0.3 ± 0.03[a]	0.2 ± 0.03[a]

Difference with control:
[a] $p < 0.001$.
[b] $p < 0.05$.
[c] $p < 0.01$.

Table 11 shows the data on catecholamine synthesis and content in the heart where they are known to be mainly localized in the adrenergic terminals. Ionol in stress can be seen to enhance dopamine synthesis tenfold and norepinephrine sixfold, and to lessen thus the decline in myocardial norepinephrine.

To appreciate the great activation of dopamine synthesis by ionol, it should be borne in mind that it is a central regulator of motor activity,[64] a vasodilator and natriuretic,[65] and at the same time has much influence on the stress reaction itself. Thus dopamine has been shown to suppress the ACTH-dependent adrenal synthesis of corticosterone[66] and therefore acts as a factor checking the hypophysial-adrenal link of the stress reaction.[66] In full conformity with this, we have found that ionol abolishes the elevation of corticosteroids in the adrenal glands and blood, which is commonly observed in stress or after administration of ACTH.[67]

Thus, the antioxidant used by us is active both in the heart proper and in the regulatory mechanisms. In the final analysis, it augments the content of such a stress-limiting factor as dopamine, prevents catecholamine depletion, and (probably through dopamine) shuts down the hypophysial-adrenal link of the stress reaction.

There are no grounds for regarding ionol as some unique drug; on the contrary, it appears to be a general issue that dealing with any antioxidant we must consider its probable central action. At any rate, in our further work aimed at using the antioxidant to avert arrhythmias in man we took account of this central action when selecting the patients. The therapy was carried out in two groups. The first one comprised patients with neurocirculatory dystonia and neurasthenic syndrome, i.e., phenomena of cardiophobia, hypochondria, and depression; the physical load test ruled out ischemic disease, and arrhythmias occurred mostly at rest. The second group was patients with moderate angina of effort, with arrhythmias elicited under load and being clearly of ischemic origin.

Ionol was administered *per os* at 20 mg/kg daily for 10 to 12 d. Arrhythmias were assessed by 24-h monitoring and counting separately the number of ventricular and atrial extrasystoles for every 3h. No positive effect was observed with angina patients, but it was quite certain in neurocirculatory dystonia (in essence — in neurogenic arrhythmias). Table 12 demonstrates the distribution of ventricular extrasystoles through the day before and after ionol treatment. As can be seen, the extrasystolia, which was most pronounced in these patients during the night, was markedly alleviated by the antioxidant; this quite reliable effect was maintained for at least 2 months after the end of the course. Simultaneously the manifestations of the neurasthenic syndrome and especially hypochondriac complaints and depressive phenomena were much abated.

TABLE 12
Effect of a Course of Ionol on the Mean Number of Supraventricular (SVE) and Ventricular (VE) Extrasystoles Throughout the Day in 21 Patients with Neurocirculatory Dystonia

Time of day (h)	Mean number of extrasystoles: Before treatment SVE	Before treatment VE	After treatment SVE	After treatment VE
00—03	651 ± 72	2156 ± 187	262 ± 37	1005 ± 95
03—06	342 ± 45	1058 ± 115	116 ± 29	651 ± 75
06—09	95 ± 10	938 ± 76	64 ± 9	405 ± 72
09—12	116 ± 11	451 ± 66	55 ± 7	156 ± 47
12—15	61 ± 7	578 ± 31	45 ± 6	256 ± 51
15—18	75 ± 8	296 ± 42	26 ± 5	105 ± 21
18—21	115 ± 10	415 ± 56	86 ± 7	156 ± 10
21—24	239 ± 23	851 ± 92	106 ± 9	211 ± 25

Thus, there is reason to believe that the antiarrhythmic action of ionol and other antioxidants in animals and man can take place both in the heart itself and through neural regulation.

Another possible and noteworthy application of antioxidants stems from the observation that the power of the natural antioxidant systems increases as the organism adapts to repeated stress and physical load (see above). On the strength of these data and in accordance with the traditions of our laboratory, we exploited the principle of mimicking the natural organismic stress-limiting systems, i.e., used the antioxidant ionol to improve physical endurance first in animals[12] and then in humans.[50]

Assays of the peroxidation product pentane, in the air exhaled by subjects have shown that submaximal and maximal veloergometric (VEL) work is accompanied with an outburst of free-radical oxidation, which can be suppressed with antioxidants.

Figure 17 shows that a prior 10-d course of 20 mg ionol daily per kilogram body weight markedly diminishes the pentane content in exhaled air upon maximal VEL. Further, it turned out that checking the outburst of peroxidation under physical load is physiologically significant since it can appreciably enhance physical endurance. According to Table 13, at submaximal load to exhaustion the antioxidant increases the total performed work by more than 40% in untrained subjects and by 80% in trained athletes.

In the aggregate the data available mean that under physical load, activated free-radical oxidation imposes a limitation on the performance. The organism can alleviate this by enhancing the synthesis of antioxidant enzymes; on the other hand, the same can be achieved by introducing antioxidants into the organism. At present, the state of free-radical oxidation and of the antioxidant systems is known to change in adaptation to many environmental factors, and we have grounds for concluding that, on the one hand, environmental adaptation determines the antioxidant status and the free-radical homeostasis in the organism as a whole and in the heart in particular; on the other, exogenous antioxidants can be used for controlling and correcting the adaptive processes.

To conclude this section, mention should be made of some promising trends in developing the antioxidant protection of the heart and the organism in whole.

The first one is studying the role of pro-oxidants and antioxidants at the genetic level, and designing such antioxidants as would act not as simple free-radical traps, but as genomic inductors. Figure 18 shows that the major natural antioxidant α-tocopherol not only scavenges free radicals, but also induces the synthesis of enzymes responsible for formation of another group of natural antioxidants and electron carriers — ubiquinones.[68] This is not a unique

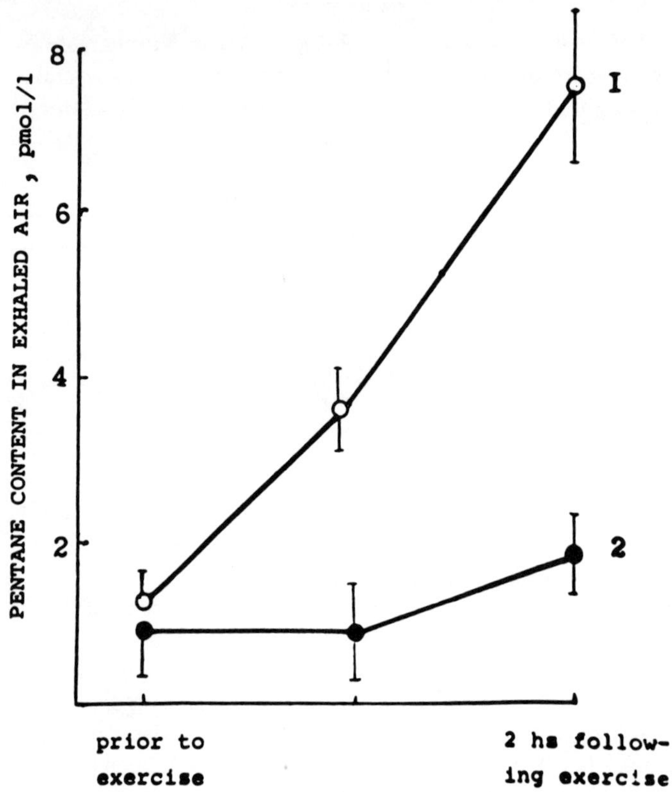

FIGURE 17. Effect of physical load and ionol on the pentane content in exhaled air in human subjects. (1) Before and (2) after administration of ionol.

TABLE 13
Effect of Ionol on Physical Endurance of Untrained and Trained Subjects

	Untrained (n = 6)		Trained (n = 24)	
	Before ionol	After ionol	Before ionol	After ionol
Duration of load, min	13.7 ± 1.9	19.6 ± 5.5[a]	23.8 ± 3.7	44.0 ± 9.6[a]
Work, N·m	2650 ± 422	3812 ± 637[a]	4666 ± 935	9245 ± 1920[a]

[a] Difference with initial indices significant at $p < 0.05$.

example: Wefers et al.[69] have reported that a synthetic antioxidant, butyl hydroxyanisol, is also a potent inductor of the antioxidant enzyme NAD(P)H: quinone reductase.

Another promising trend is elucidation of the interrelation between the antioxidant and other cell regulatory systems. Figure 19 demonstrates how the antioxidant status of the cell, in particular the myocyte of the coronary artery, can determine the balance of prostacyclin and thromboxane systhesis: in deficiency of antioxidant protection thromboxane formation prevails, with increasing probability of coronary spasm and thrombosis, whereas with optimal antioxidant protection the situation is opposite. There is good reason for studying further the relations of the cellular free-radical homeostasis with the prostaglandin (PG) system, the adenosinergic system, the receptor-dependent system of cyclic nucleotides.

The next approach of promise, to my mind, is combining antioxidants with other cardiac

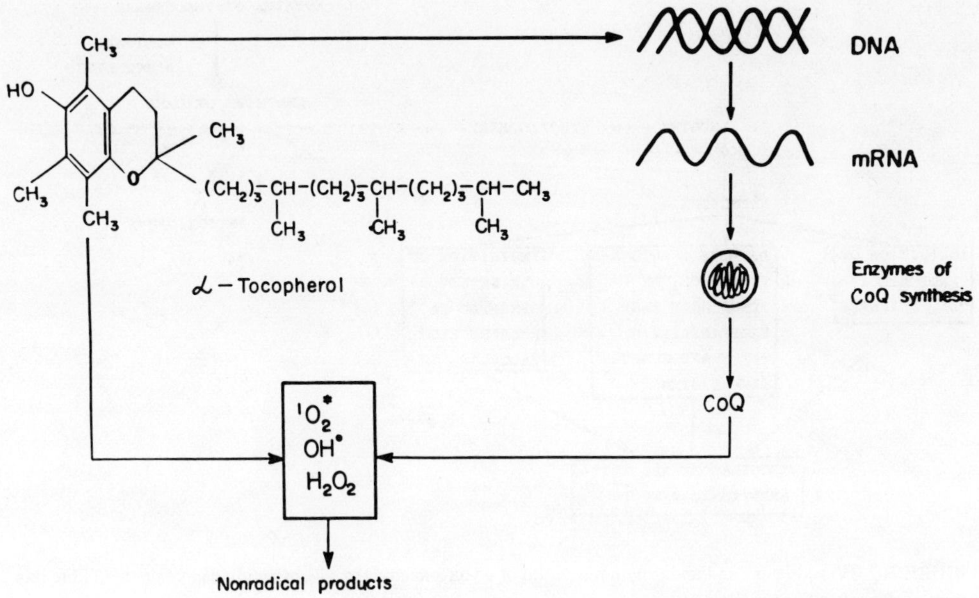

FIGURE 18. α-Tocopherol induces enzymes responsible for synthesis of ubiquinones. For explanations see text.

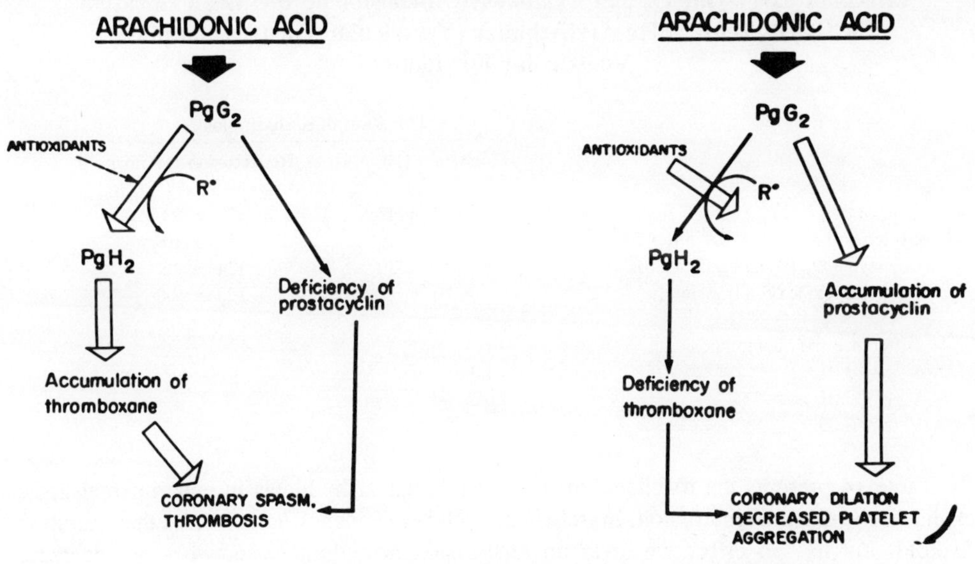

FIGURE 19. Effects of antioxidants on prostacyclin and thromboxane synthesis. PGG_2 and PGH_2, arachidonic acid endoperoxides, precursors of prostacyclin and thromboxane; R·, free radical. For explanations see text.

protectors; one of the numerous examples from this field concerns the vasodilatory and antiarrhythmic action of adenosine. Its mechanism is shown in Figure 20, yet at the same time it can be seen that the breakdown of adenosine may create a surplus of substrate for xanthine oxidase and thereby enhance generation of free radicals. It is therefore understandable that in some cases adenosine, especially in combination with inosine, may promote reperfusion arrhythmias or at any rate be not helpful against these arrhythmias. Hence it is expedient to combine the adenosine derivatives with antioxidants, e.g., of the ubiquinone group.

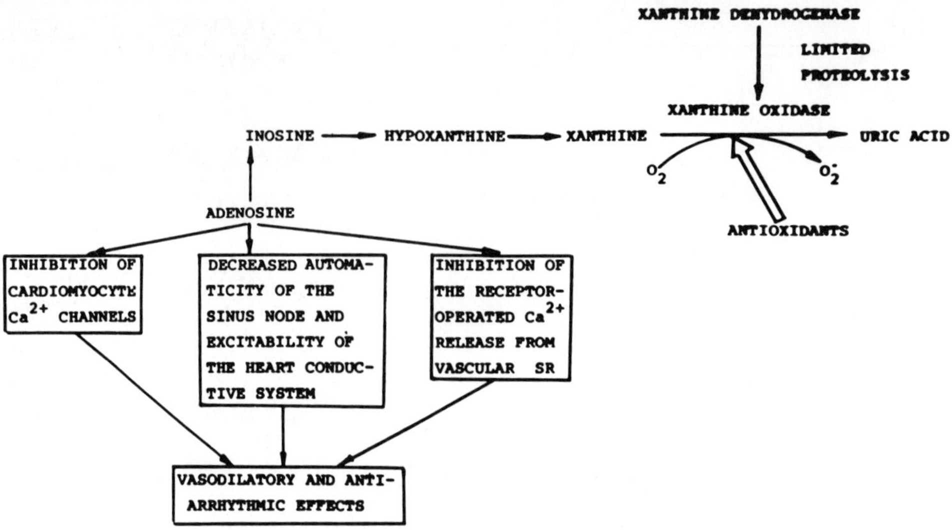

FIGURE 20. Vasodilatory and antiarrhythmic action of adenosine and the role of antioxidants in potentiating this action. For explanations see text.

TABLE 14
Effects of Coenzyme Q_9 and Cyclohexyl Adenosine on the Mean Duration of Grave Ventricular Arrhythmias (Ventricular Tachycardia plus Ventricular Fibrillation)

	Duration of arrhythmias (s)	
	Ischemia (10 min)	Reperfusion (10 min)
Control (n = 12)	150 ± 37	371 ± 57
Cyclohexyl adenosine 0.1 mmol/kg (n = 12)	33 ± 16[a]	359 ± 104
Coenzyme Q_9 10 mg/kg (n = 10)	121 ± 30	124 ± 26[b]
Q_9 plus cyclohexyl adenosine (n = 12)	26 ± 12[b]	123 ± 93[c]

Difference with control:
[a] $p < 0.02$.
[b] $p < 0.01$.
[c] $p < 0.05$.

Table 14 presents the results of treating ventricular arrhythmias in experimental acute cardiac ischemia and reperfusion. In ischemia, cyclohexyl adenosine decreases their duration fivefold, but has no effect whatever on reperfusion arrhythmias, and does not decrease animal mortality from such arrhythmias. Conversely, coenzyme Q_9 does not appreciably affect the ischemic arrhythmias, but decreases the duration of grave reperfusion arrhythmias almost fourfold and mortality threefold. When the agents are used together they are not synergistic, but an indisputable advantage of such a combination is that it is equally effective against ischemic and reperfusion arrhythmias. This may be not the most efficient combination possible, but is a most definite evidence of the prospects in this field.

Finally, the available, means of assaying the peroxidation processes in the intact organism (pentane assays in the exhaled air in various functional tests, assays of antioxidant enzymes, and other more direct approaches) appear to open the possibility of a standardized clinical evaluation of antioxidant status of the organism, which can be of certain practical importance in various diseases. Thus, our preliminary studies have shown that patients with pronounced

IHD risk factors often have lowered blood levels of antioxidant enzymes and respond to physical load with enhanced pentane production. It cannot be excluded that after a thorough analysis a reduced antioxidant status will be entered into the list of the risk factors of ischemic disease.

On the whole, the antioxidant systems of the heart itself and the use of exogenous antioxidants show much promise for heart protection.

III. PROSTAGLANDIN SYSTEM AND HEART PROTECTION FROM STRESS AND ISCHEMIC DAMAGES*

Under extensive study at present is the group of arachidonic acid derivatives, or eicosanoids, which participate as modulators in regulating the functions of various organs and tissues, from vascular tone and blood clotting mechanisms to inflammation processes and release of neuromediators and hormones.

A special place in this group is occupied by PG. Unlike other eicosanoids, PGs are capable of restricting and modulating the activation of the adrenergic link of the stress reaction, and also exhibit a cytoprotective action in the heart and other organs, which allows the PG system to be classed with the stress-limiting systems of the organism.

The initial step in formation of PG (and other eicosanoids) is the liberation of arachidonic acid from cell membrane lipids and to some extent from other lipids.[70] Formation of free arachidonic acid triggers a ''cascade'' of eicosanoid synthesis involving a number of enzymes such as prostacyclin synthetase, thromboxane synthetase, endoperoxide isomerase, and endoperoxide reductase.[71,72] It should be noted that some or other eicosanoids are preferentially produced depending on the type of cell. Thus, in blood platelets mostly thromboxanes are formed, while the yield of PG is very low,[73] whereas myocardium most typically produces prostacyclin (PGI_2)[74] and PG of the E group (PGE_1, PGE_2).[75] The coronary vascular wall yields mainly PGI_2.[73,76]

It should also be emphasized that preferential formation of particular eicosanoids in the ''arachidonic cascade'' depends on a number of factors affecting the steps of this cascade. Thus, blocking the lipoxygenase pathway gives rise mainly to PGs which are cytoprotective and vasodilatory, while leukotrienes which act in an opposite way are not formed, etc. It is noteworthy that certain steps of the cascade are associated (as already mentioned in the first section of this chapter) with LPO activation and lipid peroxide formation and are susceptible to antioxidants, and some enzymes in the cascade are sensitive to these peroxides.[71] It can thus be thought that during the stress reaction PG synthesis and the scale of their protective effect are in great measure determined by the activity of the antioxidant system and by the LPO level.

The PG system is in a certain way coupled with the stress-effecting systems: when neuromediators and stress hormones stimulate the cell functions (see Chapter 1), they may simultaneously activate eicosanoid synthesis by promoting the liberation of arachidonic acid.

Indeed, hormone and mediator action on the cell Ca^{2+}-mobilizing receptors results in activation of phospholipase C that hydrolyzes phosphatidylinositol (PI) and its derivatives to produce diacyl glycerol (DAG) and inositol triphosphate (IP_3). Thereupon DAG, on the one hand, acts together with IP_3 to raise the cytosolic Ca^{2+} and activate the cell functions, and on the other is catabolized with appropriate lipolytic enzymes to liberate arachidonic acid. Again, elevated Ca^{2+} activates the phospholipase C isozyme cleaving other membrane phospholipids (and thereby producing DAG and further arachidonic acid) and phospholipase A_2, which is the major enzyme liberating arachidonic acid from any phospholipids and phosphatidic acid.[70,77,78]

It should also be noted that enhancement of cell functions by agonists of the adenylate

* With M. G. Pshennikova.

cyclase receptors is also coupled with liberation of arachidonic acid through phospholipase A_2 activation by the cAMP-dependent protein kinase. In the heart, activation of PGE_2 and PGI_2 synthesis by catecholamines can be suppressed not only with blockers of the Ca^{2+}-mobilizing α-receptors, but also with a β-adrenoreceptor blocker.[75]

Thus, it can be supposed that during the stress reaction the increased output of hormones and mediators that are agonists of Ca^{2+}-mobilizing and adenylate cyclase-activating receptors not only changes the cell function, but at the same time can, through liberation of arachidonic acid, stimulate the biosynthesis of eicosanoids and among them PG.

The actual existence of such coupling has been to date well proved for catecholamines. There are three main lines of evidence: (1) catecholamines increase the PG output into the blood from various tissues; (2) the catecholamine-induced increase in PG output is blocked by inhibitors of catecholamine action; (3) the catecholamine-induced increase in PG output is blocked by inhibitors of PG synthesis. These data have been obtained for different organs; we shall only consider some of them pertaining to the heart.

In the late 1970s to early 1980s it has been shown that sympathetic stimulation of the isolated rabbit heart with intact innervation entails marked release of PGE and PGI_2 into the perfusate, which can be prevented by blocking the cardiac adrenoreceptors with propranolol and phentolamine.[74,79] With canine heart *in situ* administration of epinephrine and norepinephrine greatly increased the PGE content in venous blood flowing off the heart; this was completely abolished by indomethacin, which blocks cyclooxygenase, a key enzyme of the "arachidonic cascade".[80] Inhibition of the catecholamine-induced output of PG by indomethacin was also observed with the rabbit heart.[79] Finally, ^{14}C-labeled arachidonic acid has been used to demonstrate that the adrenergically stimulated PG output from the heart is the direct consequence of their enhanced synthesis.[81]

It has also been found that vasopressin activates PGI_2 synthesis in the vascular wall[82] and angiotensin II activates it in the adrenal glands.[83]

In the context of this exposition it is essential that the catecholamine-activated PG system can, through feedback, modulate the adrenergic effects on the heart and other organs by affecting norepinephrine release from sympathetic terminals and catecholamine action on the target organ cells. Most of the data available indicate that PGE_1, PGE_2, and PGI_2, usually produced by activated sympathetic regulation in the number of organs, are physiological modulators of sympathetic transmission, limiting excessive release of norepinephrine from sympathetic terminals; PGs do not affect norepinephrine reuptake, so the amount of the mediator in the action zone decreases and its influence on the effector cells is restricted correspondingly (for references see Wennmalm et al.)[75]

It is also important that PGs produce their regulatory action directly at the level of the effector cells as well. In particular, PGI_2 synthesized in the coronary vascular endothelium and intima is a coronarodilator (especially in small arteries) and a potent inhibitor of platelet aggregation, unlike thromboxane A_2 (TXA_2) produced in the platelets, which is a powerful inductor of platelet aggregation and vasoconstriction,[73,76] and unlike leukotrienes synthesized mainly by the neutrophils and having a pronounced coronaroconstrictive action.[84]

PGI_2 acquires special significance in coronary failure. In patients with coronary disease, inhibition of PGI_2 synthesis by indomethacin has been shown to attenuate the coronary sinus flow and increase the resistance in large coronary arteries despite enhanced oxygen consumption, whereas in normal coronary arteries indomethacin does not substantially reduce their diameter.[76] This phenomenon appears to be due to the prevalence of leukotrienes and their vasoconstrictive action, since there are data that show leukotriene synthesis is enhanced in coronary failure and ischemia.[87] It has also been shown that spontaneous reduction of coronary flow in partial constriction of the coronary artery, which is caused by platelet aggregation, develops as a result of the lack of PGI_2 and decreasing PGI_2/TXA_2 ratio, and is completely prevented by administration of PGI_2.[73]

Recently, a similar protective action has been found with PGE_1, which upon intracoronary infusion prevented reocclusion of coronary arteries in dogs with thrombosis of the circumflex coronary artery produced with dosed local application of electric current causing a 50% reduction of the arterial lumen; the PGE_1 effect was due to inhibition of platelet aggregation and its vasodilatory action.[85]

PGs operate through specific binding sites on the target cell membranes.[86,87] Besides, these is evidence for their cytoprotective action associated with direct influence on the cell membranes that increases membrane resistance to damaging factors. In particular, increased PGE content in gastric mucosal cells has been shown to prevent injury from concentrated solutions of ethanol, mannitol, or hydrochloric acid.[88]

In a study of the influence of PGI_2 and its stable synthetic analog quinoin-169 on isoproterenol cardiac damage, administration of PG before isoproterenol substantially attenuated the size of myocardial necrosis. Since the maximal protective effect was observed when PG was administered 1.5 to 2 h before (and within this time PGs are completely broken down in the organism), the authors concluded that the protective effect was underlain by the stabilizing action of PGs on the cardiomyocyte membranes.[89]

The mechanism of this cytoprotective action of PGs appears to be related to their lipid nature and their influence on the membrane lipid bilayer. Indeed, it has been recently[90] shown that administration of a PGI_2 analog iloprost 20 min after coronary artery ligation, when any other PG effects are unlikely to be of any help, appreciably attenuates in rats the ischemic destruction of cardiomyocyte membranes and loss of phospholipids and creatine kinase.

Hence, PGs can be supposed to prevent stress damages or diseases provoked by the stress reaction. The protective effect of PGs is most definite in stress ulceration of the gastric mucosa. Such lesions produced in rats by a 2-h immobilization stress are efficiently averted with prior administration of PGE.[91] Recently, the development of gastric stress ulcers has been found to depend on the endogenous PG level in the gastric mucosa. Ulceration in immobilization[92] and other[93] types of stress is associated with a decline in PGE_2, PGI_2, *et seq.* in the mucosa. Prior activation of PG synthesis by intragastric administration of arachidonic acid prevents both the PGE_2 drop and ulceration.[92] It has also been shown that the known antiulcerous action of the histamine H_2-receptor blocker famotidine is due to the fact that the drug prevents the stress-induced decline in gastric mucosal PG.[93] PGs provide protection against such damages by preventing gastric vasoconstriction owing to their vasodilatory properties, and by stabilizing the gastric cell membranes.

Of greatest interest for us is the role and possible protective action of PGs against stress-induced and ischemic damage to the heart. Most of the works of recent years testify that PGs display preventive and protective effects in disturbances to cardiac structure and contractility caused by stress and ischemia. Thus, we[94] have shown that reduction of myocardial extensibility and contractility after immobilization stress is prevented by prior administration of PGE_2 to animals; administration of indomethacin to inhibit PG synthesis, conversely, aggravated the stress damage to myocardial function. With the isolated rabbit heart, addition of PGI_2 to the perfusing solution starting from 10 min prior to left coronary artery ligation prevented the ischemia-induced "discharge" or norepinephrine from sympathetic terminals, as well as the drop in ATP and the creatine phosphokinase (CPK) leakage from the myocardium.[95] It can be supposed that in both works the protective effect of PG is mostly due to checking the excessive release of norepinephrine and therefore the possible adrenergic injury to the myocardium. At the same time, the above-discussed properties of PGs suggest that their coronarodilatory and cytoprotective features are also involved.

More direct evidence for this has been obtained in studies where PGs were administered not before, but after coronary occlusion, in already existing ischemia. Thus, in cats introduction of a PGI_2 analog iloprost in reperfusion 30 min and 2 h after the onset of ischemia prevented the drop in CPK activity and leakage of cathepsin D from the ischemic zone and substantially enhanced the coronary flow in the nonischemic myocardium, without changing the infarct size;[96] the authors regard these PG effects as the cytoprotective ones. The cytoprotective, membrane-stabilizing action of PG has been convincingly proved in the work[90] where a stable PGI_2 analog was administered to rats 20 min after coronary occlusion; the preparation markedly attenuated the loss of phospholipids caused by ischemic damage to cardiomyocyte membranes.

The ability of PGs to restrict the sympathetic influences and their cytoprotective properties are apparently the basis of their antiarrhythmic action in ischemic arrhythmias where, as already more than once mentioned, the stress reaction is pathogenetically important. Thus, it has been shown[97] that ligation of the left anterior descending coronary artery in anesthetized dogs led to 35% mortality within 6 h; no mortality was observed among animals receiving PGI_2 (0.32 μg/kg·min throughout the experiment). In the process, PGI_2 affected neither the infarct size nor the hemodynamic indices measured 15 and 45 min after the onset of ischemia. The authors[97] were of the opinion that the protective effect of PGI_2 was due to prevention of lethal arrhythmias. In a study with ECG recording in conscious dogs,[98] occlusion of the left circumflex coronary artery caused ventricular fibrillation in 53% (9/17) and death with 80 min in 64% of the control group; in animals receiving PGI_2 (0.1 μm/kg·min) the incidence of ventricular fibrillation was only 6% (1/17) and mortality was threefold less.

In line with these data are the results of works[99,100] showing that development of arrhythmias correlates with a decline in the PGI_2 content and the PGI_2/TXA_2 ratio. When the platelet-activating factor (PAF), which is released from leukocytes in ischemia and stress and promotes production of leukotrienes and TXA_2, was administered to guinea pigs, it substantially lowered the threshold of ouabain-induced arrhythmias and increased their lethality. This arrhythmogenic effect of PAF could be completely abolished with a selective thromboxane receptor antagonist BM 13.177 and less efficiently with the lipoxygenase inhibitor esculetin.[100] At the same time aspirin, which inhibits a key enzyme of PG and thromboxane synthesis, cyclooxygenase, did not have much influence on the PAF effect, but still showed a tendency to raising the threshold of arrhythmias, probably by attenuating the TXA_2 synthesis. Thus, in arrhythmogenic situations the PG/thromboxane ratio comes to be of great importance.

There is yet no full understanding of the localization of the antiarrhythmic effect of PG. In the glycoside model of arrhythmias, the antiarrhythmic effect is unrelated to their central action: administration of PGI_2, PGE_2, and $PGF_{2\alpha}$ into brain ventricles was ineffective against ouabain-induced extrasystoles and fibrillation, though intravenous infusion suppressed these cardiac rhythm disorders, whereas the β-blocker propranolol was effective in both cases.[101] The genesis of glycoside arrhythmias involves enhanced sympathetic influence on the heart,[102] hence it can be supposed that PGs restrict it by hindering the norepinephrine release from sympathetic terminals in the myocardium. Again, since glycoside arrhythmias involved interruption of the membrane cation pumps, the membrane-stabilizing action of PGs may also contribute to their protective effect. Further, PGs can stimulate the peripheral parasympathetic regulation of the heart which produces an antiarrhythmic effect in glycoside intoxications.[101]

In the aconitic model, on the contrary, the antiarrhythmic effect of PGs appears to be central (since it takes place upon central administration).[103]

It must be accentuated that the very question of the use of exogenous PGs in cardiac ischemic damage and arrhythmias is quite complicated and requires further serious study, because besides the above and other numerous data on the protective role of PGs there are reports[104,105] on their possible detrimental action: PGE_2 and PGI_2 can aggravate, in a dose-dependent way, the functional disturbances and arrhythmias in the isolated heart exposed to ischemia or glycosides, which is believed to result from activation of the slow Ca^{2+} channels, overloading of the cardiac cells with calcium, and mitochondrial damage.[104]

At the same time, there is a considerable body of evidence that a natural increase in the power of the PG system in the organism and normalization of the relations between PGs and other eicosanoids enhance the resistance of the organism to injurious influences. Thus, it has been convincingly demonstrated that reinforcement of the PG system in the gastric mucosa either with precursors of PG synthesis[92] or with prior adaptation to stress[88] prevents the PG deficiency and ulceration in stress[92] and increases the resistance of the gastric mucosa to chemical injury.[88]

Atherogenic dyslipoproteinemia is known as a basic cause of atherogenesis and atherosclerosis, a heavy risk factor of IHD and myocardial infarction. In recent years the blood high-/ and low-density lipoproteins (HDLP/LDLP) ratio has been found to be rather clearly related with the vascular PG synthesis. (May it be recalled that atherogenic dyslipoproteinemia evoked by stress or other causes results from impairment of the hepatic cholesterol-catabolizing enzymes and lecithin:cholesterol acyltransferase involved in HDLP formation.[106,107]) Over a decade ago, development of atherosclerosis has been shown to combine with PGI_2 deficiency.[108] Recently, certain patients with ulcerous disease of the digestive tract have been found to have hypercholesterolemia and atherogenic dyslipoproteinemia; treatment of ulcers with the PGE_2 analog enprostil was accompanied with normalization of the cholesterol status.[109] These results were supported by a special study of healthy subjects where the PGs decreased LDLP cholesterol and increased HDLP cholesterol.[109]

We[110] have shown that prior adaptation to stress elevates the blood PGE; simultaneously, such adaptation prevents the stress-induced atherogenic dyslipoproteinemia.[106] Hence, it can be concluded that PGs are capable of normalizing the lipoprotein metabolism. Since hepatocyte membrane damage is important in the pathogenesis of atherogenic dyslipoproteinemia, this protective action of PGs can be attributed to their cytoprotective effect in the liver. On the other hand, there are recent data[111] that HDLP stimulate while LDLP suppress PGI_2 synthesis in isolated coronary vessel microsomes. This implies a vicious circle: atherogenic dyslipoproteinemia may suppress the vascular PG synthesis, which in its turn reduces their hepatoprotective capacity and thereby aggravates the dyslipoproteinemia. It can thus be thought that increasing the power of the PG system enhances hepatocyte resistance to damaging factors including stress, and can therefore be a means of preventing atherosclerosis.

In the aggregate, the dat available suggest that, first, increased power of the PG system plays a certain part in the protective effect of adaptation to stress against the stress-induced and ischemic disturbances to cardiac rhythm and function, and second, there is certain promise in studying the cardioprotective properties of PGs and their analogs with a view to their use against arrhythmias.

IV. ADENOSINERGIC SYSTEM AND HEART PROTECTION FROM STRESS, ISCHEMIC, AND REPERFUSION DAMAGES*

There are three main features by which the adenosinergic system (i.e., adenosine and its receptors) can be classed with stress-limiting systems. First, adenosine has pronounced vasodilatory activity,[76,112] is not normally found in blood and peripheral tissues in acting concentrations, but is formed in the heart and other tissues and released into the blood in conditions associated with deficit of creatine phosphate (CP) and ATP and enhanced oxygen consumption in the cells: ischemia, hypoxia, physical load, action of catecholamines and hormones, etc.[112,115,117] This means that the stress reaction is naturally coupled with activation of the adenosinergic system. Second, adenosine can restrict the release of adrenergic mediators both in the central nervous system and in the periphery.[113-115] Third, it can modulate the action of neuromediators and hormones on the target organ cells.[112,116-118] Here we shall focus on these features of adenosine as applied to the heart and vessels.

* With M. G. Pshennikova.

In the myocardium, adenosine is produced from 5′-AMP by 5′-nucleotidase bound with the cardiomyocyte membrane. The enzyme is inhibited by ADP, AMP, and most strongly by CP, so normally its activity in the cell is about two orders of magnitude lower than *in vitro;* it is activated by free Mg^{2+}. Adenosine is catabolized by adenosine deaminase to inosine, this reaction being inhibited by its product.[112,119]

In a stress reaction evoked by load, hypoxia, or otherwise, under the influence of excess catecholamines and hormones and enhanced cardiac function, myocardial consumption of ATP and CP outstrips their resynthesis so that the level of these inhibitors of 5′-nucleotidase declines while the amounts of its activator Mg^{2+} (released on breakdown of ATP) and its substrate AMP increase, thus favoring formation of adenosine. The same chain of events naturally takes place in adrenergic and hormonal coronary constriction and in coronary thrombosis attending the stress reaction, especially in IHD and atherosclerosis.

It is noteworthy that catecholamines and other β- and α-adrenoreceptor agonists are themselves highly conducive to adenosine production in the heart in normoxia and ischemia.[117,120] Adenosine is released from the myocardium into the interstitial space, reaches the coronary arterioles, and acts there to restrict the detrimental action of the very factors that stimulated its formation. In other words, there is a feedback mechanism.

Two effects of adenosine are of chief importance. The first one is coronary dilation, which counteracts vasoconstriction, enhances the coronary blood flow, and thereby facilitates oxygen and substrate supplies to the myocardium and normalizes the energy balance therein. The second one is checking the excessive adrenergic influence on the cardiac muscle, which attenuates its contractile function and oxygen consumption (thus also normalizing the energy balance) and prevents the cardiotoxic action of catecholamines.

The vasodilatory effect of adenosine has been convincingly proved in experiments on animals and in clinical studies.[121-124] In particular, administration of adenosine prevents the "no-reflow" phenomenon occurring in reperfusion after ischemia, and thus prevents or substantially attenuates myocardial damage in reperfusion.[123]

Adenosine exerts its vasodilatory effect mainly by direct action on vascular myocytes, partly by interacting with the endothelium, and by suppressing the release of norepinephrine from the sympathetic terminals innervating the vessels. Now we know that the key role in contraction of the vascular smooth-muscle walls is played by the increase in calcium concentration in the myocytes owing to its entry from the outside and release from the intracellular depots. It is these mechanisms that are involved in the vasoconstrictive action of catecholamines and hormones,[77,125] and there are grounds for believing that they are also affected in the vasodilatory effect of adenosine.[76,116,126] This concept is demonstrated by the scheme in Figure 21. As can be seen, contraction of a vessel such as a coronary artery results from a chain of events triggered by increasing cytosolic Ca^{2+}. Calcium enters the cell from the outside through potential-dependent channels (II) activated upon depolarization and through receptor-dependent channels (I) activated by hormones, and is released from the SR under the influence of the inositol phosphate circuit which is activated when norepinephrine from the sympathetic terminals acts on α_1-adrenoreceptors. The last two pathways are believed to be suppressible by adenosine,[76,116,126] which is denoted by the "minus" signs in Figure 21. Though little is known as yet about the molecular mechanisms of these effects, they are likely to involve interaction of the adenosine receptors[127-129] with the Ca^{2+} channels and adrenoreceptor complexes through the G-proteins.[129] An illustration of the possible adenosine receptor-adrenoreceptor interaction is a recent study[116] with rat aortic strips showing that adenosine, while not affecting the calcium homeostasis and IP_3 content in the vascular myocytes at rest, largely checks the IP_3 synthesis and Ca^{2+} release from the SR stimulated by norepinephrine via the α_1-adrenoreceptors, and thereby prevents the norepinephrine-induced constriction of the vascular muscle. This effect is blocked with 8-phenyl theophylline, which is a selective blocker of the adenosine A_1 receptor, and potentiated with dipyridamole, which inhibits adenosine reuptake and thus sustains its effective concentration.

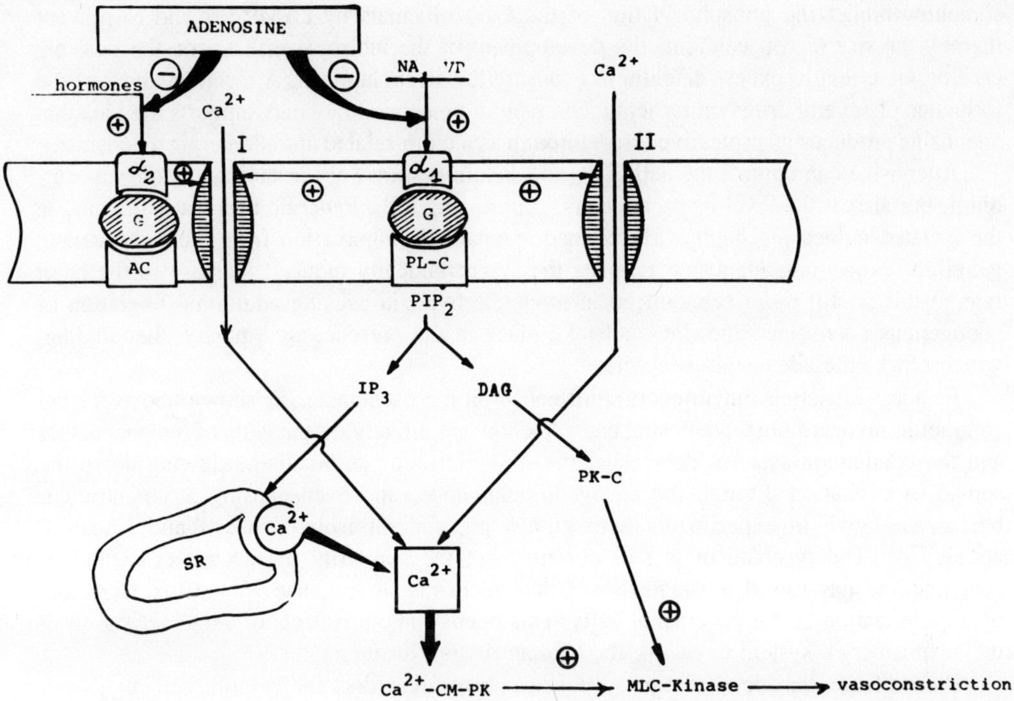

FIGURE 21. Vasodilatory action of adenosine on the stress-induced regulatory vascular spasm. (α_1, α_2), Adrenoreceptors; (I) receptor-dependent Ca^{2+} channel; (II) potential-dependent Ca^{2+} channel; (AC) adenylate cyclase; (PL C) phospholipase C; (NE) norepinephrine, (VP) vasopressin; (PIP_2) phosphatidylinositol diphosphate; (DAG) diacyl glycerol; (SR) sarcoplasmic reticulum; (PK C) protein kinase C; (Ca-CM PK) calmodulin-dependent protein kinase; (MLC kinase) myosin light chain kinase; (G) G-protein of receptor complexes. For explanations see text.

As to the interaction of adenosine with the vascular endothelium and its vasodilatory effect,[76] its nature is poorly studied, but the data that adenosine definitely (and almost as efficiently as catecholamines) stimulates PGI_2 synthesis in the isolated heart,[75] i.e., actually in coronary endothelial cells, suggest that the endothelium-dependent vasodilatory action of adenosine may involve PGs.

The second aspect of adenosine, as stated above, is its ability to restrict the influence of adrenergic regulation on the heart. Firstly, adenosine suppresses norepinephrine release from sympathetic terminals in the heart through the presynaptic A_1 receptors.[115,130] Secondly, it attenuates the positive inotropic[117,126,132,133] and chronotropic[131] effects of catecholamines on the heart.

As regards the latter, it was initially supposed that adenosine inhibits adenylate cyclase and cAMP synthesis.[132] However, further studies revealed that attenuation of the catecholamine positive inotropic effect by adenosine may be accompanied by a lesser,[117,132] the same, or even greater rise in cAMP (see Böhm et al.[126] and references therein). At the same time, adenosine and agonists of its receptors were found to suppress the positive inotropic effect of agents promoting cAMP formation or hindering cAMP breakdown, but not the positive inotropic effect of elevated extracellular calcium.[126] In other words, adenosine affects only those effects that are related to the cell cAMP content. Another line of research conducted with isolated ventricular myocytes[134] and papillary muscles[135,136] showed that adenosine inhibits the catecholamine-induced Ca^{2+} entry into the cell and checks the rise in the action potential. Thus, a concept emerging[126] is that adenosine restricts the catecholamine action on the contractile myocardium not at the step of adenylate cyclase activation and cAMP synthesis, but somewhere later in the regulatory cAMP circuit. Adenosine is supposed to somehow hinder the phosphorylation of the Ca^{2+} channels by cAMP-PK and to prevent thereby the rise in cell calcium, the development of the inotropic effect, and the possible cardiotoxic effect of excess calcium in exposure to catecholamines. A recent study[136] of the influence of several drugs on ischemic contracture in isolated rat heart supports the idea that adenosine produces its protective effect through a calcium-related antiadrenergic mechanism.

Adenosine can control the action of catecholamines not only in the contractile myocardium, but also at the level of pacemakers, suppressing the adrenergic tachycardia. Thus, in the isolated guinea pig heart with retained sympathetic innervation from the right stellate ganglion, exogenous adenosine restricts the sympathetically induced increase in the heart rate;[131] this is still more pronounced in moderate hypoxia causing additional liberation of endogenous adenosine, and does not take place in the presence of 8-phenyl theophyline, which blocks the adenosine receptors.

Besides restricting the adrenergic influence on the pacemaker (as shown above for the contractile myocardium), adenosine can somehow act directly on the cells of the pacemaker and the conduction system, decreasing the sinoatrial node automatism, slowing down the spread of excitation through the atrioventricular node, and even causing atrioventricular block, as shown in experiments with guinea pig and rat isolated hearts and sinoatrial nodes.[137-139] The mechanism is still obscure, but the similarity of this effect to that of acetylcholine has raised a suggestion[137] that adenosine may cause K^+ efflux from and hyperpolarization of the pacemaker cells. This opens some prospects of using activation of the adenosinergic system to rectify the cardiac rhythm disorders.

By and large, the adenosinergic system is a powerful cardiac and vascular self-regulatory mechanism capable of controlling the stress-induced and ischemic damage to the cardiovascular system, mainly by checking the excessive activation of the adrenergic regulation.

This concept is illustrated by the tentative scheme in Figure 22. The stress reaction, elicited by various factors including myocardial ischemia, and ensuing adrenergic activation result in depletion of the energy-rich phosphate compounds in the myocardium, which promotes liberation of adenosine. Adenosine suppresses the release of norepinephrine in the heart as well as checks the elevation of calcium in the coronary vascular myocytes (producing coronary dilation) and in the myocardiocytes (restricting the positive inotropic and chronotropic effects). This prevents or attenuates the detrimental effects of the lack of energy and calcium overloading in stress and/or ischemia. Of course the actual picture may prove much more complex than shown in the scheme. Here we only wanted to highlight the basic coupling between the stress-effecting adrenergic and the stress-limiting adenosinergic systems in the regulation of the heart.

At the same time it is important to remember that adenosine not only modulates the regulation of the executive organs, but is also active in the central nervous system as well, where it is present at high concentrations and its receptors and binding sites are abundant in various brain regions: hippocampus, cerebellum, hypothalamus, etc.[114,115,134] At present the adenosinergic system is regarded as a chief modulator of neuronal function. It mainly acts to impede neurotransmission by suppressing the release of neuromediators through the A_1 and A_2 receptors located on the axonal presynaptic membrane.[113,114,127,140] Besides, neuronal inhibition by adenosine has also been observed at the postsynaptic membrane level.[127,140] These data come from experiments with exogenous adenosine and its receptor agonists; however, convincing evidence is available that the same holds true for the endogenous mechanism (see Jackisch[113] for references).

Many researchers are of the opinion that both A_1 and A_2 receptors are coupled to adenylate cyclase; engagement of A_1 suppresses the enzyme and therefore Ca^{2+} entry through the neuronal presynaptic membrane, thus blocking the release of mediator; A_2, conversely, activates the cyclase, Ca^{2+} entry, and mediator release.[114,141] However, A_2 requires agonist concentrations three orders of magnitude higher than A_1, i.e., micromolar rather than na-

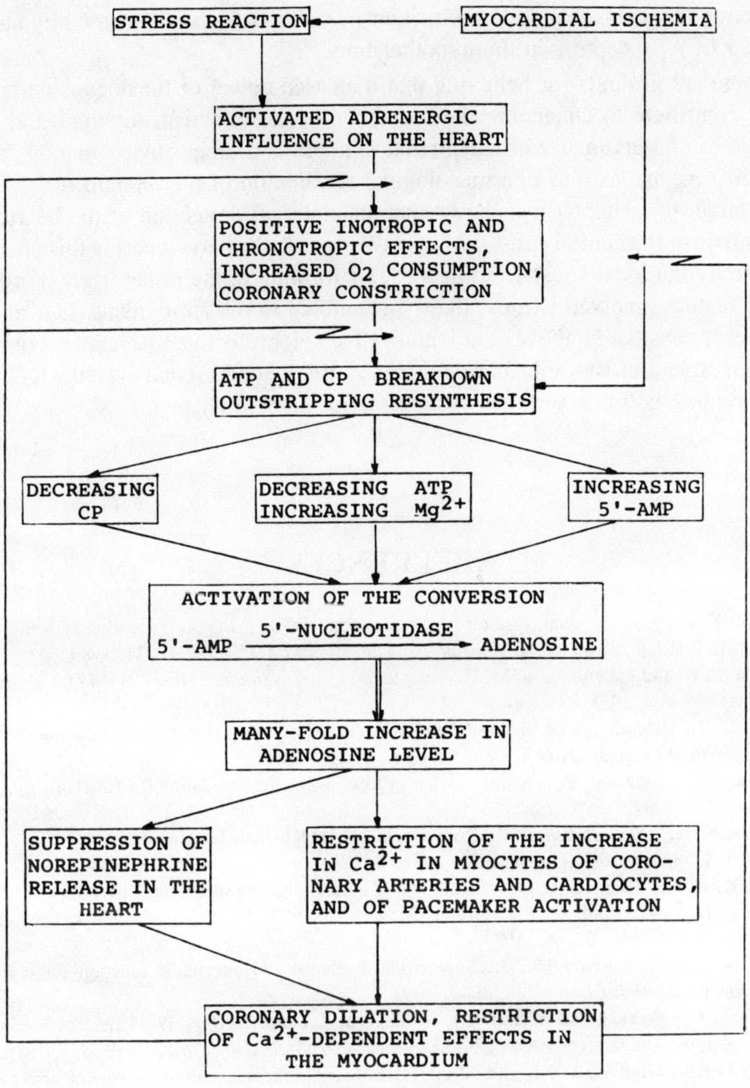

FIGURE 22. Coupling of the adenosinergic system to the stress reaction, and the cardioprotective effect of adenosine. For explanations see text.

nomolar levels (see Anderson et al.[127] for references). This apparently explains the mostly inhibitory, depressant action typical of adenosine in the central nervous system.[114] On the other hand, there are data that show adenosine can act through its receptors directly on the Ca^{2+} channels of the neuronal membrane regardless of the adenylate cyclase activity.[114,140] Taking account of what has been said above of the adenosine mechanisms in the heart and vessels, one can think that in the neurons adenosine affects the calcium homeostasis in much the same way, through receptor interaction with the Ca^{2+} channels and intracellular stores.

For us here it is essential that the central action of adenosine may be a weighty component of its stress-limiting function. Besides the data on inhibition of norepinephrine release in the brain, this idea is also favored by the fact that agonists of adenosine receptors and blockers of adenosine reuptake in the brain produce strong inhibition of the cardiovascular sympathetic tone and, in particular, have an antihypertensive effect.[114] Further, adaptation to repeated brief exposures to immobilization and electric pain stress, which is an important factor restricting the stress reaction and its injurious effects,[2] is accompanied by an increase in the number of A_1 receptors in the hypothalamus.[127]

Thus, there are grounds for believing that increased power of the adenosinergic system may greatly contribute to enhancing the resistance of the organism to stress and ischemic damage. This can be attained with adaptation to stress and other environmental factors, or with alternative means such as pharmacological stimulation of this system.

By and large, this chapter has shown that adaptational protection of the heart is not an exclusive domain of the central stress-limiting systems. An important part in this phenomenon can be played by the local stress-limiting systems forming in the organ itself. Furthermore, the scope of factors involved is most likely not limited to the antioxidant, PG, and adenosinergic systems considered above, but includes the cytoprotective mechanisms operative in the subcellular structures (myofibrillar membranes, mitochondria) and even the DNA genetic template. How true is this assertion we shall see in the next chapter.

REFERENCES

1. **Meerson, F. Z.,** Stress-limiting systems of the organism and their role in preventing ischemic damage to the heart (in Russian), *Byull. Vses. Kardiol. Nauchn. Tsentra AMN SSSR,* 1, 34, 1985.
2. **Meerson, F. Z. and Pshennikova, M. G.,** *Adaptation to Stress Situations and Physical Loads* (in Russian), Meditsina, Moscow, 1988.
3. **Hearse, D. J., Humphrey, S. M., and Chain, E. B.,** Abrupt reoxygeneration of the anoxic potassium-arrested perfused rat heart, *J. Mol. Cell. Cardiol.,* 5, 395, 1973.
4. **Bakh, A. N.,** On the role of peroxides in the process of medical oxidation (in Russian), *Zh. Russ. Fiz. Khim.* 29, 373, 1987.
5. **Semenov, N. N.,** *Chain Reactions* (in Russian), Goskhimtekhizdat, Leningrad, 1934.
6. **Fridovich, I.,** Superoxide and evoluation, *Horisons Biochem. Biophys.,* 1, 37, 1974.
7. **Mason, K. E. and Emmel, A. F.,** Vitamin E and muscle pigment in the rat, *Anat. Res.,* 92, 33, 1945.
8. **McBroon, J., Sunderland, D. A., Mote, J. R., and Jonen, T. D.,** Effect of acute scurvy on the guinea pig heart, *Arch. Pathol.,* 23, 20, 1973.
9. **McCord, J. M. and Fridovich, I.,** Superoxide dismutase: an enzymatic function for erythrocuprein (hemocuprein), *J. Biol. Chem.,* 244, 6049, 1969.
10. **Guarniery, C., Ferrari, R., Visioli, O., Caldarera, C., and Nayler, W.,** Effect of α-tocopherol on hypoxic-perfused and reoxygenated rabbit heart muscle, *J. Mol. Cell. Cardiol.,* 10, 893, 1978.
11. **Kogan, A. Kh., Kudrin, A. N., and Nikolaev, S. M.,** On the question of the role of lipid peroxidation in the mechanism of epinephrine injury to the myocardium, in *Free-Radical Lipid Oxidation in the Norm and in Pathology* (in Russian), Petrusevich, Yu. M., Ed., Nauka, Moscow, 1976, 68.
12. **Meerson, F. Z.,** *Pathogenesis and Prevention of Cardiac Stress and Ischemic Damage* (in Russian), Meditsina, Moscow, 1984.
13. **Meerson, F. Z., Didenko, V. V., Belkina, L. M., and Manukhina, E. B.,** Lipid peroxidation and antioxidant protection of the heart in stress, ischemia, and arrhythmias, in *Cellular Antioxidant Defense Mechanisms,* Chow, Ch. K., Ed., CRC Press, Boca Raton, FL, 1988, 215.
14. **Arkhipenko, Yu. V., Kagan, V. E., and Kozlov, Yu. P.,** Modification of the enzymic system of Ca^{2+} transport in the sarcoplasmic reticulum upon lipid peroxidation, molecular mechanisms of the changes in Ca ATPase activity (in Russian), *Biokhimiya,* 3, 433, 1983.
15. **McCord, J. M. and Roy, R.,** The pathophysiology of superoxide: role in inflammation and ischemia, *Can. J. Physiol. Pharmacol.,* 60, 1346, 1982.
16. **Chambers, D., Parks, D., and Patterson, G.,** Xanthine oxidase as a source of free radical damage in myocardial ischemia, *J. Mol. Cell. Cardiol.,* 17, 145, 1985.
17. **Hess, M., Manson, N., and Okabe, E.,** Involvement of free radicals in the pathophysiology of ischemic heart disease, *Can. J. Physiol. Pharmacol.,* 60, 1382, 1982.
18. **Schaper, J., Pasyk, S., Hoffman, M., and Schaper, W.,** Early ultrastructural changes in myocardial ischemia and infarction, in *Ischemic Myocardium and Antianginal Drugs,* New York, 1979, 3.
19. **Hammond, B., Kontos, H., and Hess, M.,** Oxygen radicals in the adult respiratory distress syndrome, in myocardial ischemia and reperfusion injury, and cerebral vascular damage, *Can. J. Physiol. Pharmacol.,* 63, 173, 1985.

20. **Gutkin, D. V. and Petrovich, Yu. A.,** Activity of myocardial antioxidant enzymes in myocardial ischemia (in Russian), *Byull. Eksp. Biol. Med.,* 1, 33, 1982.
21. **Didenko, V. V. and Dosmagambetova, R. S.,** Activation of lipid peroxidation and depression of antioxidant enzymes of the myocardium in experimental infarction, and prevention of these phenomena with inderal, ionol, verapamil, in *Actual Problems of Disease and Reconvalescence* (in Russian), Kryzhanovskii, G. N., Eds., AMN SSSR, Moscow, 1983, 12.
22. **Julicher, R., Tujburg, L., and Sterrenberg, L.,** Decreased defense against free radicals in rat during normal reperfusion after hypoxic ischemic and calcium-free perfusion, *Life Sci.,* 35, 1281, 1984.
23. **Barsacchi, R., Camici, P., Bottigli, H., Salvadori, P., Pelosi, G., Mairino, M., and Ursinsi, F.,** Correlation between hydroperoxide-induced chemiluminescence of the heart and its function, *Biochim. Biophys. Acta,* 762, 241, 1983.
24. **Meerson, F. Z.,** The role of lipid peroxidation in the myocardium in stress and the antioxidant protection of the heart, in *Oxygen Radicals in the Pathophysiology of Heart Disease,* Signdl, P. K., Ed., Kluwer, Academic Press, Boston, 1988.
25. **Sazontova, T. G., Arkhipenko, Yu. V., and Meerson, F. Z.,** Increased activity of the enzymes of antioxidant heart protection in adaptation of rats to short stress exposures (in Russian), *Byull. Eksp. Biol. Med.,* 10, 411, 1987.
26. **Luck, H.,** Catalase, in *Methods of Enzymatic Analysis,* Bergmayer, H., Ed., Pergamon Press, New York, 1963, 885.
27. **Fridovich, I.,** Superoxide dismutase, *Acc. Chem. Res.,* 5, 321, 1972.
28. **Emerson, C. M., Mason, D. I., and Guthberg, G. E.,** Erythrocyte glutathion peroxidase content and serum tocopherol levels in newborn infants, *Br. J. Haematol.,* 22, 667, 1972.
29. **Lankin, V. Z., Gurevich, S. M., Kotelevtseva, N. V., Tikhadze, A. K., and Gerasimova, E. N.,** Role of lipid peroxides in the pathogenesis of atherosclerosis. Lipoperoxide detoxication by the glutathione peroxidase system in the aorta (in Russian), *Vopr. Med. Khim.,* 22, 392, 1976.
30. **Okhawa, H., Ochishi, N., and Yagi, K.,** Assay for lipid peroxides in animal tissues by thiobarbituric acid reaction, *Analyt. Biochem.,* 95, 351, 1979.
31. **Meerson, F. Z. and Katkova, L. S.,** Effect of prior adaptation to short stress exposures on the resistance of the spontaneously contracting myocardium to an LPO inducer (in Russian), *Byull. Eksp. Biol. Med.,* 10, 397, 1985.
32. **Dubinina, E. E., Sal'nikova, A. A., Ramenskaya, N. P., and Efimova, L. E.,** Peroxidation and the blood antioxidant system in the ontogeny (in Russian), *Vopr. Med. Khim.,* 5, 28, 1984.
33. **Higuchi, M., Cartier, L.-J., and Holloszy, J.,** The effect of endurance training on free radical scavenging enzymes in rats, *Med. Sci. Sports Exerc.,* 15, 93, 1983.
34. **Jenkins, R., Martin, D., and Goldberg, E.,** Lipid peroxidation in skeletal muscle during atrophy and acute exercise, *Med. Sci. Sports Exerc.,* 15, 93, 1983.
35. **Quantanilha, A.,** Effects of physical exercise and/or vitamin E on tissue oxidative metabolism, *Biochem. Soc. Trans.,* 12, 403, 1984.
36. **Guarniery, C., Flamigni, F., and Caldarera, C. M.,** Role of the oxygen in the cellular damage induced by reoxygenation of hypoxic heart, *J. Mol. Cell. Cardiol.,* 12, 797, 1980.
37. **Yellon, D. M., Downey, J. M., and Hearse, D. J.,** Myocardial infarct-size limitation. Principles, problems and possibilities, *G. Ital. Cardiol.,* 14, 892, 1984.
38. **Akizuki, S., Yoshida, S., Chambers, D., Eddy, L., Parmley, L., Yellon, D., and Downey, J.,** Infarct size limitation by the xanthine oxidase inhibitor allopurinol in closed-chest dogs with small infarcts, *Cardiovasc. Res.,* 19, 686, 1985.
39. **Miura, T., Yellon, D., Kingma, J., and Downey, J.,** Protection afforded by allopurinol in the first 24 hours of coronary occlusion is diminished after 48 hours, *Free Radical Biol. Med.,* 5, 25, 1988.
40. **Reimer, K. and Jennings, K.,** Failure of xanthine oxidase inhibitor allopurinol to limit infarct size after ischemia and reperfusion in dogs, *Circulation,* 77, 1069, 1985.
41. **Jolly, S., Kane, W., Bailie, M., Abrams, G., and Lucchesi, B.,** Canine myocardial reperfusion injury. Its reduction by the combined administration of superoxide dismutase and catalase, *Circ. Res.,* 54, 277, 1984.
42. **Przyklenk, K. and Kloner, R.,** Effect of oxygen-derived free radical scavengers on infarct size following six hours of permanent coronary artery occlusion: salvage or delay of myocardial necrosis, *Basic Res., Cardiol.,* 82, 146, 1987.
43. **Romson, J., Hook, B., Kunkel, S., Abrams, G., Schork, A., and Lucchesi, B.,** Reduction in the extent of myocardial ischemic injury by neutrophil depletion in the dog, *Circulation,* 67, 1016, 1983.
44. **Jolly, S., Kane, W., Bruce, G., Hook, B., Abrams, G., Kunkel, S., and Lucchesi, S.,** Reduction of myocardial infarct size by neutrophil depletion: effect of duration of occlusion, *Am. Heart J.,* 112, 682, 1986.
45. **Kirlin, Ph., Romson, J., and Pitt, B.,** Ibuprofen-mediated infarct size reduction: effects on regional myocardial function in canine myocardial infarction, *Am. J. Cardiol.,* 50, 849, 1982.

46. **Reimer, K. and Jennings, R.,** Failure of xanthine oxidase inhibitor allopurinol to limit infarct size after ischemia and reperfusion in dogs, *Circulation,* 71, 1069, 1985.
47. **Savov, V. M., Didenko, V. V., Dosmogambetova, R. S., Meerson, F. Z., and Kagan, V. E.,** Lipid peroxidation in the myocardium in experimental infarction (in Russian), *Biol. Nauki,* 5, 30, 1985.
48. **Evsev'eva, M. E., Shinkarenko, V. S., Didenko, V. V., and Meerson, F. Z.,** Limitation of ischemic necrosis with the antioxidant ionol (in Russian), *Byull. Eksp. Biol. Med.,* 8, 152, 1989.
49. **Meerson, F. Z. and Evsevieva, M. E.,** Disturbances of the heart structure and function in chronic haemolytic anemia, their compensation with increased coronary flow and their prevention with ionol, an inhibitor of lipid peroxidation, *Adv. Myocardiology,* 5, 201, 1984.
50. **Meerson, F. Z., Kagan, V. E., Beresneva, Z. V., Boev, V. M., and Prilipko, L. L.,** Effect of antioxidant on cardiac contractile function and physical endurance in man (in Russian), *Teor. Prakt. Fiz, Kul't.,* 8, 14, 1983.
51. **Meerson, F. Z., Belkina, L. M., Ugolev, A. A., Golubeva, L. Yu., Abdikaliev, N. A., and Solomatina, E. S.,** Use of antioxidants to prevent experimental myocardial infarction and reoxygenation disturbances to the heart (in Russian), *Kardiologiya,* 10, 81, 1980.
52. **Meerson, F. Z.,** Stress damage to nonischemic divisions of the heart in experimental infarction and its prevention, *Clin. Cardiol.,* 6, 163, 1983.
53. **Meerson, F. Z., Belkina, L. M., Sazontova, T. G., Arkhipenko, Yu. V., and Saltykova, V. A.,** The role of the lipid peroxidation in pathogenesis of arrhythmias and prevention of the cardiac fibrillation with antioxidants, *Basic Res. Cardiol.,* 82, 123, 1987.
54. **Rona, G., Chappel, C. I., Balazs, R., and Gaudry, R.,** An infarct-like myocardial lesion and other toxic manifestations produced by isoproterenol in rat, *Arch. Pathol.,* 67, 443, 1959.
55. **Lepran, I., Koltai, M., Siegmund, W., and Szekeres, L.,** Coronary artery ligation, early arrhythmias and determination of the ischemic area in conscious rats, *J. Pharmacol. Methods,* 9, 219, 1983.
56. **Manning, A., Coltart, D., and Hearse, D.,** Ischemic and reperfusion-induced arrhythmias in the rat. Effects of xanthine oxidase inhibition with allopurionol, *Circ. Res.,* 55, 545, 1984.
57. **Parrat, J. and Wainwright, C.,** Failure of allpurinol and a spin-trapping agent N-t-butyl-α-phenyl nitrone to modify significantly ischemic and reperfusion-induced arrhythmias, *Br. J. Pharmacol.,* 91, 49, 1987.
58. **Woodward, B. and Zakaria, M.,** Effect of some free radical scavengers on reperfusion-induced arrhythmias in the isolated rat heart, *J. Mol. Cell. Cardiol.,* 17, 485, 1985.
59. **Bernier, M., Hearse, D., and Manning, A.,** Reperfusion-induced arrhythmias and oxygen-derived free radicals. Studies with "anti-free radical" interventions and a free radical-generating system in the isolated perufsed rat heart, *Circ. Res.,* 58, 331, 1986.
60. **Agozzino, S., Peruszi, M., Cremonesi, P., and Sarret, M.,** Correlation between plasmatic and cardiac malondialdehyde levels and arrhythmias induced by regional ischemia and reperfusion in anesthetized rat. Effect of some antioxidants, *J. Mol. Cell. Cardiol.,* 19 (Suppl. III), S2, 1987.
61. **Takamura, T., Fukushima, A., Kondo, T., Ajioka, M., Sugiyama, S. and Ozawa, T.,** The effect of coenyzme Q_{10} derivates on reperfusion arrhythmias, *J. Mol. Cell. Cardiol.,* 19 (Suppl. 1), 42, 1987.
62. **Manning, A., Bernier, M., Crome, R., Little, S., and Hearse, D. J.,** Reperfusion-induced arrhythmias: a study of the role of xanthine oxidase-derived free radicals in the rat heart, *J. Mol. Cell. Cardiol.,* 20, 35, 1988.
63. **Singal, P. K., Kapur, N., Beamish, R. E., Das, P. K., and Dhalla, N. S.,** Antioxidant protection against epinephrine-induced arrhythmias, in *Stress and Heart Disease,* Beamish, R. E., Singal, P. K., and Dhalla, N. S., Eds., Martinus Nijhoff, Boston, 1985, 190.
64. **Doda, M. and Gyorgy, L.,** Dopaminergic inhibition of sympathetic activity in the cat, *Pol. J. Pharmacol.,* 37, 397, 1985.
65. **Schwartz, J.,** The dopaminergic system in the periphery, *J. Pharmacol.,* 15, 401, 1984.
66. **Matsuki, M., Nishida, S., Kashiwa, J., Horio, M., Joneda, M., Enoh, M., Satoh, A., and Oyama, H.,** Effect of dopamine on ACTH-induced glucocorticoid secretion in rat adrenal suspended cells, *Horm. Metab. Res.,* 17, 429, 1985.
67. **Meerson, F. Z., Malyshev, V. V., Petrova, V. A., and Manukhina, E. B.,** The antioxidant ionol suppresses ACTH-induced secretion of corticosterone (in Russian), *Byull. Eksp. Biol. Med.,* 107, 42, 1989.
68. **Donchenko, G. V., Metal'nikova, N. P., and Kruglikova, A. A.,** Interconnection of changes in RNA and ubiquinone syntheses in rat liver under the influence of tocopherol (in Russian), *Vopr. Pitan.,* 5, 63, 1982.
69. **Wefers, H., Komai, T., Talalay, P., and Sies, H.,** Protection against reactive oxygen species by NAD(P)H: quinone reductase induced by the dietary antioxidant butylated hydroxyanisole (BHA). Decreased hepatic low-level chemiluminescence during quinone redox cycling, *FEBS Lett.,* 169, 63, 1984.
70. **Levine, L., Xiao, D., and Little, C.,** Increased arachidonic acid metabolites from cells in culture after treatment with the phosphatidylcholine-hydrolyzing phospholipase C from Bac. cereus, *Prostaglandins,* 34, 633, 1987.

71. **Carpenter, M. P.,** Antioxidant effect on the prostaglandin endoperoxide synthetase product profile, *Fed. Proc., Fed. Am. Soc. Exp. Biol.,* 40, 189, 1981.
72. **Samuelsson, B.,** Leukotrienes: mediators of immediate hypersensitivity reactions and inflammation, *Science,* 220, 568, 1983.
73. **Tada, M., Ezumi, K., Yamagushi, M., Kuzuya, T., Matsuda, H., Abe, H., Uchida, Y., and Murao, S.,** Reduction of prostacyclin synthesis as a possible cause of transient flow canine coronary artery, *J. Mol Cell. Cardiol.,* 16, 1137, 1984.
74. **Shaffer, J. E. and Malik, K. U.,** Enhancement of prostaglandin output during activation of beta-1-adrenoceptors in the isolated rabbit heart, *J. Pharmacol. Exp. Ther.,* 223, 729, 1982.
75. **Wennmalm, M., Fitzgerald, G. A., and Wennmalm, A.,** Prostacyclin as neuromodulator in the sympathetically stimulated rabbit heart, *Prostaglandins,* 33, 675, 1987.
76. **Young, M. A. and Vatner, S. F.,** Regulation of large coronary arteries, *Circ. Res.,* 59, 579, 1986.
77. **Abdel-Latif, A. A.,** Calcium-mobilizing receptors, polyphosphoinositides, and the generation of second messengers, *Pharmacol. Rev.,* 38, 227, 1986.
78. **Cao, Y.-Z., Choy, K. O. P. C., and Chan, A. C.,** Regulation by vitamin E of phosphatidylcholine metabolism in rat heart, *Biochem. J.,* 247, 135, 1987.
79. **Hedqvist, P.,** Basic mechanisms of prostaglandin action on autonomic neurotransmission, *Annu. Rev. Pharmacol. Toxicol.,* 17, 259, 1977.
80. **Boroyan, R. G.,** Changes in prostaglandin release in the heart under various experimental conditions (in Russian), *Krovoobrashchenie,* 6, 9, 1977.
81. **Wennmalm, A.,** Prostaglandin-mediated inhibition of noradrenaline release, *Prostaglandins,* 15, 113, 1978.
82. **Hassid, A. and Oudinet, J.-P.,** Relationship between cellular calcium and prostaglandin synthesis in cultured vascular smooth muscle cells, *Prostaglandins,* 32, 457, 1986.
83. **Delarne, C., Perrotean, I., Lirhmann, I., Netchitailo, P., Homo-Delarche F., and Vandry, H.,** Role of prostacyclin in steroidogenesis by frog interrenal gland *in vitro, Prostaglandins,* 31, 5, 1986.
84. **Ertl, G.,** Eikosanoid effects on coronary bloodflow and ischemic myocardium, *Eur. Heart J.,* 8 (Suppl. i), 457, 1987.
85. **Benedict, C. R., Sheng, W. L., and Todd, G. E.,** Prostaglandin E prevents coronary occlusion by thrombus formation, *Circulation,* 76 (Suppl. II), 4, II-37, abs. 0145, 1988.
86. **Caparoffa, L., Ceserani, R., Mongelli, N., Sauti-Soncin, E., Ragazzi, E., and Fassina, G.,** Depression and excitation induced in mice by two geometric isomers of (+)13,14-didehydro-20-methylcarboprostacyclin, FCE 22177 and FCE 22176. Comparison with effects on blood pressure and platelet aggregation, *Prostaglandins,* 33, 35, 1987.
87. **Coleman, R. A., Humphrey, P. P. A., Kennedy, I., and Lumley, P.,** Prostanoid receptor — the development of a working classification, *TIPS,* 5, 303, 1984.
88. **Wallace, J. and Cohen, M.,** Gastric mucosal protection with chronic mild restraint: role of endogenous prostaglandins, *Am. J. Physiol.,* 247, 6127, 1984.
89. **Körmöszy, P. Sz., Vértesi, Cs., Mikns, E., Tardos, L., and Kovács, G.,** Cardioprotective effect of prostacyclin and 7-oxo-PGI_2 in rats against chronic isoproterenol damage, *Prostaglandins,* 33, 505, 1987.
90. **Darius, H., Osborne, J. A., Reibel, D. K., and Lefer, A. M.,** Protective action of stable prostacyclin analogue in ischemia-induced membrane damage in rat myocardium, *J. Mol. Cell. Cardiol.,* 19, 243, 1987.
91. **Kawarada, Y., Lambek, J., and Matsumoto, T.,** Pathophysiology of stress ulcer and its prevention. II. Prostaglandin E and microcirculatory responses in stress ulcers, *Am. J. Surg.,* 129, 217, 1975.
92. **Auguste, L.-J., Augus, C., Stein, T. A., and Wise, L.,** Arachidonic acid protection of rat mucosa against stress ulceration, *J. Surg. Res.,* 43, 103, 1987.
93. **Takanok, K., Sugiyama, S., Goto, H., Nakazawa, S., and Ozawa, T.,** Effect of the H_2-blocker famotidine on gastric mucosal prostaglandin levels in water immersion stress in rats, *Arzneim. Forsch.,* 38(I), 364, 1988.
94. **Shimkovich, M. V. and Pshennikova, M. G.,** Effect of prior administration of prostaglandin E_2 and prostaglandin synthesis inhibitor indomethacin on disturbance of heart contractile function in stress (in Russian), *Byull. Eksp. Biol. Med.,* 5, 536, 1986.
95. **Schrör, K., Darius, H., Addiks, K., Köster, R., and Smith, E. F.,** PGI_2 prevents ischemia-induced alterations in cardiac catecholamines without influencing nerve stimuation-induced catecholamine release in nonischemic conditions, *J. Cardiovasc. Pharmacol.,* 4, 741, 1982.
96. **Smith, E. F., Gallenkämper, W., Beckmann, R., Thomsen, T., Mannesmann, G., and Schrör, K.,** Early and late administration of PGI_2 analogue, ZK-36374: effects on myocardial preservation, collateral blood flow and infarct size, *Cardiovasc. Res.,* 18, 163, 1984.
97. **Ribeiro, L. G. T., Brandon, T. A., Hopkins, D. G., Reduto, L. A., Taylor, A. A., and Miller, R. R.,** Prostacyclin in experimental myocardial ischemia: effects on hemodynamics, regional myocardial blood flow, infarct size and mortality, *Am. J. Cardiol.,* 47, 835, 1981.
98. **Starnes, V. A., Primm, R. K., Woosley, P. L., Oate, J. A., and Hammon, J. W.,** Administration of prostacyclin prevents ventricular fibrillation following coronary occlusion in conscious dogs, *J. Cardiovasc. Pharmacol.,* 4, 765, 1982.

99. **Friedrich, T., Lichey, J., Nigam, S., Priesnitz, M., and Wegscheider, K.,** Follow-up of prostaglandin plasma levels after acute myocardial infarction, *Am. Heart J.*, 109, 218, 1985.
100. **Riegel, A. and Mest, H.-J.,** The effect of PAF (platelet-activating factor) on experimental cardiac arrhythmias and its inhibition by substances influencing arachidonic acid metabolites, *Prostagland. Leuk. Med.*, 28, 103, 1987.
101. **Rao, T. S., Seth, S. D., Mauchauda, S. C., and Nayer, U.,** The lack of involvement of central nervous system in the antiarrhythmic effect of prostaglandins E_2, $F_{2\alpha}$ and I_2 in cat, *Prostaglandins*, 33, 339, 1987.
102. **Gillis, R. A. and Quest, J. A.,** The role of the nervous system in the cardiovascular effects of digitalis, *Pharmacol. Rev.*, 31, 19, 1980.
103. **Mest, H. J. and Winkler, J.,** Significance of sympathetic nervous system for the central antiarrhythmic effect of prostaglandin E_2, $F_{2\alpha}$, I_2 on aconitic-induced cardiac arrhythmias in rats, *Biomed. Biochim. Acta*, 43, 143, 1984.
104. **Moffat, M. P., Karmazyn, M., and Ferrier, G. R.,** Prostaglandins as a key modulator of reperfusion-induced cardiac injury. Initial studies into possible mechanisms, in *Pathogenesis of Stress-Induced Heart Disease*, Martinus Nijhoff, Boston, 1985, 320.
105. **Moffat, M. P., Karmazym, M., and Ferrier, G. R.,** Role of prostaglandins in the arrhythmogenic effects of ouabain on isolated guinea pig hearts, *Eur. J. Pharmacol.*, 141, 383, 1987.
106. **Meerson, F. Z., Tverdokhlib, V. P., and Nikonorov, A. A.,** Prevention of atherogenic dyslipoproteinemias and of the complex of metabolic disturbances in the liver in emotional pain stress (in Russian), *Vopr. Med. Khim.*, 6, 104, 1988.
107. **Tverdokhlib, V. P., Ozerova, I. N., Tvorogova, M. G., Olfer'ev, A. M., and Meerson, F. Z.,** Influence of emotional pain stress on lipid level and cholesterol esterification in rat blood (in Russian), *Patol. Fiziol. Eksp. Ter.*, 4, 27, 1988.
108. **Gryglewski, R. J., Dembinskakiec, A., Zmuda, A., and Gryglewska, T.,** Prostacyclin and thromboxane A_2 biosynthesis capacities of heart, arteries and platelets at various stages of experimental atherosclerosis in rabbits, *Atherosclerosis*, 31, 385, 1978.
109. **Schwartz, K. E., Zaro, B., Burton, P., Hunt, J., Pennelly, Is., and Sevelins, H.,** Reduction of serum lipoproteins in man by the oral administration of prostaglandin analogue (enprostil), *Atherosclerosis*, 71, 9, 1988.
110. **Meerson, F. Z., Pshennikova, M. G., Kuznetsova, B. A., and Shimkovich, M. V.,** Effect of adaptation to stress on the relation between catecholamines and prostaglandins in blood in acute stress exposure (ASE), *J. Mol. Cell. Cardiol.*, 21, (Suppl. II), 105, 1989.
111. **Haghighi, A. Z. and Pynadath, T. J.,** Stimulation of prostacyclin synthesis in rats treated with phenobarbital, *Prostagland. Leuk. Med.*, 28, 267, 1987.
112. **Berne, R. M.,** The role of adenosine in the regulation of coronary blood flow, *Circ. Res.*, 47, 807, 1980.
113. **Jackisch, R., Fehr, R., and Hertting, G.,** Adenosine: an endogenous modulator of hippocampal noradrenaline release, *Neuropharmacology*, 24, 499, 1985.
114. **Marangos, P. J.,** Biochemical and pharmacologic properties of brain adenosine receptors and uptake sites, *Pfluegers Arch.*, 407 (Suppl. 1), S5, 1986.
115. **Fuder, H.,** Selected aspects of presynaptic modulation of noradrenaline release from heart, *J. Cardiovasc. Pharmacol.*, 7 (Suppl. 5), S2, 1985.
116. **Long, C. J. and Stone, T. W.,** Adenosine reduces agonist-induced production of inositol phosphates in rat aorta, *J. Pharm. Pharmacol.*, 39, 1010, 1987.
117. **Dobson, J. G., Fenton, R. A., and Romano, F. D.,** The antiadrenergic action of adenosine in the heart, *Pfluegers Arch.*, 407 (Suppl. 1), S15, 1986.
118. **Böhm, M., Bruckner, R., Meger, W., Nose, M., Schmitz, W., Starbatty, J., and Scholz, H.,** Evidence for adenosine receptor-mediated isoprenaline-antagonistic effects of the adenosine analogs PIA and NECA on force of contraction in guinea-pig atrial and ventricular cardiac preparations, *Naunyn-Schmiedeberg's Arch. Pharmacol.*, 331, 131, 1985.
119. **Heller, L. J., Sherin, J. C., and Mohrman, D. E.,** Exogenous inosine increases interstitial [adenosine] of isolated perfused rat hearts, *Circulation*, 78 (Suppl. II), Abstr. 2212. 1988.
120. **Kikakaze, M., Hori, M., Tamai, J., Koretsunge, Y., Imai, K., Iwakura, K., Kitabatake, A., Inoue, M., and Kamada, T.,** Alpha$_1$-adrenergic activity regulates adenosine release during myocardial ischemia, *Pfluegers Arch.*, 407 (Suppl. I), S50, 1986.
121. **Van Wylson, D. G. L., Willis, J., Lasley, R. O., and Mentzer, R. M.,** Dobutamine increases myocardial interstitial fluid adenosine concentration and coronary blood flow as measured by cardiac microdialysis, *Circulation*, 78 (Suppl. II), abs. 0680, 1988.
122. **Babbitt, D. G., McCroskey, D., Virmani, R., and Forman, M. B.,** Preservation of vasodilatory reserve by intracoronary adenosine in the canine reperfusion model, *Circulation*, 78 (Suppl. II), abs. 1350, 1988.
123. **Babbitt, D. G., Virmani, R., McCroskey, D., and Forman, M. B.,** The "no reflow" phenomenon: an important mechanism in the evolution of reperfusion injury, *Circulation*, 78 (Suppl. II), Abstr. 1482, 1988.

124. **Vita, J. A., Cox, D. A., Treasure, Ch. B., Fish, R. D., McLanachan, J. M., Gauz, P., and Selwyn, A.,** Response of human coronary arteries to adenosine, *Circulation,* 78 (Suppl. II), Abstr. 2214, 1988.
125. **Timmermans, P. B., Chiu, A. T., and Thoolen, M. J. M.,** Calcium handling in vasoconstriction to stimulation of alpha$_1$- and alpha$_2$-adrenoceptor, *Can. J. Physiol. Pharmacol.,* 65, 1649, 1987.
126. **Böhm, M., Brückner, R., Neumann, J., Nose, M., Schmitz, W., and Scholz, H.,** Adenosine inhibits the positive inotropic effect of 3-isobutyl-1-methylxanthine in papillary muscles without effect on cyclic AMP or cyclic GMP, *Br. J. Pharmacol.,* 93, 729, 1988.
127. **Anderson, S. M., Leu, J. R., and Kant, G. J.,** Chronic stress increases the binding of the A_1 adenosine receptor agonist, [^{3}H]cyclohexyladenosine, to rat hypothalamus, *Pharmacol. Biochem. Behav.,* 30, 169, 1988.
128. **Liang, B. T.,** Desensitization of cardiac A_1 adenosine receptor, *Circulation,* 78 (Suppl. II), Abstr. 2227, 1988.
129. **Longabaugh, J. P., Didsbury, J. R., and Stiles, G. L.,** G-Protein mRNA levels during A_1-adenosine receptor desensitization, *Circulation,* 78 (Suppl. II), Abstr. 2228, 1988.
130. **Hedquist, P. and Fredholm, B. B.,** Inhibitory effect of adenosine on adrenergic neuroeffector transmitter in the rabbit heart, *Acta Physiol. Scand.,* 105, 120, 1978.
131. **Tessari, F., Prosdocimi, M., Coleman, H., Boykin, M. T., and Belardinelli, L.,** Modulation of the effects of sympathetic nerve stimulation by adenosine and hypoxia in guinea pig heart, *Circulation,* 78 (Suppl. II), Abstr. 1411, 1988.
132. **Schrader, J., Baumann, G., and Gerlach, E.,** Adenosine as inhibitor of myocardial effects of catecholamines, *Pfluegers Arch.,* 371, 29, 1977.
133. **Lammeraut, J. and Becsei, I.,** Left ventricular contractility and developed tension in the intact dog submitted to an intracoronary infusion of adenosine, *J. Physiol. (London),* 229, 41, 1979.
134. **Isenberg, G. and Belardinelli, L.,** Ionic basis for the antagonism between adenosine and isoproterenol on isolated ventricular myocytes, *Circ. Res.,* 55, 309, 1984.
135. **Schmitz, W., Böhm, M., Brückner, R., Burmann, H., Meyer, W., Neumann, J., Nose, M., and Scholz, H.,** Relationship between the effects of cAMP-increasing agents and adenosine in the mammalian heart, in *Adenosine Receptors and Modulation of Cell Function,* Stefanovich, V., Rudolphi, K., and Schubert, P., Eds., IRL Press, Oxford, 1985, 295.
136. **Lasley, R. D., Rhee, J. W., Van Wylen, D. G. L., and Mentzer, R. M.,** Adenosine enhances tolerance to myocardial ischemia via an A_1 receptor mechanism, *Circulation,* 78 (Suppl. II), abs. 1049, 1988.
137. **Belardinelli, L., West, G. A., and Clemo, H. F.,** Modulation of sinoatrial and atrio-ventricular node function by adenosine, *Pfluegers Arch.,* 407 (Suppl. I), S26, 1986.
138. **Belardinelli, L., Tenton, R. A., West, G. A., Linden, J., Althaus, J. S., and Berne, R. M.,** Extracellular action of adenosine and the antagonism by aminophylline on the atrioventricular conduction of isolated perfused guinea pig and rat heart, *Circ. Res.,* 51, 569, 1982.
139. **Halperin, C. and Belardinelli, L.,** Adenosine mediates ischemia-induced bradycardia in isolated perfused canine atria, *Circulation,* 78 (Suppl. II), abs. 2550, 1988.
140. **Dunwiddle, T. V. and Proctor, W. P.,** Mechanisms underlying responses to adenosine in the central nervous system, *Pfluegers Arch.,* 407 (Suppl. 1), S15, 1986.
141. **Snyder, S. H.,** Drug and neurotransmitter receptors in the brain, *Science,* 224, 22, 1984.

Chapter 6

THE PHENOMENON OF ADAPTIVE STABILIZATION OF STRUCTURES AND HEART PROTECTION

I. INTRODUCTION

The question in what measure the adaptational protection of the heart is due to changes in neurohormonal regulation and in what measure to changes in the heart muscle cells has remained open until quite recently. A most simple approach to this problem was obviously to elucidate whether or not the cardioprotective effect of adaptation observed in the whole organism is retained when the isolated hearts of adapted animals are exposed to injurious factors. In accordance with this, we have studied the effect of adaptation on the resistance of the isolated heart to ischemia and reperfusion, to high catecholamine and calcium concentrations, and finally its effect on the inactivation of some cardiomyocyte structures during autolysis.

II. EFFECT OF ADAPTATION TO REPEATED STRESS ON ISOLATED HEART RESISTANCE TO ISCHEMIC AND REPERFUSION DAMAGE

Our experiments[1] have shown that a fruitful model for studying the effects of adaptation is offered by ischemic and reperfusion arrhythmias.

The diagram in Figure 1A demonstrates that in a 20-min acute ischemia produced with coronary artery ligation, the total duration of grave arrhythmias (ventricular tachycardia and ventricular fibrillation) is the greatest in conscious closed-chest animals, 40% less in anesthetized ones ($p<0.01$), and 25 times less in isolated hearts ($p<0.001$). At present this is not at all surprising, being quite in line with the concept of the decisive role of cardiac neural regulation disturbances, and first of all of the excessive adrenergic effect on the heart, in the pathogenesis of ischemic arrhythmias.

In other words, we are again facing the obstinate fact that in local ischemic injury to the heart the evolving arrhythmias are of central genesis. Figure 1B shows that the picture is different in reperfusion arrhythmias developing in response to restitution of blood flow through the ischemic myocardium. Here the differences in the arrhythmic response of the heart in the whole organism and in isolation are smaller than and opposite to those in ischemia: the duration of reperfusion arrhythmias in isolated hearts is 60% greater than in conscious animals ($p<0.05$). This also should not be surprising, since complete prolonged clamping of the coronary artery followed by its abrupt reopening brings on simultaneously the oxygen and the calcium paradoxes.[2] This gives rise to at least two phenomena that are often fatal for the heart. The first one is marked activation of lipid peroxidation (LPO) and other components of the lipid triad, with massive destruction of the cell membranes and ensuing calcium entry into the cell. The second one is the cardiotoxic effect of calcium: myofibrillar contracture, uncoupling of oxidative phosphorylation in mitochondria, activation of phospholipases and proteases, and breakdown of cell structures. In the whole organism these essentially local effects can be to some extent additionally checked by the extracardiac antioxidant and calcium-binding agents, whereas in the isolated heart there are only local cell mechanisms to oppose them. As a result, both the injury as such and its arrhythmogenic effect turn out to be greater.

These data prompt a conclusion that *the ischemic arrhythmias are elicited mainly through the central regulatory mechanisms, while the reperfusion ones through the local cardiac*

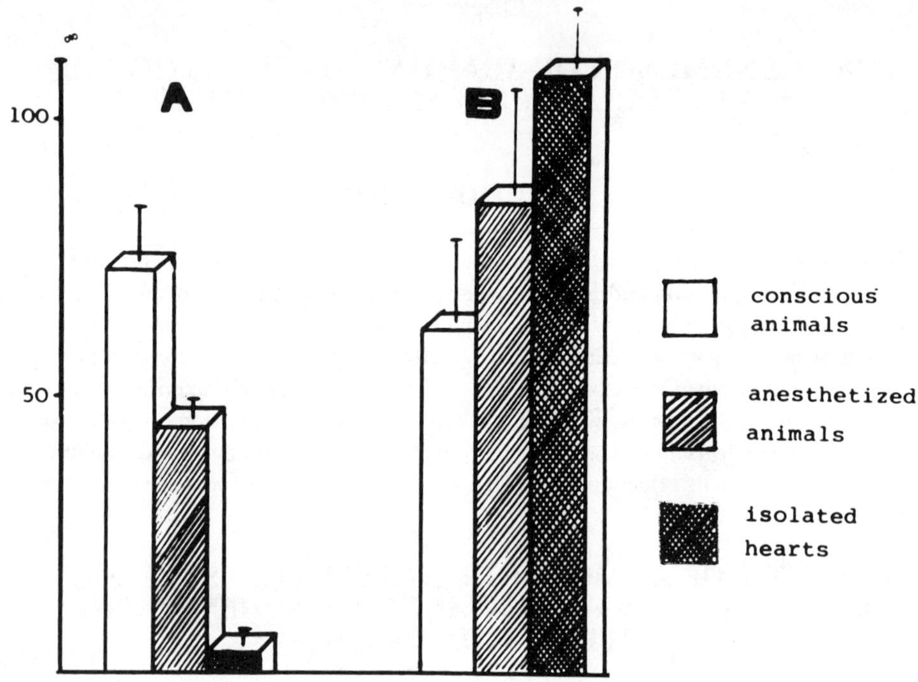

FIGURE 1. Overall duration of (A) ischemic and (B) reperfusion arrhythmias (ventricular tachycardia plus ventricular fibrillation) in conscious and anesthetized animals and in isolated hearts.

mechanisms, and consequently in the adaptational self-defense of the heart the ischemic arrhythmias can be attenuated or abolished mainly owing to activation of the central stress-limiting systems, while the reperfusion arrhythmias mainly by activation of the local systems.

To assess the validity of this assertion, we have conducted experiments to elucidate how the protective antiarrhythmic effect of adaptation to stress is realized in the ischemic and reperfused isolated heart, i.e., under conditions where the central stress-limiting systems can certainly be of no appreciable importance.

Rat hearts were isolated according to Langendorf; ischemia was produced by ligating the left descending coronary artery for 20 min, then the ligature was loosened and the heart monitored in reperfusion for 10 min. The main results are presented in Table 1.

One can see that through 20 min of ischemia all control and adapted hearts retained their contractile activity, but the total duration of arrhythmias in adapted hearts was 36% less than in controls; the ischemic arrhythmias were represented mostly by extrasystoles.

Reperfusion elicited much more grave arrhythmias in both groups, and the protective effect of adaptation proved much more pronounced. Thus, the total duration of arrhythmias in the adapted hearts decreased almost by half. The most serious form — fibrillation — developed in 8 out of 10 control hearts, but only in four adapted ones. The total duration of fibrillation in the adapted group was smaller than in the control group by a factor of 7.3. Finally, seven adapted hearts, but only three control hearts, were still working by the 10th min of reperfusion.

The general issue is that *in the course of adaptation to short stress exposures a local mechanism is established in the heart that efficiently protects it from reperfusion arrhythmias and is less effective against the ischemic ones.*

In further studies, it was important to find out whether or not this local antiarrhythmic mechanism can have direct cytoprotective action, i.e., whether it protects the myocardial cells from reperfusion injury. To this end, we made use of the ''reperfusion paradox''

TABLE 1
Effect of Prior Adaptation to Stress on Ischemic and Reperfusion Arrhythmias in Isolated Hearts

	Acute ischemia		Reperfusion	
Indices	Control (n = 10)	Adapted (n = 10)	Control (n = 10)	Adapted (n = 10)
Extrasystole				
Number of hearts	7	6	10	10
Total duration (s)	215	129	753	1079
Ventricular tachycardia				
Number of hearts	6	4	10	10
Total duration (s)	22	24	1317	1374
Mean duration	2.2 ± 1.1	2.4 ± 1.1	132 ± 42	137 ± 67
Ventricular fibrillation				
Number of hearts	0	0	8	4
Total duration (s)	0	0	3198	440
Mean duration	0	0	319 ± 55	44 ± 42[a]
All arrhythmias				
Number of hearts	7	6	10	10
Total duration (s)	273	153	5268	2893
Mean duration	27 ± 9	15 ± 9	526 ± 26	289 ± 69[b]
Number of hearts arrested	0	0	7	3

[a] $p < 0.05$.
[b] $p < 0.01$.

discovered by Hearse et al.[2] Figure 2 shows the response of isolated control and adapted hearts to reperfusion following a 15-min total ischemia. Adaptation can be seen to largely check the depression of contraction amplitude and to decrease the extent of contracture in the reperfusion paradox. Of especial interest are the curves in part C, which reflect the leakage of creatine phosphokinase (CPK) into the perfusate owing to sarcolemmal damage. The enzyme leakage and hence the membrane damage are much less in the adapted hearts. Thus, there is unambiguous evidence that adaptation of the whole organism to stress results in formation in the heart proper of some mechanism that protects the cardiac cells (in particular, their sarcolemmal membrane) from reoxygenation damage.

III. LOCAL ADAPTATIONAL PROTECTION OF THE HEART AGAINST TOXIC CATECHOLAMINE LEVELS AND EXCESS CALCIUM

After ischemia and reperfusion, the next important factor damaging the heart in natural conditions is the excess of catecholamines and the catecholamine-induced excessive entry of calcium into the sarcoplasm. Accordingly, our experiments were aimed at evaluating the resistance of isolated adapted hearts to both of these.

When the isolated heart is perfused with toxic doses of epinephrine (5×10^{-5} *M*), there evolves sinus tachycardia with marked impairment of contractility (a severalfold decrease in contraction amplitude and contraction and relaxation velocities, and large contracture) as well as rhythm disorders such as numerous extrasystoles and atrioventricular (AV) block (Figure 3). Prior adaptation to stress largely attenuates the epinephrine-induced arrhythmias, as well as the adrenotoxic contracture and impairment of cardiac contractility. In this context, it is essential that the adrenergic heart injury is in great measure due to cAMP-mediated activation of the slow Ca^{2+} channels through which excess calcium enters the cardiomyocytes. Therefore, detailed studies were then carried out on the resistance of isolated control and adapted hearts to contractural and arrhythmogenic effects of high calcium.

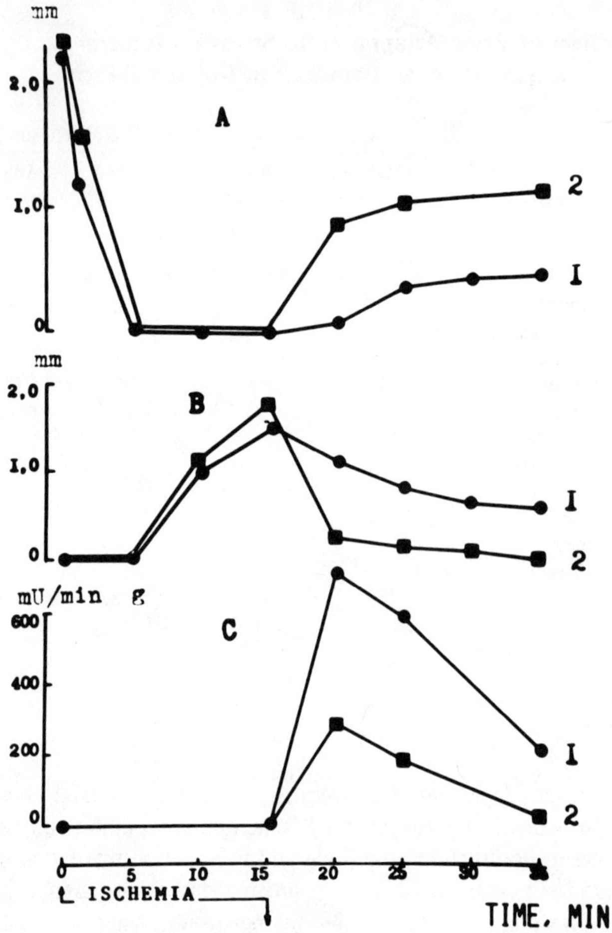

FIGURE 2. Effect of adaptation to stress on (A) contraction amplitude, (B) extent of contracture, and (C) leakage of CPK from isolated rat hearts in ischemia and reperfusion. (1) Control, (2) adapted.

With isotonically contracting hearts from control and adapted animals, the calcium concentration in the perfusing solution was raised from normal 1.36 to 10 m*M*. Changes in pH and osmolarity were insignificant and therefore not compensated for. The hypercalcium perfusion was carried out for 2 min. The contracture was determined by relating the diastolic apicobasal length of the heart to its length at rest before the calcium shift-up. Three types of ventricular arrhythmias — extrasystole, tachycardia, and fibrillation — were characterized by (1) the number of hearts with each type; (2) the total duration of the given type in the whole group; and (3) the mean duration of the given type per one heart in the group (taking into calculation the total number of hearts in the group regardless of the occurrence of arrhythmias).

The recordings in Figure 4 allow a qualitative assessment of the action of excess calcium on the control and the adapted hearts. The ECGs show that ventricular extrasystoles appear in 15 to 20 s of high calcium in the control heart, but not in the adapted one. As to isotonic contractility, the calcium shift-up first produced a positive inotropic effect in both groups, then in the control the diastolic relaxation was impaired, giving rise to large transient contracture and a pronounced decrease in the contraction amplitude, which were both negligible in the adapted hearts.

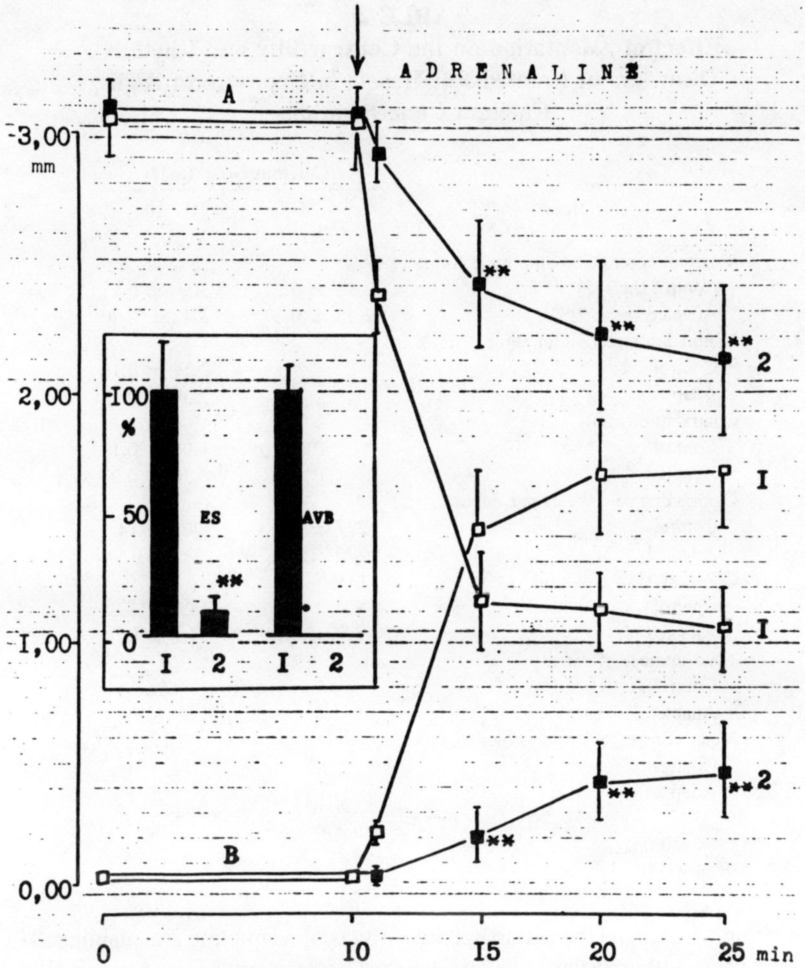

FIGURE 3. Effect of adaptation to stress on (A) contraction amplitude, (B) contracture, and (inset) arrhythmias in isolated hearts exposed to cardiotoxic doses of epinephrine (5×10^{-5} *M*). (1) Control, (2) adapted. (ES) Extrasystole, (AVB) atrioventricular block.

The quantitative evaluation of the antiarrhythmic and anticontractural effect of adaptation can be found in Table 2. At first, in both groups the excess of calcium increases the contraction amplitude by 30%, but then the amplitude declines in the control, but remains high in the adapted hearts, where the contracture proves to be three times less. The number of extrasystoles in adaptation is fivefold lower than in the control.

Thus, *prior adaptation of animals to short, noninjurious exposures to stress markedly attenuates the contractural and arrhythmogenic action of excess calcium on the isolated heart.*

At the next stage of our work, calcium was removed from the perfusing solution for 5 min and then returned to normal. As shown in Figure 5, removal of calcium disrupts the electromechanical coupling in both control and adapted hearts; as it does so, in adaptation the AV block develops after a longer latent period (222 ± 30 s vs. 132 ± 24 s in the control, $p < 0.05$). The major differences between the two groups are seen as the calcium concentration is restituted, and the control hearts develop contracture attended with decreased contraction amplitude and pronounced group extrasystolia, whereas the adapted hearts display practically such phenomena.

TABLE 2
Effect of Adaptation on the Contractility and Rhythm Disorders of Isolated Rat Hearts in Exposure to High Calcium Concentrations

	Calcium conc. (m*M*)	
Indices	**1.36**	**10**
Maximal contraction amplitude (mm)		
Control (n = 7)	2.78 ± 0.21	3.59 ± 0.21
Adapted (n = 7)	2.56 ± 0.17	3.42 ± 0.20
Minimal contraction amplitude (mm)		
Control		2.54 ± 0.19
Adapted		3.30 ± 0.18[a]
Contracture (mm)		
Control	0	1.04 ± 0.19
Adapted	0	0.36 ± 0.09[b]
Contraction rate (beats per minute)		
Control	277 ± 10	291 ± 14
Adapted	270 ± 7	313 ± 15
Coronary flow (ml/min)		
Control	9.6 ± 0.7	13.7 ± 1.0
Adapted	8.7 ± 0.6	13.5 ± 0.7
Total number of extrasystoles		
Control	0	76
Adapted	0	13
Mean number of extrasystoles		
Control		11 ± 4
Adapted		2 ± 1[a]

[a] $p < 0.05$.
[b] $p < 0.01$.

The anticontractural and the antiarrhythmic effects of adaptation are quantitated in Tables 3 and 4. One can see that at the same spontaneous contraction rate and coronary flow after returning calcium to the perfusing solution, in adapted hearts the contracture is 2.5 times less and, conversely, the contraction amplitude is twice higher than in the controls (Table 3). Concurrently, within the first 5 min after calcium restitution the number of ventricular extrasystoles per heart in the adapted group is about half that in the control, the incidence of ventricular tachycardia is 2.5 times less, and its mean duration is over 14 times less (Table 4).

In the aggregate these data provide convincing evidence for the greater capacity of the membrane mechanisms of calcium homeostasis in the adapted hearts with regard to abolishing such detrimental effects of excess calcium as contracture and arrhythmia. This in all probability is achieved through faster removal of Ca^{2+} from the sarcoplasm. There are three main mechanisms responsible for this process, namely the sarcoplasmic reticulum (SR) calcium pump, the sarcolemmal calcium pump, and the Na^{+}/Ca^{2+} exchanger.

To assess the probable role of each of these mechanisms in the protective effect of adaptation, at the next stage of our work we loaded the papillary muscle cells with calcium using a low-sodium solution. Rat right ventricular papillary muscle was placed into a temperature-controlled (30°C) chamber with carbogen-saturated Krebs-Henseleit solution at pH 7.3 to 7.4. The perfusion rate was 10 to 12 ml/min. One end of the muscle was fixed rigidly and the other was connected to a TD-112 isotonic sensor. The experiment was preceded by a 1-h stabilization period when the muscle was stimulated with rectangular 5-m electric impulses with an amplitude equal to 1.5 to 2 threshold values at a frequency of 0.5 Hz.

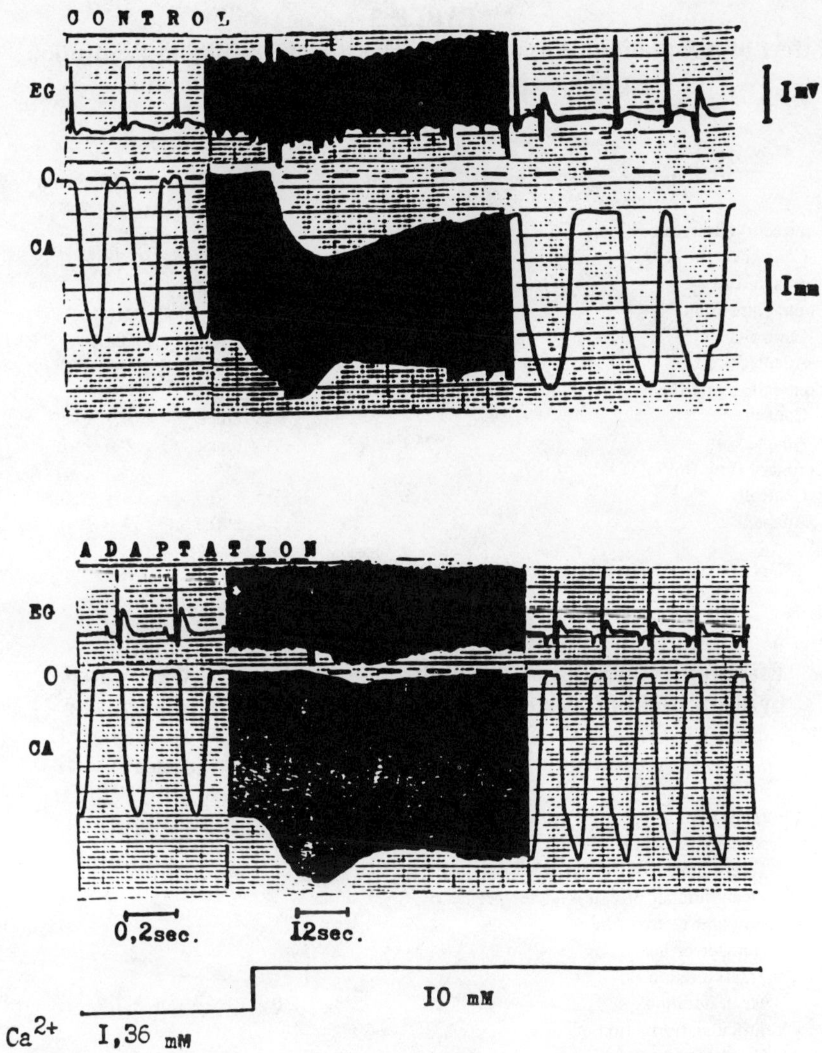

FIGURE 4. Effect of adaptation to stress on the electric and mechanical activity of the isolated rat heart at high Ca^{2+} concentration. (EG) Electrogram, (CA) isotonic contraction amplitude. For explanations see text.

The stimulation was carried out with silver chloride electrodes and a SEN 3201 stimulator (Nihon Kohden, Japan). The recording equipment was the same as in previous works.

The bioelectric activity of myocardial cells was measured with the use of ''floating'' microelectrodes made from glass capillaries filled with 3 *M* KCl and connected via a 30 μm tungsten wire to a Nihon Kohden MEZ 8201 preamplifier, wherefrom the signal was supplied to an oscilloscope and/or into the memory of Nihon Kohden RAT 1100 for subsequent analysis.

Before the experiment the muscle was stretched to a length providing the maximal contraction amplitude. The muscle was stimulated for 2 min at a frequency of 3 Hz, then stimulation was discontinued and the normal solution was replaced with the low-sodium one (9 m*M* sodium with sucrose as a substitute); the development of hyponatrium contracture was monitored for 10 min with recording of the rest potential (RP).

In such an experiment, calcium enters the cell through the Na^+/Ca^{2+} exchange mechanism and accumulates in the sarcoplasm to a very high concentration; this cannot be

TABLE 3
Effect of Adaptation on Isolated Rat Heart Contractility in Restitution of Normal Calcium after Calcium-Free Perfusion

	Calcium conc. (m*M*)		
Indices	**1.36**	**0, 5 min**	**1.36, 5 min**
Contraction amplitude (mm)			
Control (n = 7)	2.63 ± 0.18	0	0.73 ± 0.18
Adapted (n = 7)	2.50 ± 0.19	0	1.53 ± 0.30[a]
Contracture (mm)			
Control	0	0.58 ± 0.04	1.09 ± 0.09
Adapted	0	0.41 ± 0.10	0.44 ± 0.19[a]
Contraction rate (beats per minute)			
Control	277 ± 12	AV block	237 ± 20
Adapted	269 ± 10	AV block	240 ± 7
Coronary flow (ml/min)			
Control	9.5 ± 0.6	13.5 ± 0.7	8.5 ± 0.8
Adapted	8.3 ± 0.6	13.4 ± 0.7	7.6 ± 0.6

[a] $p < 0.05$.

TABLE 4
Effect of Adaptation on Arrhythmias in Isolated Hearts Caused by Restitution of Normal Calcium after Calcium-Free Perfusion

Indices	**Control (n = 7)**	**Adapted (n = 7)**
Extrasystole		
Number of hearts	7	7
Total number of extrasystoles	315	175
Mean number of extrasystoles per heart	45 ± 7	25 ± 5[a]
Ventricular tachycardia		
Number of hearts	5	2
Total duration (s)	41	3
Mean duration	5.8 ± 2.0	0.4 ± 0.6[a]
Ventricular fibrillation		
Number of hearts	2	0
Total duration (s)	18	0

[a] $p < 0.05$.

abolished or attenuated by the sarcolemmal Ca ATPase, which is responsive in the low calcium range and normally participates only in the final stage of diastole.[3] Hence the main burden is to be taken by the SR calcium pump.

Figure 6 shows that in the initial solution the muscles from control and adapted animals contract with approximately the same amplitude (10 to 12% of their diastolic length). The low-sodium solution elicits great differences between them: in the control, within 10 min contracture reaches a plateau, with a stable shortening of the muscle close to its contraction amplitude under stimulation in the Krebs-Henseleit solution; with the adapted muscle the contracture is insignificant.

The quantitative results of the whole series of these experiments are presented in Figure 7: in the control group the contracture in 10 min of low-sodium perfusion approximates the normal contraction amplitude, whereas in the adapted group it is fivefold less. Accordingly, the RP declines to 57 mV in the control, but remains at 68 mV in the adapted group. This is most probably explained by the fact that adaptation enhances the efficiency of the SR calcium pump.

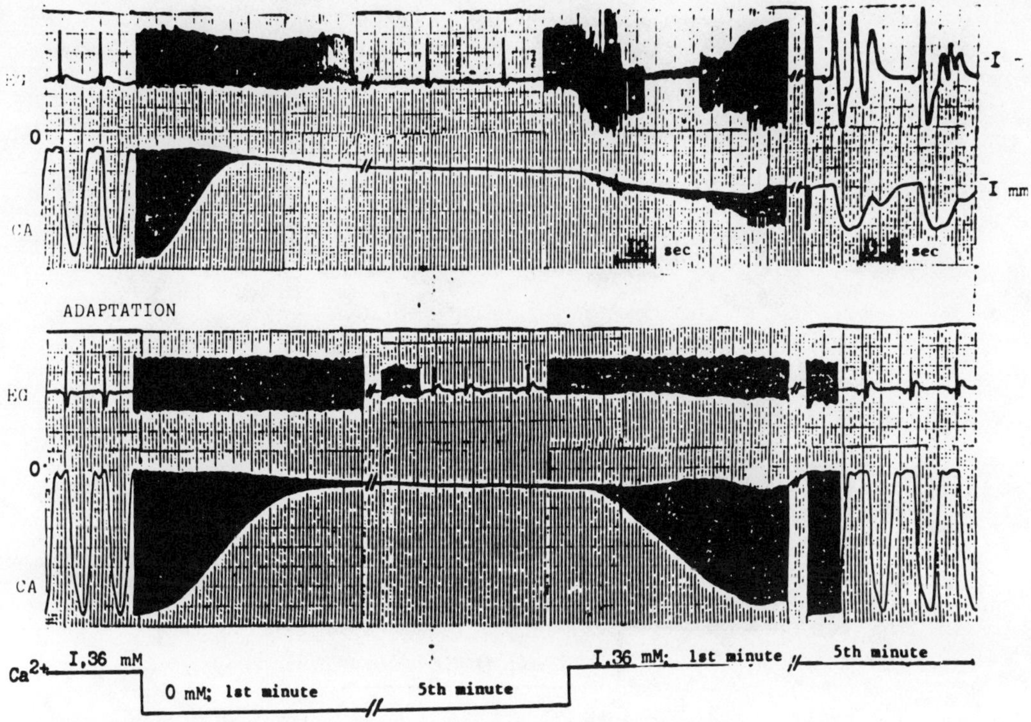

FIGURE 5. Effect of adaptation to stress on the electric and mechanical response of the isolated heart to calcium-free perfusion and restitution of calcium. Designations are as in Figure 4. For explanations see text.

To study further the mechanisms of the antiarrhythmic effect of adaptation, we used the same technique with papillary muscle to evaluate the main electrophysiological parameters of the myocardial cells under an increase of such a physiological determinant of calcium loading as the contraction frequency at normal or elevated calcium.

There are several issues from Table 5. First, at increasing contraction rate and high calcium the RP is reliably lower in control than in adaptation (69 mV vs. 82 mV), i.e., the difference is qualitatively the same as with low sodium. Since in combined action of high calcium and imposed contraction rate the calcium load is mainly created owing to its entry through the sarcolemma, this is real evidence for the adaptively enhanced ability of the cardiomyocytes to maintain the RP in calcium overload that may be caused by different mechanisms.

Second, owing to the normal RP retained at maximal calcium load (high calcium and 3 Hz) the amplitude of the action potential (AP) in adapted specimens exceeds the control one by 25%, which should favor the maintenance of a high enough conduction velocity under such conditions.

Third, the most consistent observation is that the well-known phenomenon of shortening RP with increasing contraction rate at physiological and high calcium levels is much less pronounced in the papillary muscle from adapted animals. As a result, at 180 contractions per minute the duration of the AP was twice longer in the adapted group at 10 to 90% repolarization. Thus, prior adaptation to repeated stress undoubtedly prolongs the AP and hence the effective refractory period at near-physiological contraction rates; this change by itself must diminish the probability of premature depolarization.

The data on papillary muscle contractility obtained in the same experiments are presented in Table 6 and show that at physiological calcium concentrations accelerated contractions

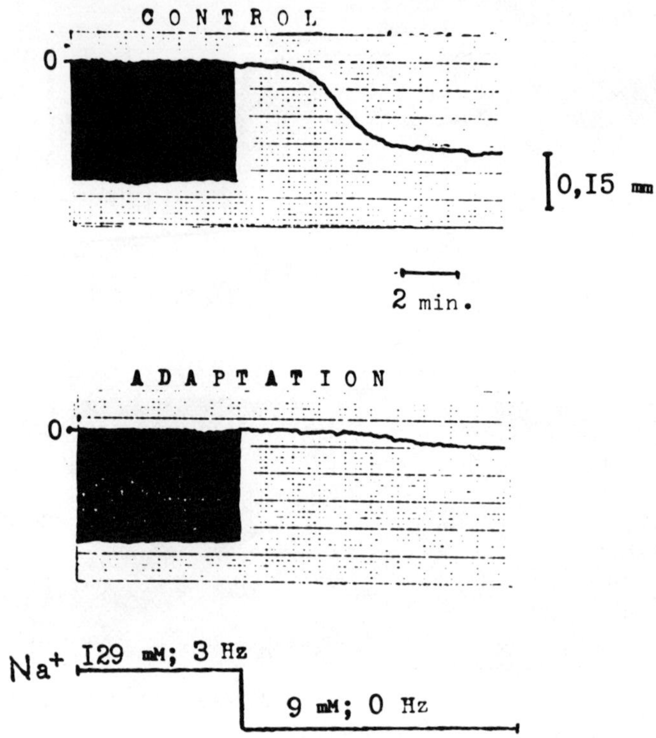

FIGURE 6. Effect of adaptation to stress on the hyponatrium contracture of papillary muscle. The tracings present the changes in muscle length; the "0" level corresponds to complete diastolic relaxation.

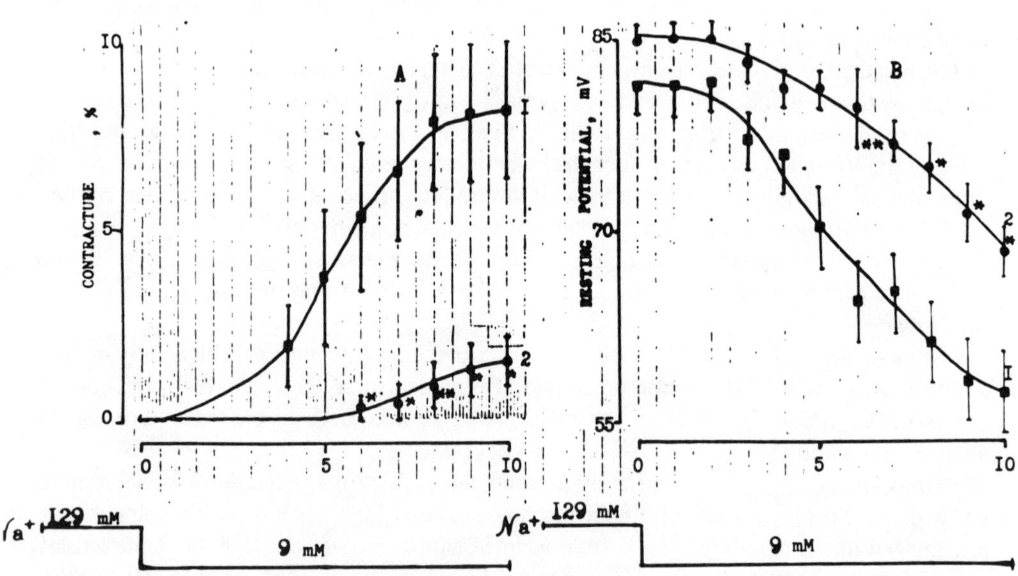

FIGURE 7. Effect of adaptation to stress on (A) contracture and (B) rest potential of the rat papillary muscle exposed to low-sodium solution (9 mM Na^+).

TABLE 5
Effect of Adaptation on the Bioelectric Activity of Papillary Muscle Cells

Indices		2.5 m*M* Ca^{2+} Pacing Frequency (Hz)			18 m*M* Ca^{2+} Pacing frequency (Hz)		
		0.5	1.0	3.0	1.0	3.0, 5 min	3.0, 10 min
Overshoot (mV)							
Control		28.3 ± 1.6	30.0 ± 3.8	14.1 ± 1.9	33.0 ± 3.0	4.3 ± 5.6	5.4 ± 5.8
Adapted		23.4 ± 3.4	21.0 ± 3.2	13.1 ± 2.4	27.7 ± 3.9	13.0 ± 4.4[a]	18.0 ± 5.1[a]
Rest potential (mV)							
Control		75.3 ± 2.9	77.5 ± 3.0	69.0 ± 1.2	87.5 ± 2.0	75.8 ± 3.0	69.0 ± 5.0
Adapted		79.8 ± 1.1	76.8 ± 2.2	74.3 ± 2.7	83.8 ± 2.8	75.4 ± 3.4	82.0 ± 3.0[a]
Action potential (mV)							
Control		104.4 ± 1.8	107.5 ± 3.4	83.2 ± 4.3	120.3 ± 1.8	80.6 ± 6.6	74.0 ± 8.9
Adapted		103.3 ± 3.5	97.8 ± 3.2	87.4 ± 3.1	111.0 ± 2.4[a]	88.0 ± 4.0	99.8 ± 4.0[a]
Duration of repolarization (m)							
10%	Control	6.0 ± 0.8	5.0 ± 0.7	3.5 ± 0.7	6.2 ± 0.8	1.6 ± 0.2	1.4 ± 0.2
	Adapted	7.6 ± 0.6	7.0 ± 0.7	6.2 ± 0.8[a]	6.7 ± 0.6	3.7 ± 0.8[a]	2.8 ± 0.3[b]
30%	Control	15.0 ± 1.6	14.0 ± 1.9	6.2 ± 1.0	11.0 ± 1.0	3.2 ± 0.3	2.5 ± 0.3
	Adapted	16.5 ± 1.1	15.7 ± 1.4	12.0 ± 1.5[b]	12.7 ± 0.8	6.2 ± 1.4[a]	4.9 ± 0.4[b]
50%	Control	25.8 ± 3.0	23.4 ± 3.3	9.8 ± 1.5	16.3 ± 1.4	5.2 ± 0.6	3.8 ± 0.4
	Adapted	29.3 ± 2.1	30.2 ± 2.7	18.3 ± 2.4[b]	18.9 ± 0.7	8.8 ± 1.9	7.1 ± 0.7[b]
70%	Control	81.4 ± 16.0	63.0 ± 12.0	17.7 ± 3.7	29.5 ± 2.9	8.1 ± 0.9	5.7 ± 0.5
	Adapted	110.0 ± 16.9	98.0 ± 11.0	38.1 ± 7.9[a]	47.8 ± 4.0[b]	13.8 ± 3.0	11.1 ± 1.4[b]
90%	Control	215.0 ± 16.0	196.0 ± 22.0	50.0 ± 13.0	107.0 ± 24.0	22.1 ± 5.2	13.1 ± 3.2
	Adapted	235.0 ± 13.0	220.0 ± 7.0	106.4 ± 18.5[a]	185.0 ± 12.7[a]	59.0 ± 13.0[a]	35.0 ± 5.1

[a] $p < 0.05$.
[b] $p < 0.01$.

TABLE 6
Effect of Adaptation on the Contractility Parameters of Rat Papillary Muscle

Indices	2.5 m*M* Ca^{2+} Pacing frequency (Hz)			18 m*M* Ca^{2+} Pacing frequency (Hz)		
	0.5	**1.0**	**3.0**	**1.0**	**3.0, 5 min**	**3.0, 10 min**
Contraction amplitude (% initial muscle length)						
Control (n = 7)	21.8 ± 1.2	20.8 ± 1.4	11.0 ± 2.0	18.0 ± 1.4	4.3 ± 1.1	1.1 ± 0.1
Adapted (n = 7)	19.5 ± 1.0	18.9 ± 0.8	12.8 ± 1.2	17.8 ± 0.9	10.2 ± 2.2[a]	4.7 ± 1.2[a]
Contraction rate (muscle length units/s)						
Control	1.46 ± 0.07	1.43 ± 0.06	0.77 ± 0.14	1.06 ± 0.10	0.28 ± 0.08	0.09 ± 0.01
Adapted	1.27 ± 0.07	1.27 ± 0.07	0.93 ± 0.04	1.13 ± 0.05	0.66 ± 0.13[a]	0.35 ± 0.09[a]
Relaxation rate (muscle length units/s)						
Control	1.14 ± 0.06	1.10 ± 0.09	0.64 ± 0.13	0.79 ± 0.09	0.20 ± 0.05	0.09 ± 0.01
Adapted	0.98 ± 0.05	0.98 ± 0.05	0.74 ± 0.08	0.80 ± 0.07	0.58 ± 013[a]	0.32 ± 0.08[a]
Contracture (% initial muscle length)						
Control	0	0	0	1.5 ± 1.5	15.4 ± 1.3	28.4 ± 2.1
Adapted	0	0	0	0	4.6 ± 2.3[b]	12.5 ± 2.8[c]
Contracture (% initial contraction amplitude)						
Control	0	0	0	13	140	258
Adapted	0	0	0	0	36[a]	97[b]

[a] $p < 0.05$.
[b] $p < 0.01$.
[c] $p < 0.001$.

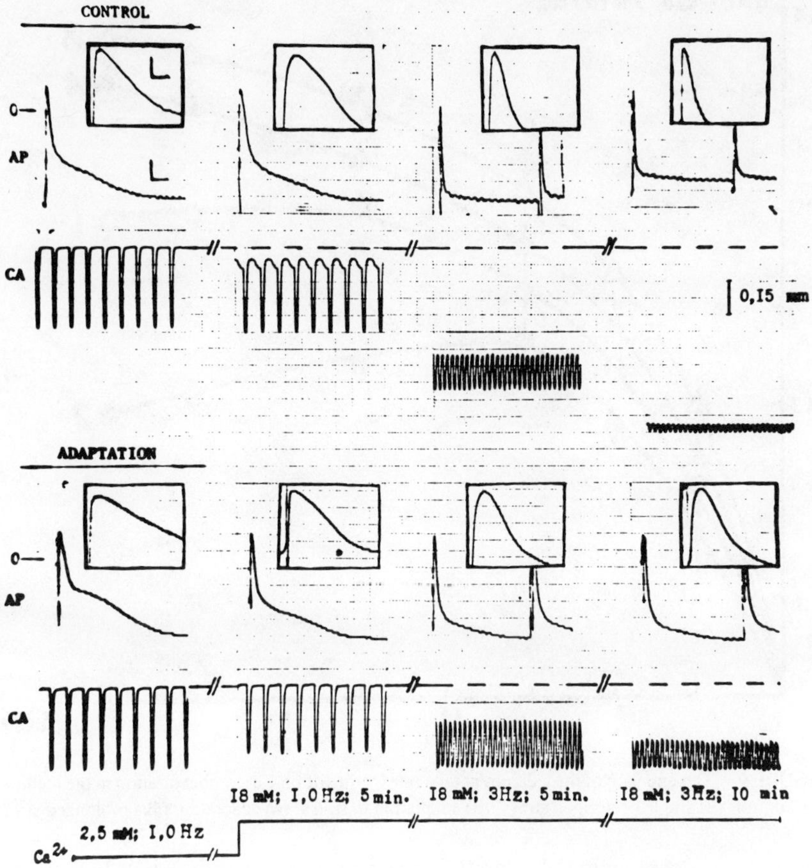

FIGURE 8. Effect of adaptation to stress on the electric activity (action potential, AP) and isotonic contraction (contraction amplitude, CA) of the papillary muscle exposed to high calcium and increased pacing frequency. The insets show the AP tops at higher sweep.

result in a negative inotropic effect, with no differences between the two groups. At high calcium and 180 contractions per minute, the adapted muscles exceed the controls twofold to fourfold in the contraction amplitude and contraction and relaxation velocities; this is so because upon adaptation the calcium-induced contracture proves to be 2.5 times less. Thus, in our experiments adaptation was equally effective against the hypercalcium contracture in ventricles and papillary muscles of isolated hearts. This obviously could only be due to enhanced calcium binding and removal.

The data summarized in Tables 5 and 6 are illustrated by experimental recordings in Figure 8. As can be seen, the high calcium load at a stimulation frequency of 180 min^{-1} greatly "narrows" the AP of myocardial cells and almost completely suppresses the contractility of the papillary muscle. In a specimen from adapted animal, the AP duration is much less affected and contractility is retained at the same calcium load.

Thus, on the one hand we have earlier shown that adaptation to stress is effective against adrenergic, ischemic, and reperfusion arrhythmias, and on the other, here we see that it has antiarrhythmic and anticontractural effects against calcium overloading of the cardiac muscle, whatever its cause. This is not likely to be just a coincidence, and is most probably due to the fact that an excess of calcium accumulates in the cardiac cells and acts arrhythmogenically in all types of heart damage against which adaptation has proved effective (acute ischemia

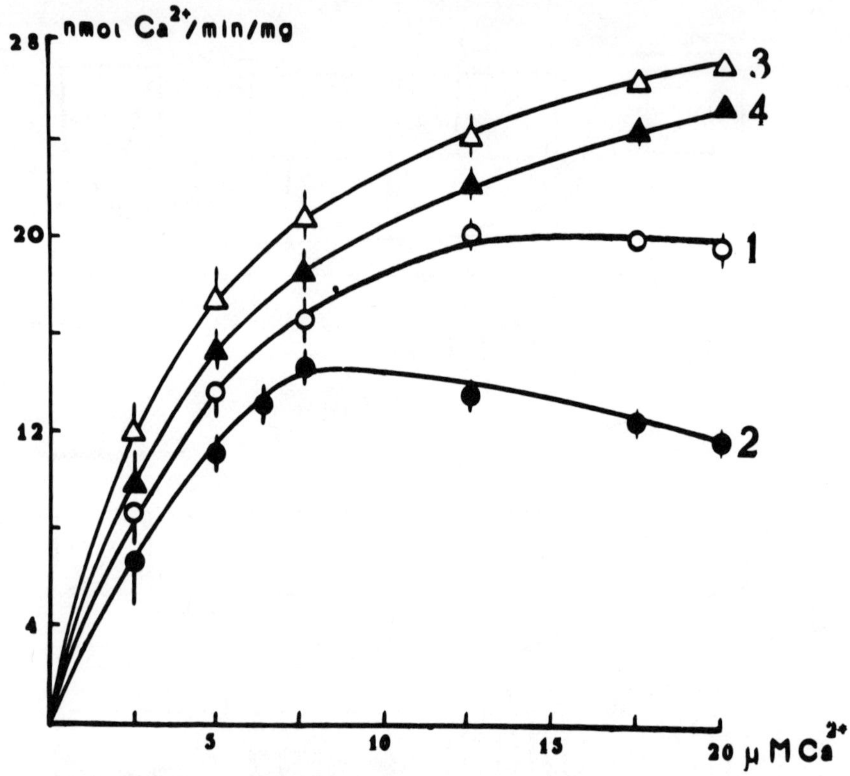

FIGURE 9. Dependence of the calcium uptake rate by the SR on Ca^{2+} concentration in the medium. (1) Control, (2) single prolonged stress, (3) adaptation to stress, (4) adaptation plus prolonged stress.

and reperfusion, acute myocardial infarction, emotional pain stress [EPS]). Indeed, increased calcium entry into the cell or its excess in the sarcoplasm have been demonstrated in ischemia and reperfusion,[4] and in EPS[5] attended with a drop in the fibrillation threshold. In all such cases enhanced calcium-removing capacity would diminish the probability of arrhythmias. Our data on the direct protective effect of adaptation against excess calcium provide unequivocal support to this suggestion.

Along this line, we next assessed the effect of adaptation on the capacity of the calcium-transporting mechanisms, and on the resistance of these and other cell components to autolysis, which is a major necrobiotic factor.

IV. EFFECT OF ADAPTATION TO STRESS ON THE FUNCTION OF THE SARCOPLASMIC RETICULUM CALCIUM PUMP AND MITOCHONDRIA AND ON THEIR RESISTANCE TO AUTOLYSIS

The studies on the SR calcium pump[7] included four series of experiments on rats: (1) control, (2) prolonged (6 h) immobilization stress, (3) adaptation to short (1 h) stresses, and (4) prolonged immobilization stress on the next day after completion of adaptation. Rats were sacrificed by decapitation 2 h after stress or 1 d after the end of adaptation. Hearts were extracted, washed with saline, and frozen in liquid nitrogen. Homogenates were prepared and Ca^{2+} uptake by the SR vesicles was measured ionometrically as described in Chapter 1, Section VIII.

Figure 9 demonstrates the dependence of the calcium uptake rate on its concentration in the medium. It can be seen that in control SR the uptake rate increases with the ion

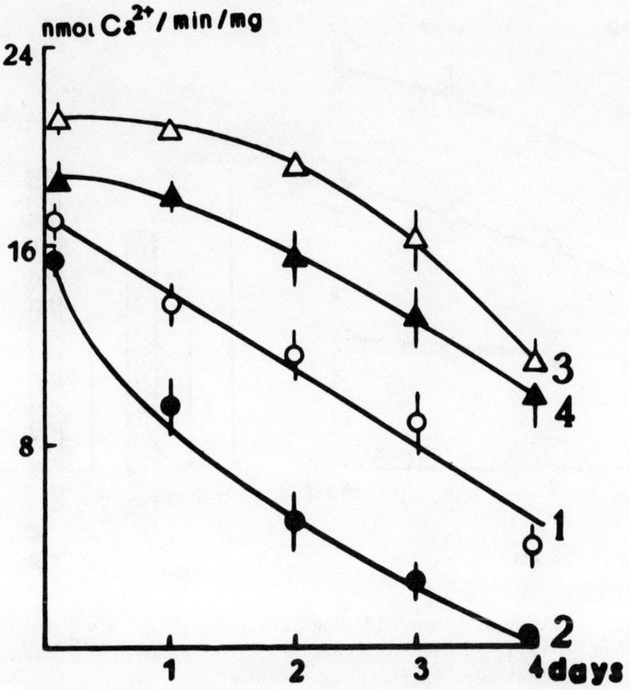

FIGURE 10. Decline in the rate of calcium uptake by rat myocardial SR vesicles during storage of the homogenates at 4°C. (1) Control, (2) single prolonged stress, (3) adaptation to stress, (4) adaptation plus prolonged stress.

concentration, reaching a plateau at 1 to $2 \cdot 10^{-5}$ *M* Ca^{2+}. Upon prolonged stress the uptake is slower and its rate reaches a maximum already at 7.5 μ*M*; moreover, at higher calcium concentrations it is inhibited so that at 20 μ*M* it is almost twice lower than in the control.

It can further be seen that adaptation to short stresses results in substantial enhancement of calcium uptake (e.g., a 30% surplus at 5 μ*M* Ca^{2+}), and the uptake rate still increases at high calcium concentrations without reaching a plateau. The same pattern is observed in stress after adaptation, so that after prolonged stress the uptake rate in adapted animals is reliably higher than in nonadapted ones at both physiological and elevated calcium concentrations. Thus, prior adaptation not only itself enhances the calcium-accumulating ability of cardiac-cell SR, but certainly protects the SR membranes from the adverse influence of prolonged immobilization stress.

It is known that the state of the SR calcium pump depends in great measure on its lipid microenvironment which is exposed to such endogenous cell factors as lipases, phospholipases, LPO, etc. Since the activity of such factors has been proved to change in stress and adaptation to stress, these changes may affect the SR calcium transport. Therefore, we have studied the dynamics of inactivation of the SR calcium pump during storage of homogenates, whereby the cell structures have been exposed to endogenous degrading factors.

Figure 10 shows the decline in the calcium uptake rate in SR as the preparations are kept at 4°C. In the control this process is linear and about 20% of initial activity is retained in 4 d. After stress the inactivation is much faster and in 4 d no uptake is observable. Adaptation, besides enhancing the initial uptake rate, greatly retards its decline; even after stress following adaptation the SR retains half of its activity in 4 d. Thus, adaptation makes the SR membrane so much more resistant to degrading factors that, even upon stress, its calcium pump remains markedly more stable than in the control.

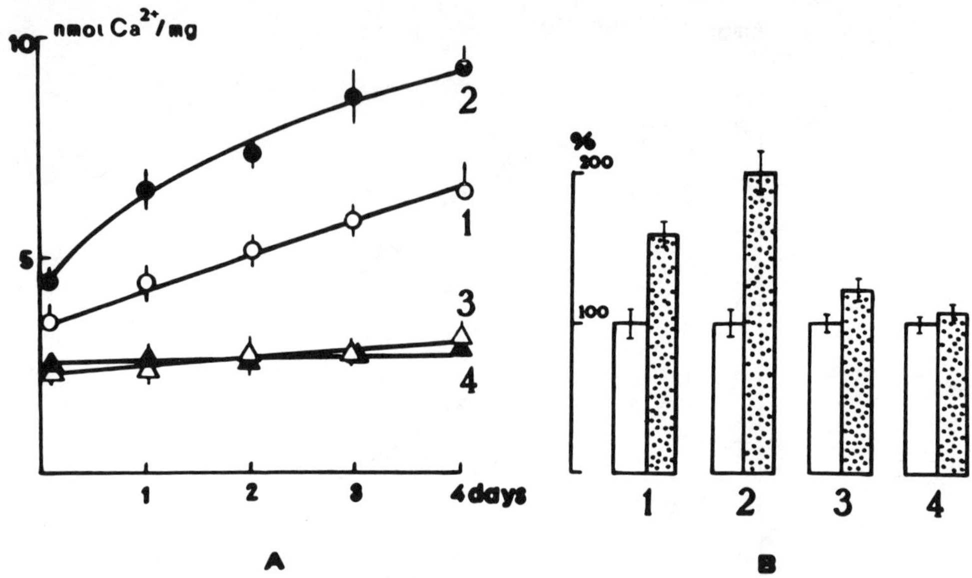

FIGURE 11. Release of calcium in myocardial homogenates during storage at 4°C. (A) Free Ca^{2+} content at tissue to medium ratio of 1:4. (B) Relative increase in free calcium content in 3 d. (1) Control, (2) single prolonged stress, (3) adaptation to stress, (4) adaptation plus prolonged stress.

Another criterion for assessing the state of myocardial membrane structures can be the dynamics of accumulation in the homogenates of free calcium released from the SR and mitochondria. As shown in Figure 11, such leakage is clearly observable in the control and still more pronounced upon stress; after adaptation, the release of free calcium is greatly diminished, and upon stress following adaptation there are no appreciable changes throughout the 4 d of incubation. *This striking fact of practically no leakage of calcium from the intracellular depots in the myocardium of animals exposed to stress after prior adaptation testifies to a radically enhanced stability of membrane structures due to adaptation, which can thus block the action of endogenous injuring factors.*

The stress-induced impairment of the SR calcium pump and its faster inactivation in storage appear to be associated, since much the same natural degrading factors are involved in stress damage and autolysis. Indeed, stress is attended with activation of phospholipases[8] and LPO,[9] lysosomal labilization and release of proteases,[10] and ensuing damage to membranes and their enzymes — Na,K ATPase[11] and SR Ca ATPase.[12] Activation of LPO,[13,14] phospholipases[15-17] and proteases,[18] lysosomal labilization,[19] and decreasing activity of membrane-bound enzymes[20,21] have also been shown in autolysis. It is therefore understandable that the stress damage not only depresses the function of the SR calcium pump, but also precipitates its inactivation in autolysis. It is essential that in our experiment stress increased the free calcium content in the homogenate and aggravated its leakage in autolysis. This is quite in line with the *in vivo* accumulation of calcium in the cardiomyocytes damaged by stress or ischemia. Since Ca^{2+} can activate phospholipases and at certain concentratios also LPO, this may complete a "vicious circle" in groups of cells, in which the natural degrading factors increase the leakage of Ca^{2+} from the intracellular depots and the free Ca^{2+} in its turn potentiates their cytotoxic action. In prolonged stress this corresponds to formation of micronecroses and then focal cardiosclerosis (see Chapter 1).

The ability of adaptation to short stress exposures to prevent the impairment of cardiac structure, function, and electric stability in stress-induced, ischemic, and reperfusion damage has been found in 1985 and confirmed in further works.[22,23] Now it has for the first time

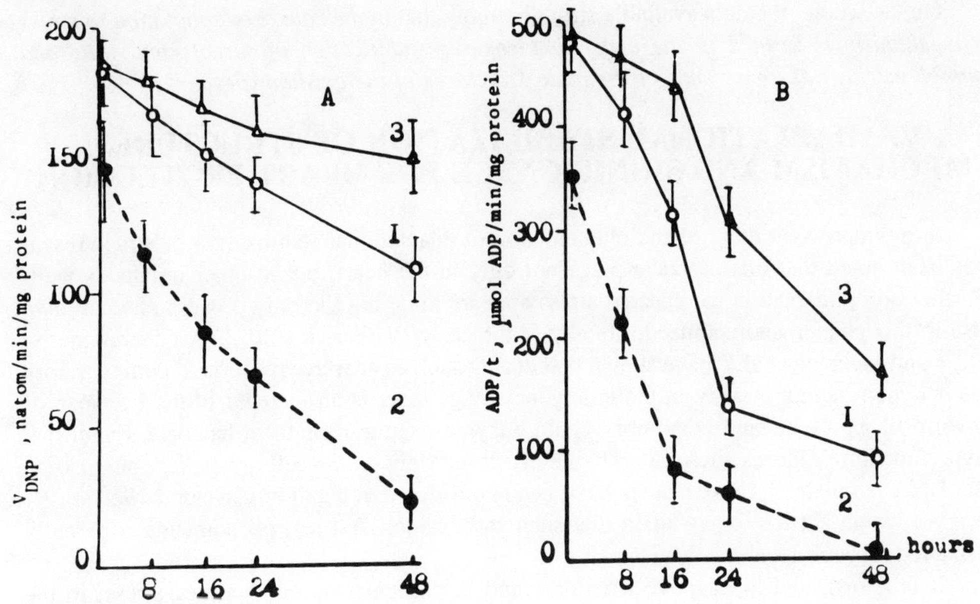

FIGURE 12. Effect of stress and adaptation on the changes in mitochondrial respiration and phosphorylation during storage. (A) Dinitrophenol-uncoupled respiration, (B) phosphorylation rate with succinate as substrate. (1) Control, (2) stress, (3) adaptation.

been elucidated that an important component of the adaptational protection of the heart at the cell level is the enhanced efficiency of the SR calcium pump and the greater ability of the SR membrane to withstand the action of degrading factors.

The fact that adaptation to repeated stress protects the heart from calcium-induced damage at physiological and biochemical levels is in our opinion of principal importance. Indeed, on the one hand calcium is a universal activator of the organismic physiological functions, and on the other it is now well known that excess calcium is the central link of most different types of heart damage. This link is blocked by the mechanisms evoked in adaptation to repeated stress. Hence, development of kinds of adaptation to stress suitable for humans, or isolation and pharmaceutical use of metabolites formed in adaptation, hold much promise for heart protection in a wide range of diseases.

In an attempt to unravel the mechanisms involved in such cardioprotective stabilization, it was first of all necessary to ascertain whether we were dealing with a peculiar phenomenon only specific for the SR membranes or with a general pattern encompassing all cellular structures. In a step along this line, we studied the inactivation of respiration and phosphorylation in mitochondria during prolonged storage and the effect of stress and adaptation on this process, by measuring the generally accepted parameters of respiration and phosphorylation after various times (up to 48 h) of incubation of mitochondrial suspensions at 4°C.

Figure 12A demonstrates the decline in the maximal rates of oxygen consumption upon complete uncoupling with dinitrophenol. As can be seen, in the mitochondria from animals exposed to EPS this index is 15% lower immediately upon isolation and further decreases to a much greater extent. Inactivation of mitochondria from adapted animals is much slower than in the control. Qualitatively, the same pattern is observed with the phosphorylation rate as shown in Figure 12B.

Thus, upon adaptation to repeated stress the ability of mitochondria to withstand natural degradation during autolysis is as certainly enhanced as that of the SR membranes. The experiments considered earlier on the leakage of CPK in reperfusion make it likely that the same stabilization takes place in the sarcolemma.

On the whole, the data available strongly imply that *in the course of adaptation to stress a mechanism is formed in the heart that ensures stabilization of sarcolemma, SR, and mitochondria, i.e., in essence of the main structures of the cardiomyocyte.*

V. ADAPTATIONAL STABILIZATION OF STRUCTURES; MECHANISM AND SIGNIFICANCE FOR HEART PROTECTION

In a wider assessment of the phenomenon of adaptational stabilization of structures, it has been noted that this can take place not only in the heart, but in other organs as well. Furthermore, adaptation to repeated stress appears to be not the only process that can give rise to this phenomenon. Indeed, already in the early 1970s Zak et al.,[24] Aschenbrenner et al.,[25] and Meerson et al.[26] have shown that during such an adaptive reaction as compensatory heart hyperfunction already in the emergency stage there is an increase in the life span of myofibrillar proteins and respiratory chain enzymes. Quite recently it has been found that hyperfunction produces such a stabilizing effect not only on the cell organelles, but also on the DNA template.[27] These studies have been considered in detail in Chapter 1, Section V. Here it would suffice to say again that such stabilization is a real phenomenon apparently achieved through local mechanisms.

It is known that in adaptive reactions, and in particular during repeated stress, in the heart there is an increase in the activity of antioxidant enzymes[28,29] and in the number of adenosine receptors,[30] and the membrane phospholipid composition changes towards a lower content of unsaturated fatty acids.[31] Maybe all these factors somehow contribute to the adaptational stabilization of structures. However, the most intriguing interpretation of this phenomenon emerges if we combine the concept of the regulatory system "inositol triphosphate-diacylglycerol" (IP_3-DAG) with the concept of so-called heat-shock proteins (HSP).

As applied to our experiments, it can be envisaged (scheme in Figure 13) that reiteration of stress episodes results in reiterated action of stress hormones on the Ca^{2+}-mobilizing receptors, which via phospholipase C activate the IP_3-DAG regulatory circuit. IP_3 acts on special receptors on the SR to cause release of calcium and is thus the intracellular messenger for immediate adaptive reactions. On the other hand, DAG is a messenger for long-term adaptation: it can act via protein kinase C and the sarcolemmal Na^+/H^+ exchange to activate transcription, cell growth, and proliferation.[35] Such activation of the genetic apparatus in hyperfuction and hypertrophy,[36] heat exposure,[37] hypoxia,[36] i.e., in diverse but certainly stressful situations, is attended with accumulation of HSP_{70}, HSP_{68}, and HSP_{58}. These stress proteins reputedly normalize the function of damaged cell nuclei and abolish disturbances of mRNA splicing and protein synthesis.[37] The scheme reflects the assumption that in repeated stress the increasing concentration of DAG activates, among others, the genes coding for the stress proteins. These proteins, in their turn, stabilize the structures both at the organellar and the genetic template levels.

In testing the suggestion that stress proteins are involved in the adaptational stabilization of structures, account should be taken of the recent data that the thermal stability of tissues from animals preadapted to heat is proportional to the accumulation of HSP in these tissues.[38,39] On the strength of these data, we decided to evaluate the heat tolerance of isolated hearts from stress-adapted animals (i.e., the hearts clearly exhibiting the phenomenon of adaptational stabilization). As shown in Figure 14, their thermostability proved to be markedly enhanced. Perfusion with a solution warmed up to 42°C caused severe depression of contractility, pronounced contracture, and massive leakage of CPK in the control hearts, but only slightly affected the adapted ones. This experiment conducted by Malyshev argues in favor of a role of stress proteins in such stabilization. On the whole, however, the hypothesis of the genetic mechanism of the phenomenon of adaptational stabilization of

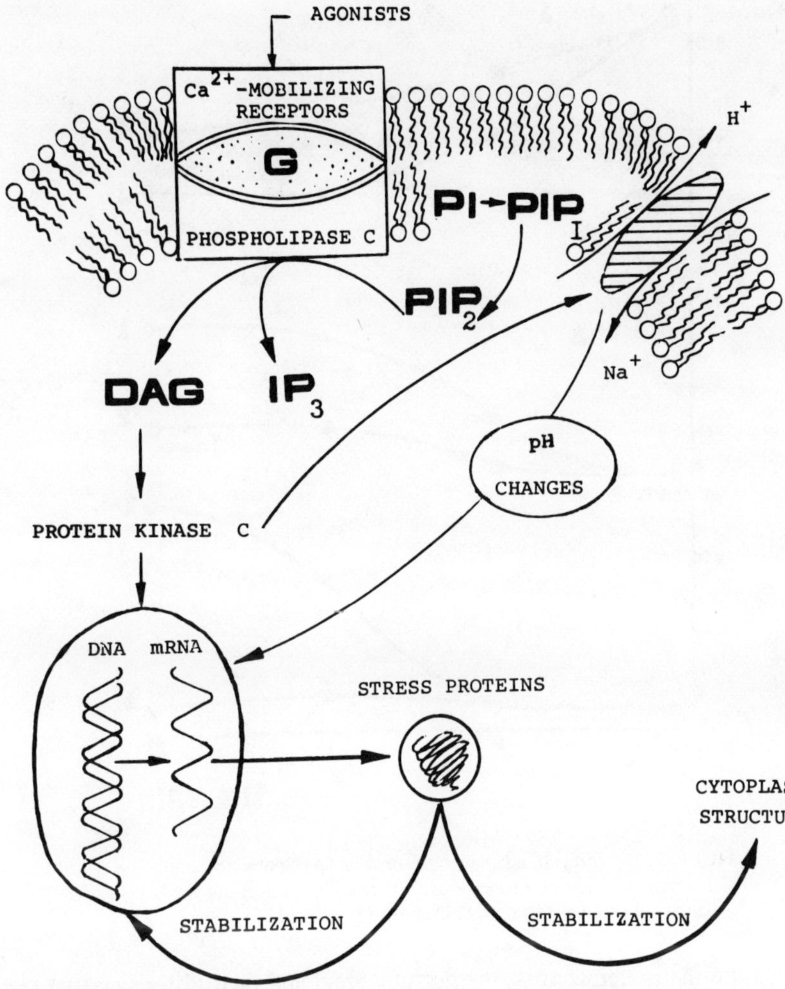

FIGURE 13. A hypothetical mechanism of stabilization of cell structures in repeated stress exposures. (G) G-protein, (PI) phosphoinositol, (PIP) phosphoinositol phosphate, (PIP_2) phosphoinositol diphosphate, (IP_3) inositol triphosphate, (DAG) diacyl glycerol.

structures poses many more questions than it does solve: what is the gene-control mechanism underlying the enhanced formation of the stress proteins? do these proteins indeed stabilize the structures? and, finally, is such stabilization achieved through suppressing the natural degrading factors such as phospholipases and proteases or through directly enhancing the resistance of membranes and other cell structures to these factors? Notwithstanding, the phenomenon itself raises no doubt; moreover, it is actually operative, protecting the heart against direct damage from ischemia and ensuring reduction of the infarct size.

This has been demonstrated in a special morphometric study that we carried out together with Shneider and Ustinova. In so doing, we took account of the already classical works of Lowe et al.,[40] who have shown that despite artery ligation in one strictly definite place, the size of ischemic myocardium may greatly vary with individual animals; at the same time the size of necrosis determined histologically 3 d after artery ligation is directly dependent on and always smaller than the ischemic area, since part of the cells in the periphery of the ischemic region — in the ''risk area'' — restore their structure and function.[41] As all these zones can be affected by the individual peculiarities of the coronary bed, we thought it

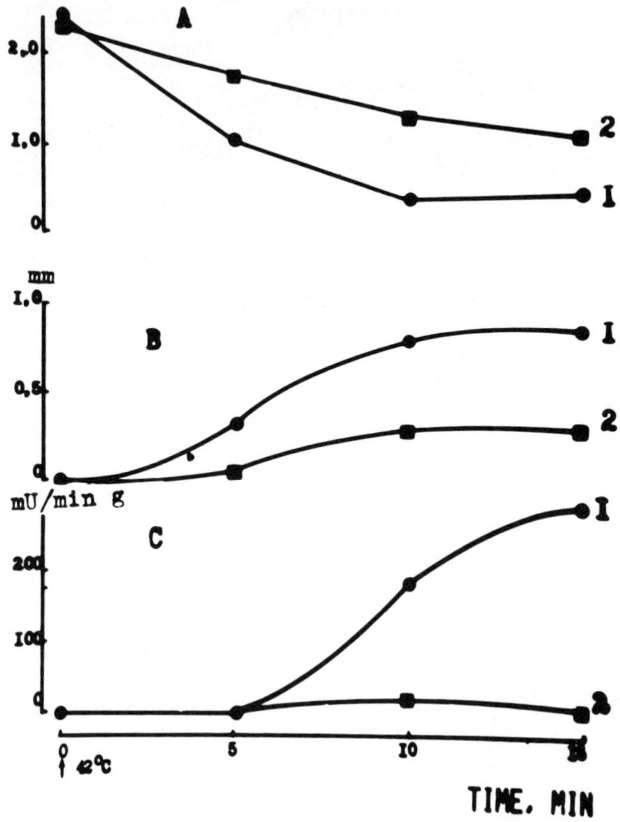

FIGURE 14. Effect of adaptation to stress on (A) contraction amplitude, (B) contracture, and (C) leakage of CPK from isolated hearts exposed to elevated temperature (42°C). (1) Control, (2) adapted.

optimal to measure the ischemic area, the necrotic area, and their difference (the recovery area) in the same animal.

To this end we used a modified method of Lepran et al.[42] which makes it possible, without opening the chest, to tighten the ligature applied on the coronary artery for 30 min, then to loosen it and 1 d after, when the necrosis has already formed in the myocardium, to tighten it again to reproduce acute ischemia; immediately upon ligation an emulsion of lipid microspheres is rapidly introduced into the left ventricular cavity.[43] The heart is then removed, frozen, and sectioned; nonfixed sections are stained with nitroblue tetrazolium to reveal the necrotic area, and sections from formaldehyde-fixed material are stained for lipid to reveal the ischemic area, which is not penetrated by the emulsion. The results are then quantitated into percentages of volume in accordance with the principles of stereological analysis.[44]

Table 7 demonstrates that prior adaptation to stress does not appreciably affect the volume of myocardium that becomes ischemic upon acute coronary artery ligation. At the same time, the adaptation more than doubles the recovery zone in the ischemic myocardium, so that the necrotic volume as related to the ischemic and total myocardial volume decreases nearly by half.

Consequently, adaptation to stress lacks anti-ischemic action, but has a pronounced cytoprotective effect, which can be thought of as a direct manifestation of the phenomenon of the adaptational stabilization of structures. This allows one to think that studies of the genetic mechanisms of this phenomenon are not a purely academic issue; there are two appraoches which hold promise for expanding the possibilities of heart protection.

TABLE 7
Effect of Prior Adaptation to Stress on the Ischemic, Recovery, and Necrotic Volumes in Experimental Myocardial Infarction

Series	Percentage			
	Ischemic to total	Necrotic to ischemic	Recovered ischemic to ischemic	Necrotic to total
Control (n = 14)	36.8 ± 3.6	73.5 ± 3.8	26.5 ± 1.7	27.0 ± 1.4
Adapted (n = 11)	34.3 ± 4.1	44.7 ± 4.1	55.3 ± 2.0	15.3 ± 1.4
p		<0.01	<0.01	<0.05

First, it has been found in recent years that a cardioprotective effect in many instances resembling that of adaptation to repeated stress can be experimentally achieved with transauricular acupuncture, in which pulsed currents are passed through subcortical formations of the animal brain to cause moderate catalepsy. In the long run, such courses prevent the impairment of cardiac metabolism and electric stability commonly observed in EPS,[45] and largely restrict the ischemic and reperfusion arrhythmias.[46] Recent experiments in our laboratory show that electroacupuncture, like adaptation to stress, brings on myocardial alterations that enhance the direct cardiac resistance to damaging factors. Similar results have been obtained in combined adaptation of animals to moderate intermittent hypoxia and cold. In the aggregate, the data now available suggest that the phenomenon of the adaptational stabilization of structures constitutes the foundation of the currently developing methods for protecting the heart with adaptation.

Second, the stress proteins, some similar factors, or stable synthetic analogs thereof may in future be used to artificially reconstruct this phenomenon (just as the inductor of angiogenesis discovered by Schaper et al.[47] has now proved capable of being used to cause growth of coronary vessels). In other words, it cannot be excluded that some factors involved in the adaptational stabilization mechanism will find their place among pharmacological means of gene regulation.

The contents of Chapters 3 and 4 have provided unequivocal evidence that the adaptational heart protection is not at all restricted to local cell mechanisms. The next chapter, considering the protection of the heart and of the whole organism with prior adaptation to intermittent hypoxia, offers a good example of efficacious coordination of neurohumoral and cellular factors in the integrated mechanism of long-term adaptation and natural prophylaxis.

REFERENCES

1. **Meerson, F. Z., Ustinova, E. E., and Manukhina, E. B.,** Prevention of cardiac arrhythmias by adaptation to hypoxia: regulatory mechanisms and cardiotropic effect, *Biomed. Biochem. Acta,* 48, 83, 1989.
2. **Hearse, D. J., Humphrey, S. M., and Chain, E. B.,** Abrupt reoxygenation of the anoxic potassium-arrested perfused rat heart, *J. Mol. Cell. Cardiol.,* 5, 395, 1973.
3. **Meerson, F. Z., Malyshev, I. Yu., and Sazontova, T. G.,** Adaptation to stress exposure prevents arrhythmogenic and contractural effects of the excess of Ca^{2+} on the heart by the increased activity of sarcoplasmic reticulum, *Basic Res. Cardiol.,* in press.
4. **Opie, L. H.,** Myocardial ischemia — metabolism and its modification, *SAMT,* 72, 740, 1987.
5. **Meerson, R. Z., Samosudova, N. V., Glagoleva, E. V., Shimkovich, M. V., and Belkina, L. M.,** Impairment of the myocardial contractile function and cardiomyocyte ultrastructure upon emotional pain stress (in Russian), *Arkh. Anat. Gistol. Embriol.,* 84, 43, 1983.
6. **Witt, A. and Rosen, M.,** Pathophysiologic mechanisms of cardiac arrhythmias, *Am. Heart J.,* 106, 798, 1983.

7. **Meerson, F. Z., Sazontova, T. G., and Arkhipenko, Yu. V.,** Adaptation to short-term stress exposure activates Ca-pump in sarcoplasmic reticulum and reduces the rate of its inactivation during autolysis, *J. Mol. Cell. Cardiol.*, in press.
8. **Guski, H., Meerson, F. Z., and Wassilew, G.,** Comparative study of ultrastructure and function of the rat heart hypertrophied by exercise or hypoxia, *Exp. Pathol.*, 2, 108, 1981.
9. **Meerson, F. Z., Kagan, V. E., Prilipko, L. L., Rozhitskaya, I. I., Giber, L. M., and Kozlov, Yu. P.,** Activation of lipid peroxidation in emotional pain stress (in Russian), *Byull. Eksp. Biol. Med.*, 10, 404, 1979.
10. **Meerson, F. Z., Pavlova, V. I., Kamilov, F. Kh., and Yakushev, V. S.,** Use of sodium gamma-hydroxybutyrate for prevention of damages caused by emotional pain stress (in Russian), *Patol. Fiziol. Eksp. Ter.*, 3, 26, 1979.
11. **Meerson, F. Z., Sazontova, T. G., Kagan, V. E., Tverdokhlib, V. P., and Arkhipenko, Yu. V.,** Role of lipid peroxidation in the inhibition of cardiac Na,K ATPase in stress (in Russian), *Byull. Eksp. Biol. Med.*, 12, 42, 1983.
12. **Meerson, F. Z., Arkhipenko, Yu. V., Rozhitskaya, I. I., and Kagan, V. E.,** Impairment of cardiac Ca^{2+}-transporting systems in emotional pain stress (in Russian), *Byull. Eksp. Biol. Med.*, 4, 60, 1981.
13. **Bondarenko, N. A., Devyatkina, T. A., Voskresenskii, O. N., and Val'dman, A. V.,** Influence of chronic emotional stress on the state of lipid peroxidation in emotional and unemotional rats (in Russian), *Byull. Eksp. Biol. Med.*, 6, 12, 1985.
14. **Dzhafarov, A. I.,** Kinetics of lipid peroxidation in cell organelles that had undergone anoxia under various conditions (in Russian), *Byull. Eksp. Biol. Med.*, 10, 425, 1981.
15. **Gribanov, G. A. and Sergeev, S. A.,** Rat myocardial lipids in autolysis (in Russian), *Vopr. Med. Khim.*, 4, 33, 1983.
16. **Kozel'tsev, V. L., Golubev, V. I., and Volodina, T. V.,** Protective role of phospholipids in enzymic degradation of mitochondrial membrane proteins (in Russian), *Vopr. Med. Khim.*, 5, 680, 1980.
17. **Boime, I., Smith, E. E., and Hunter, F. E.,** The role of fatty acids in mitochondrial changes during liver ischemia, *Arch. Biochem. Biophys.*, 139, 425, 1970.
18. **Rebrov, L. B., Kozel'tsev, V. A., Shishkin, S. S., and Debov, S. A.,** Some enzymatic aspects of postmortem autolysis (in Russian), *Vestn. Akad. Med. Nauk SSSR*, 10, 82, 1983.
19. **Wildenthal, K.,** Lysosomal alterations in ischemic myocardium: result or cause of myocellular damage?, *J. Mol. Cell. Cardiol.*, 10, 595, 1978.
20. **Suyatna, F. D., van Voldhoven, P. P., Borgers, M., and Mannaerts, G. P.,** Phospholipid composition and amphiphile content of isolated sarcolemma from normal and autolytic rat myocardium, *J. Mol. Cell. Cardiol.*, 20, 47, 1980.
21. **van Jaarsveld, H., Potgieter, G. M., and Lochner, A.,** Enzymatic and structural modifications of mitochondrial NADH-ubiquinone reductase with autolysis as experimental model, *Enzyme*, 39, 151, 1988.
22. **Meerson, F. Z., Belkina, L. M., Dyusenov, S. S., Saltykova, V. A., and Shabunina, E. V.,** Prevention of impairment of cardiac electric stability in experimental myocardial infarction with prior adaptation to short stress exposures and with antioxidant ionol (in Russian), *Kardiologiya*, 8, 19, 1986.
23. **Meerson, F. Z. and Pshennikova, M. G.,** *Adaptation to Stressful Situations and Physical Loads* (in Russian), Meditsina, Moscow, 1988.
24. **Zak, R., Aschenbrenner, V., and Rabinowitz, M.,** Synthesis and degradation of myocsin in cardiac hypertrophy, *J. Clin. Invest.*, 50 (Abstr.), 102a, 1971.
25. **Aschenbrenner, V., Druyan, R., Albin, R., and Rabinowitz, M.,** Haem *a*, cytochrome *c* and total protein turnover in mitochondria from rat heart and liver, *Biochem. J.*, 119, 157, 1970.
26. **Meerson, F. Z., Yavich, M. P., Lapteva, R. I., and Lerman, M. I.,** Dynamics of RNA and protein breakdown in compensatory heart hyperfunction (in Russian), *Vopr. Med. Khim.*, 1, 9, 1973.
27. **Meerson, F. Z., Yavich, M. P., Rozhitskaya, I. I., and Golubeva, L. Yu.,** Abolishment of stress activation of DNA reparative synthesis in the myocardium in heart hyperfunction (in Russian), *Byull. Eksp. Biol. Med.*, 7, 655, 1989.
28. **Sazontova, T. G., Arkhipenko, Yu. V., and Meerson, F. Z.,** Enhanced activity of antioxidant enzymes in adaptation to short stress exposures (in Russian), *Byull. Eksp. Biol. Med.*, 10, 411, 1987.
29. **Meerson, F. Z.,** The role of lipid peroxidation in the stress and the antioxidant protection of the heart, in *Oxygen Radicals in the Pathophysiology of Heart Disease*, Singal, P. K., Ed., Kluwer Academic, Boston, 1988, 285.
30. **Andersson, S. M., Levy, J. R., and Kant, C. R.,** Chronic stress increases the binding of the A_1 adenosine receptor agonist, [^{3}H] cyclohexyladenosine, to rat hypothalamus, *Pharmacol. Biochem. Behav.*, 30, 169, 1988.
31. **Gudbjarnasson, S., Doel, B., Oskurselottir, G., and Hullgrimsson, J.,** Modification of cardiac phospholipids and catecholamines stress tolerance, in *α-Tocopherol, Oxygen and Biomembrane*, De Duve, C. and Hayashi, O., Eds., Elsevier/North-Holland Biomed. Press, Amsterdam, 1978, 297.
32. **Michell, B.,** Inositol phosphates. Profusion and confusion [news], *Nature*, 319, 176, 1986.

33. **Berridge, M. J.,** Inositol triphosphate and diacylglycerol as second messenger, *Biochem. J.,* 220, 345, 1984.
34. **Gorelick, F. S.,** Second messenger systems and adaptation, *Gut,* 28, 79, 1987.
35. **Hammond, G. L., Lai, Y. K., and Markert, C. L.,** Diverse forms of stress lead to a new pattern of gene expression through a common and essential metabolic pathway, *Proc. Natl. Acad. Sci. U.S.A.,* 79, 3485, 1982.
36. **Currie, R. W. and White, F. P.,** Trauma-induced protein in rat tissues: a physiological role for a ''heat shock protein''?, *Science,* 214, 72, 1981.
37. **Yost, H. G. and Lindquist, S.,** RNA splicing is interrupted by heat shock and is protected by heat shock protein synthesis, *Cell,* 45, 185, 1986.
38. **Landry, J., Bernier, D., Cretien, P., Nicole, L. M., Tanguay, R. M., and Marrean, N.,** Synthesis and degradation of heat shock proteins during development and decay of thermotolerance, *Cancer Res.,* 42, 2456, 1982.
39. **Li, G. S. and Werb, Z.,** Correlation between synthesis of heat shock proteins and development of thermotolerance in Chinese hamster fibroblasts, *Proc. Natl. Acad. Sci. U.S.A.,* 79, 3219, 1982.
40. **Lowe, J. E., Reimer, K. A., and Jennings, R. R.,** Experimental infarct size as a function of the amount of myocardium at risk, *Am. J. Pathol.,* 90, 363, 1978.
41. **Reimer, K. A.,** Myocardial infarct size. Measurements and predictions, *Arch. Pathol. Lab. Med.,* 104, 225, 1980.
42. **Lepran, I., Koltai, M., Siegmund, W., and Szekeres, L.,** Coronary artery ligation, early arrhythmias and determination of the ischemic area in conscious rats, *J. Pharmacol. Methods,* 9, 219, 1983.
43. **Lillie, R. D.,** *Histopathologic Technique and Practical Histochemistry,* McGraw-Hill, New York, 1965.
44. **Avtandilov, G. G., Yabluchanskii, N. I., and Gubenko, V. G.,** *Systemic Stereometry and Study of Pathological Processes* (in Russian), Mir Publ., Moscow, 1981.
45. **Radzievskii, S. A., Chuvil'skaya, L. M., Vorontsova, E. Ya., Ustinova, E. E., and Meerson, F. Z.,** Prevention of the stress drop in the cardiac fibrillation threshold with transauricular acupuncture (in Russian), *Byull. Eksp. Biol. Med.,* 8, 151, 1987.
46. **Meerson, F. Z., Radzievskii, S. A., Vorontsova, E. Ya., Golubeva, L. Yu., and Chuvil'skaya, L. M.,** Possibility of reflex activation of stress-limiting systems and prevention of cardiac rhythm disorders with acupuncture (in Russian), *Kardiologiya,* 1, 88, 1989.
47. **Schaper, W., Quinkler, W., and Scharma, H. S.,** Heart adaptation to the ischemic stress, *J. Mol. Cell. Cardiol.,* 21 (Suppl. 3), S23, 1989.

Chapter 7

ADAPTATION TO INTERMITTENT HYPOXIA AND ITS USE FOR PROTECTING THE HEART FROM STRESS AND ISCHEMIC DAMAGE

I. INTRODUCTION

Adaptation to hypoxia follows the general patterns typical of adaptation to any other environmental factor and briefly considered in Chapter 1 (see the scheme in Figure 1 therein). Accordingly, adaptation to hypoxia goes through four main stages. Yet, in the *initial stage* there is some difference, which is first of all due to the fact that unlike the factors causing motor, behavioral reactions, the lack of oxygen initially does not act on extroreceptors, but gradually invades the inner milieu of the organism to cause hypoxemia and to upset thus its homeostasis. Only through hypoxemia the oxygen deficit stimulates the chemoreceptors of the aortal-carotid zone and the centers regulating respiration, circulation, and other organs, eliciting at least three substantial shifts.

First, hypoxemia enhances the function of the systems specifically responsible for oxygen transport from the outer milieu and its distribution in the organism, i.e., causes lung hyperventilation, higher cardiac output, and dilation of brain and cardiac vessels with concomitant narrowing of muscle and abdominal vessels and ensuing rise in blood pressure. Second, there is a fully pronounced stress reaction, in particular a marked catabolic effect, negative nitrogen balance, etc. (see Chapter 1). Third, acute hypoxia directly limits the function of the mitochondrial respiratory chain and thereby the ATP synthesis in various organs and tissues and first of all in the higher divisions of the central nervous system, which entails a more or less pronounced impairment of motor and intellectual activity.

Of course the extent of such shifts may vary depending on the genetically determined individual tolerance of the organism and the depth of hypoxia. Nevertheless, it is just this syndrome attended with large losses of energy and structures that characterizes the initial, emergency stage of adaptation to hypoxia.

In the *second, transitional stage,* the mechanism considered in detail elsewhere[1] activates nucleic acid and protein synthesis in the cells of the systems carrying the main load in adaptation to hypoxia. This results in selective growth of structures that have been limiting oxygen transport and ATP production, i.e., growth of vessels, enhanced erythropoiesis, proliferation of mitochondria, etc.

In the *third stage,* that of stable long-term adaptation, these processes give rise to a complex of structural changes which we have some time ago termed the "systemic structural trace" and which constitutes the material basis of stable long-term adaptation.

In certain cases, e.g., in adaptaion to excessive altitude, hypoxia, or in genetic intolerance to this factor, the process may develop into the *fourth, unnecessary stage* of wear-out when the systemic structural trace is gradually destroyed and adaptation turns into disease.

The aim of this Chapter is to demonstrate, first experimentally and then clinically, that adaptation to moderate, rationally dosed hypoxia can be used to protect the heart against stress-induced and ischemic damage. This means that we tried in the most economical way to form the systemic structural trace that constitutes the basis of the third stage of the process and of all the prophylactic and therapeutic effects described henceforth. As we shall see, in adaptation to hypoxia the systemic structural trace has quite ramified architectonics, encompassing many neural centers, endocrine glands, and working organs. Such a broad structural basis of adaptation to hypoxia should not be surprising, since in the whole organism hypoxia may arise not only from reduced oxygen content in the inhaled air and is not an exclusive domain of pathology. On the contrary, in the healthy organism hypoxemia or relative tissue hypoxia inevitably and most commonly occurs in significant loads on the whole organism or on particular organs and systems. Accordingly, the organism has evolved an efficient apparatus for antihypoxic defense, and to hypoxia caused by load or reduced oxygen content in the air it responds first with immediate but unstable and then with stable long-term adaptation.

Many years of experimental studies have now led to the concept that such stable adaptation is based on at least five complexes forming an integrated systemic structural trace.

The *first complex* develops in the oxygen uptake and transport system, which responds to the lack of oxygen in the milieu with regulatory hyperfunction. In the very first days of exposure to hypoxia the formation of the systemic structural trace manifests itself as enhanced RNA and protein synthesis in the lungs,[1] heart,[2] bone marrow which generates erythrocytes,[3,4] coronary vessels,[5] and in the sympathetic neurons innervating the heart.[6] This results in increased respiratory surface and number of lung alveoli, moderate hypertrophy and increased functional capacity of the heart, increased capacity of the coronary bed, polycythemia and increased oxygen capacity, and hypertrophy of the neurons of the respiratory centers and respiratory muscles.

Simultaneously, the power of the energy-providing system is augmented in the cells of the heart and other organs, as evidenced by the greater number of mitochondria and elevated glycolytic enzyme activity.[5] Concurrently, changes develop in the cardiac neural regulation: hypertrophy of the sympathetic neurons of stellate ganglia and elevated adrenal content of norepinephrine with a balanced rise in cardiac phosphodiesterase.[7] These changes, by increasing the power and efficiency of respiration and circulation and enforcing the possibility of their adrenergic mobilization, not only definitely enhance the resistance of the organism to hypoxia, but also produce the well-known cross-protective effect against physical load and potentiate training to this factor. Furthermore, adaptation to hypoxia protects the heart in myocardial infarction. It produces (1) an anti-ischemic effect, i.e., owing to collaterals the ischemic area is attenuated,[8] and (2) a direct cytoprotective effect, i.e., a larger portion of the primarily ischemic tissue then recovers and does not undergo necrosis (see below). As a result, 1 d after infarction the infarct size proves smaller and heart contractility is better retained than in the control.

The *second complex* comprises quite a number of shifts at the higher level of neuroendocrine regulation, and involves activation of RNA and protein synthesis in the brain. In the large hemispheres this process is most pronounced in the cortex, where the RNA concentration rises by 50% and protein synthesis is doubled; in the lower brain divisions, less sensitive to the lack of oxygen, the activation is much smaller, but proves pronounced again in the vegetative centers of the medulla oblongata.[9] In the process, the diameter of cell nuclei increases in the cortical pyramid neurons and decreases in the glial cells, i.e., there is a shift in the neuroglial relations probably associated with the donor functions of the glia.[10]

Simultaneously, serotonin and dopamine accumulate in the brain, while the norepinephrine content decreases somewhat; and in the adrenal glands the amount of opioid peptides, first of all beta-endorphin, increases many times over,[11] whereas the blood levels of serotonin and histamine decline.[12] As expected, this broad complex of stable changes in the neuroendocrine regulation has consequences that go far beyond just enhancing the tolerance to hypoxia. They show as quicker formation of conditioned reflexes and especially their better preservation,[13] radical changes in the animal behavior in conflict situations (like rats acquiring the ability to carry out a vital drinking reflex at such electric-pain stimulation as has previously kept them away from the drinking bowl),[14] or increased resistance to the epileptogenic action of a strong audio stimulus.[15]

Besides, the regulatory changes brought on in adaptation restrict the stress reaction and protect the heart, stomach, and liver from stress damage.[16,17] Such protection takes place in

TABLE 1
Effect of Adaptation to Intermittent Hypoxia on the Hepatic Cytochrome P_{450} System

Indices	Control	Adapted
N-Demethylase activity (nmol/min·mg)	4.23 ± 0.19	5.57 ± 0.13[a]
Cytochrome b_5 (nmol/mg)	0.50 ± 0.02	0.81 ± 0.03[a]
Cytochrome P_{450} (nmol/mg)	0.63 ± 0.03	1.10 ± 0.04[a]

[a] $p < 0.01$.

a rather generalized form and is revealed, in particular, as complete prevention of marked attenuation of stress enzymemia (i.e., release of cytosolic and lysosomal enzymes into the blood commonly observed upon severe stress).[18]

Accordingly, with adaptation to intermittent hypoxia it proves possible to prevent not only the stress-induced drop in cardiac contractility and fibrillation threshold,[19] but also ischemic arrhythmias whose neurogenic origin has been proved in numerous modern studies.[20,21]

The *third complex* reveals itself as stable enough shifts in the regulation of water-salt metabolism and the myogenic tone of resistive vessels. Adaptation is attended with partial atrophy of the hypothalamic supraoptic nucleus and of the adrenal glomerular zone, i.e., structures that through aldosterone and the antidiuretic hormone ensure retention in the organism of a certain reserve of water and sodium chloride.[1,22] This is accompanied by a decline in the myogenic component of the vascular tone and decreased rigidity of arteria and arterioles, which should attenuate the extent of pressor reflexes. Clearly, such shifts must cause the organism to lose the excess of water and salt and, other things being equal, must diminish the probability of hypertension. Indeed, in spontaneously hypertensive rats adaptation to hypoxia largely impedes the development of hypertension, which is rather close to the hypertensive disease of man.[23] A similar effect of adaptation is observed with deoxycorticosterone-salt hypertension.[24]

The *fourth complex* of changes is found in the immune system, where B lymphocytes become predominant over T lymphocytes in the lymphoid organs such as spleen. An important consequence of this is partial depression of the T-mediated immune reaction and a concomitant enhancement of the humoral immune response as judged by the number of antibody-producing cells and the antibody levels in the blood.[25,26] These adaptive changes in the immune system are the cause of certain modulatory protective effects of adaptation, namely (1) suppression of such an allergic phenomenon as adjuvant arthritis;[27,28] (2) attenuation of the stress-induced enhancement of delayed-type hypersensitivity,[28] and (3) prevention of the stress depression of normal killers which are an important element of antitumor immunity.[29]

Finally, the *fifth complex* consists in that adaptation to intermittent hypoxia substantially increases the hepatic content of cytochrome P_{450}-linked enzymes, acting paradoxically like chemical inducers. Table 1 shows the data of Nikonorov et al. on this issue.

This novel fact implies that the detoxicating capacity of the liver must increase in adaptation to hypoxia, and agrees nicely with the earlier reports that such adaptation appreciably enhances the tolerance to hallucinogens and epileptogens.[5] It also explains the important data that such adaptation prevents the impairment of reflex activity and the enzymemia of injury in animals acutely or chronically exposed to hydrogen sulfide-containing gas condensate.[30] Further, it is essential that, besides increasing the overall cytochrome P_{450} content, adaptation to intermittent hypoxia enhances the hepatic activity of cholesterol 7-α-hydroxylase, the enzyme responsible for cholesterol oxidation to bile acids. This factor,

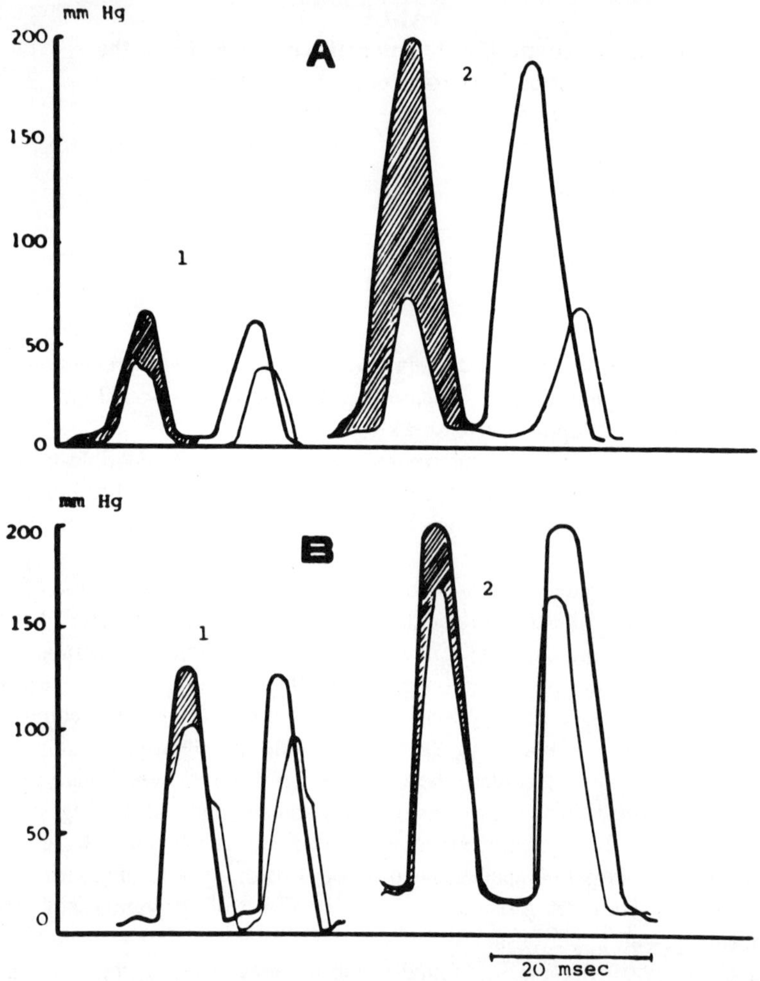

FIGURE 1. Curves of left ventricular pressure in (A) nonadapted rats and (B) rats adapted to altitude hypoxia. (1) Physiological rest, (2) aortic clamping. The shaded zone reflects the defect of contractility caused by ischemic necrosis.

together with the higher stress resistance of the organism, would naturally prevent the stress damage to the liver and thereby the stress-induced atherogenic dyslipidemia,[17] which can play a weighty role in development of coronary atherosclerosis.

This presentation does not involve a detailed consideration of all possible protective effects of adaptation to hypoxia. In accordance with the main line of the book, we shall first consider two examples of the use of adaptation to intermittent hypoxia in an altitude chamber, to protect the heart from stress-induced, ischemic, and reperfusion damage, and to prevent hepatic damage and atherogenic dyslipidemia.

II. ADAPTATION TO HYPOXIA PREVENTS MYOCARDIAL STRESS AND ISCHEMIC DAMAGE AND CARDIAC ARRHYTHMIAS

It is almost 20 years since it has been quantitatively established that prior adaptation to hypoxia in an altitude chamber appreciably protects the heart against direct ischemic injury caused by coronary artery ligation.

Figure 1 shows the results of our experiments in which the cardiac contractile function

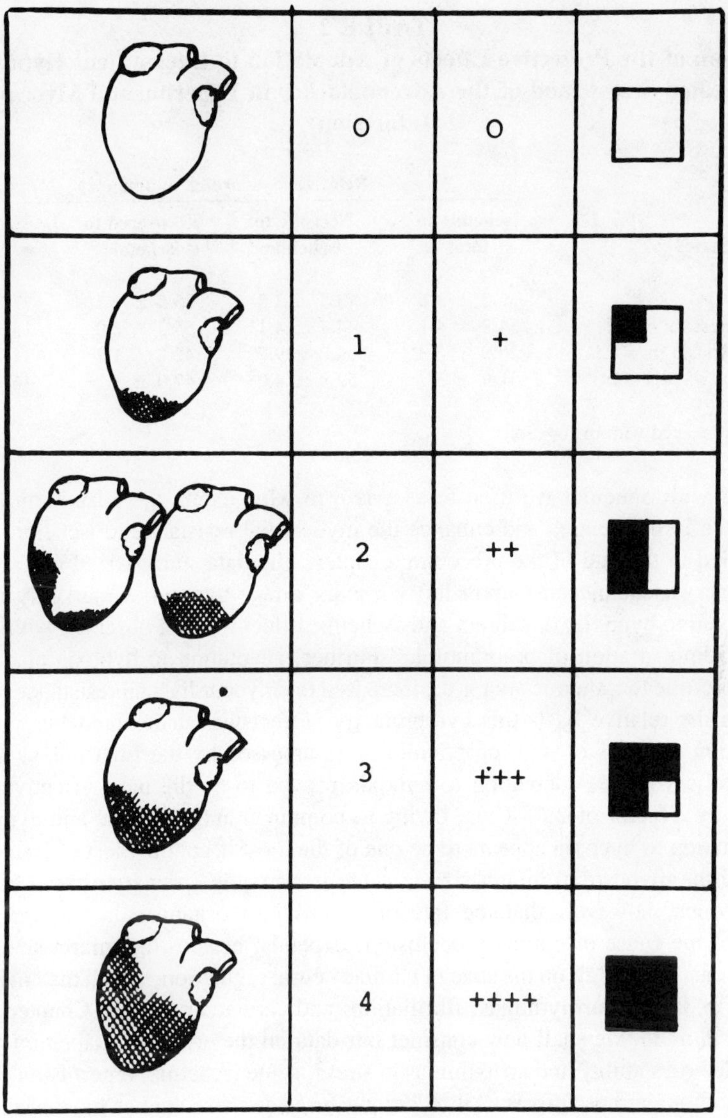

FIGURE 2. Evaluation of the extent of sympathomimetic myocardial necrosis. (Adapted from Poupa, O., Krofta, K., and Prochazka, J., *Fed. Proc., Fed. Am. Soc. Exp. Biol.*, 25, 1243, 1966. With permission.)

and the myocardial infarct size were determined 2 d after coronary artery ligation in non-adapted rats and in rats adapted to intermittent hypoxia for 1.5 months.[8] In these experiments the necrotic area (which at that time could be only roughly estimated) in adapted animals was reduced by 27%, whereas the depression of the maximal contraction force was three times less. Here we can recall the still earlier data of Poupa et al.;[31] in this work the size of isoproterenol-induced myocardial necroses was expressed in arbitrary points as shown in Figure 2, and was found to be threefold smaller in hypoxia-adapted animals.

These facts per se made one optimistic in respect of using adaptation to moderate intermittent hypoxia to protect the heart from stress-induced and adrenergic damage. In all our experiments described above and henceforth the adaptation was carried out as follows: during the first 4 to 5 d the animals were "raised" first to 500, then to 1000, 2000, 3000, and 5000 m. At this "plateau" the animals had 20 to 25 hypoxic exposures of 5 to 6 h each, 6 times per week.

TABLE 2
Comparison of the Protective Effects of Adaptation to Intermittent Hypoxia and to Repeated Stress, and of the Adrenoblocker in Experimental Myocardial Infarction

	Relative myocardial volume (%)			
Series	Ischemic to total	Necrotic to ischemic	Recovered to ischemic	Necrotic to total
Control (n = 14)	36.8 ± 3.6	73.5 ± 3.8	26.5 ± 1.7	27.0 ± 1.4
Adapted to stress (n = 11)	34.3 ± 4.1	44.7 ± 4.1[a]	55.3 ± 2.0[a]	15.3 ± 1.4[a]
Adapted to hypoxia (n = 11)	20.9 ± 3.3[a]	56.0 ± 9.7[a]	42.2 ± 1.2[a]	11.7 ± 1.2[a]
Propranolol (n = 14)	31.9 ± 3.7	52.9 ± 4.0[a]	47.0 ± 1.7[a]	16.9 ± 1.3[a]

[a] $p < 0.05$ compared with the control.

Together with Shneider we tried to ascertain to what extent the adaptation to hypoxia can restrict the ischemic area and enhance the myocardial resistance to ischemia, in experiments detailed in the end of the preceding chapter. The data summarized in Table 2 show that the primary ischemic area upon left coronary artery ligation is markedly reduced in animals adapted to hypoxia; this direct anti-ischemic effect was not observed with adaptation to stress or administration of propranolol.[32] Further, adaptation to hypoxia also decreased the relative necrotic to ischemic area, i.e., increased the myocardial cell resistance to ischemia (although on the relative basis this cytoprotective effect was understandably smaller than with adaptation to stress or with propranolol). As assessed by the final index, namely the relative necrotic volume, adaptation to hypoxia proved to be the most effective, reducing the necrosis by a factor of 2.5. Thus, owing to combined anti-ischemic and cytoprotective action, adaptation to hypoxia appears to be one of the most if not the most efficacious means of restricting the myocardial infarct size in acute irreversible coronary artery occlusion.

It is obvious, however, that the fate of a conscious organism in such an infarction (regardless of the cause of coronary occlusion) depends, besides the infarct size, on many other factors, and first of all on the state of cardiac neural regulation, which may predetermine or, conversely, prevent arrhythmias, fibrillation, and cardiac arrest (see Chapters 3 and 4). Bearing this in mind, we shall now consider our data on the effect of adaptation to hypoxia on cardiac electric stability and arrhythmias in stress, acute ischemia, reperfusion, infarction, and postinfarction cardiosclerosis. All techniques used in these studies have been described earlier.

In the control animals, the ventricular fibrillation threshold (VFT) varied within 6.8 to 8.1 mA; vagal stimulation with quadruple-threshold currents lead to bradycardia (the heart rate dropped from 330 to 120 beats per minute, i.e., by more than 60%) attended with only occasional extrasystoles. After an immobilization stress, the VFT dropped more than twofold, to 3.4 to 3.7 mA; bradycardia was aggravated without any appreciable increase in the number of extrasystoles; there was no impairment of the contractile function. In animals preadapted to hypoxia the VFT was the same as in controls, whereas the vagal bradycardia was less than 40% and was not attended with extrasystoles; their VFT and contractility were in no way affected by the immobilization stress. Thus, the widely known phenomenon of a poststress decline in the cardiac fibrillation threshold[33] was completely prevented by prior adaptation to hypoxia.

The antiarrhythmic action of adaptation to hypoxia in acute ischemia is most pronounced in conscious animals, less pronounced under anesthesia, and insignificant in isolated hearts (Figure 3); in reperfusion, it decreases the duration of grave arrhythmias by half in all three cases. These data prompt the idea that its protective action involves mainly central mech-

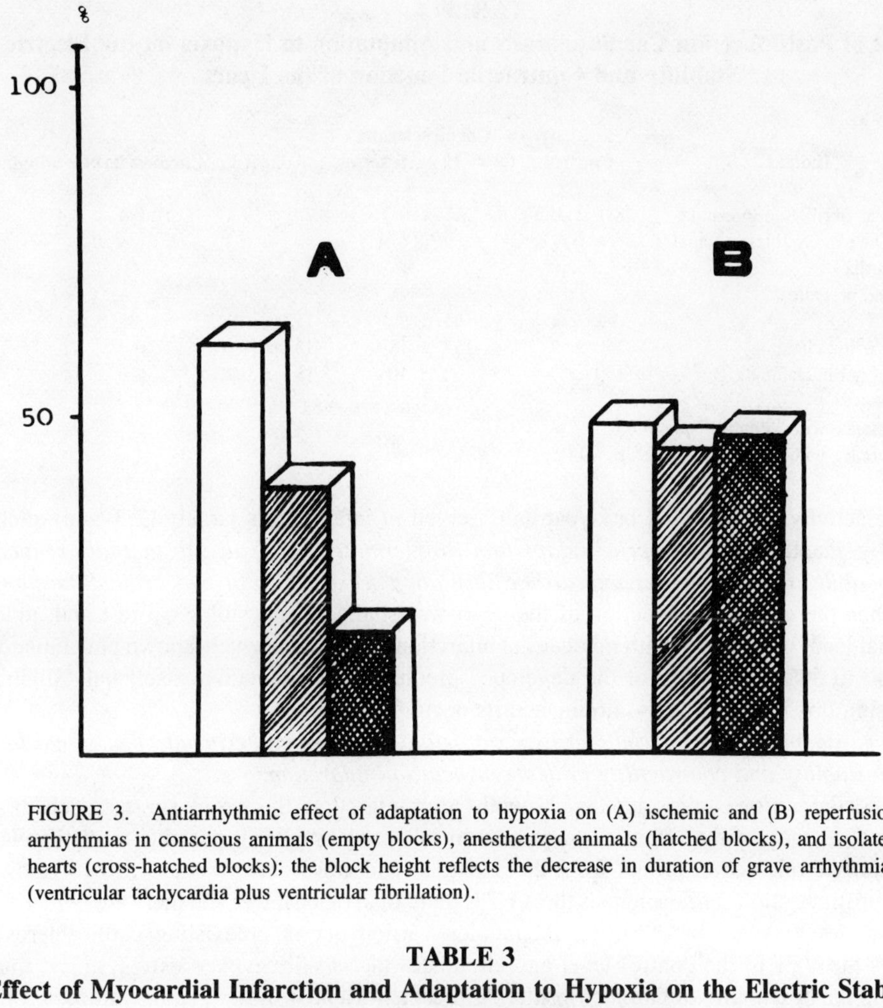

FIGURE 3. Antiarrhythmic effect of adaptation to hypoxia on (A) ischemic and (B) reperfusion arrhythmias in conscious animals (empty blocks), anesthetized animals (hatched blocks), and isolated hearts (cross-hatched blocks); the block height reflects the decrease in duration of grave arrhythmias (ventricular tachycardia plus ventricular fibrillation).

TABLE 3
Effect of Myocardial Infarction and Adaptation to Hypoxia on the Electric Stability and Contractile Function of the Heart

Indices	Control	Infarction	adapted (n = 10 each series)	Adapted + infarction
Ventricular fibrillation threshold	5.3 ± 0.2	2.0 ± 0.3[a]	5.2 ± 0.3	4.6 ± 0.4[b]
Number of extrasystoles in vagal bradycardia	0	124	0	54
Developed pressures				
At rest	110 ± 9	52 ± 10[a]	117 ± 8	77 ± 7[b]
5 s of aortic clamping	208 ± 18	121 ± 17[a]	215 ± 35	181 ± 20[b]
30 s of aortic clamping	220 ± 21	116 ± 17[a]	240 ± 21	193 ± 14[b]

[a] Difference with "control" $p < 0.05$.
[b] Difference with "infarction" $p < 0.05$.

anisms in ischemia and mainly local cardiac mechanisms in reperfusion (see also Chapter 6, Section II).

The data presented in Table 3 demonstrate the influence of prior adaptation to hypoxia on the electric stability and the contractile function of the heart in infarction. As can be seen, adaptation virtually completely prevents the drop in the VFT. Further, the pronounced

TABLE 4
Effect of Postinfarction Cardiosclerosis and Adaptation to Hypoxia on the Electric Stability and Contractile Function of the Heart

Indices	Control	Cardiosclerotic (n = 10 each series)	Adapted	Cardiosclerotic adapted
Ventricular fibrillation threshold	8.1 ± 0.3	3.7 ± 0.7[a]	7.9 ± 0.4	6.4 ± 0.4[b]
Number of extrasystoles in vagal bradycardia	0	78	0	0
Developed pressure				
At rest	95 ± 4	65 ± 9[a]	113 ± 4[a]	88 ± 8[b]
5 s of aortic clamping	150 ± 7	137 ± 18	181 ± 9[a]	163 ± 12
30 s of aortic clamping	159 ± 7	62 ± 10[a]	181 ± 10[a]	149 ± 14[b]

[a] Difference with "control" $p < 0.05$.
[b] Difference with "cardiosclerotic" $p < 0.05$.

ectopic activity during vagal bradycardia observed in infarction is largely (2.3-fold) attenuated by adaptation. Thus, *prior adaptation to intermittent hypoxia substantially reduces the probability of extrasystoles and cardiac fibrillation in experimental myocardial infarction.*

When the contractile function of the heart was studied at physiological rest and under maximal load, the animals with myocardial infarction displayed the well-known phenomenon — a 40 to 50% depression of the developed pressure. The adaptation, itself only slightly increasing this index, reliably diminished its decline in infarction.

Thus, adaptation to intermittent hypoxia definitely restricts the impairment of cardiac electric stability and contractility in acute myocardial infarction.

In postinfarction cardiosclerosis, 2 months after infarction, there is no stress or ischemia; therefore, a study of the effect of adaptation in this model makes it possible to distinguish its antiarrhythmic action proper from the antistress and anti-ischemic ones. Table 4 shows that in postinfarction cardiosclerosis the VFT is more than twice lower and there are numerous extrasystoles in vagal bradycardia. Adaptation carried out in preexisting cardiosclerosis restores the VFT to the control level and eliminates the vagally evoked extrasystoles, thus reducing the probability of cardiac fibrillation. Further, Table 4 shows that in cardiosclerotic animals adapted to hypoxia the developed pressure after 30 s of aortic clamping remains as high as at the fifth second.

Thus, adaptation to hypoxia abolishes the disturbances of cardiac electric stability and contractility typical of postinfarction cardiosclerosis.

To elucidate the structural basis of this therapeutic effect, we undertook a morphometric study of the relative scar volume, relation of formed elements in the cicatrix, and vascularization of the adjacent myocardial tissue.

Vascularization and formed elements were quantitated using stereometric grids.[34] The scar size was determined with serial histotopographic sections of the heart cut at every 2 mm starting from the apex. The relative scar volume was calculated in accordance with the principle of Dellesse that the cross-section areas of structures relate as their volumes.[35]

These results are shown in Table 5: adaptation to hypoxia reduces the relative scar volume by about one third, the cicatrix itself becomes denser with a greater proportion of collagen fibers and a lesser proportion of edematous stroma and all formed elements. Simultaneously, the amount of vessels in the myocardial tissue adjacent to the cicatrix increases by one third.[36]

By and large, *adaptation to hypoxia restricts the infarct size in acute coronary artery occlusion, and reduces the size of the preexisting postinfarction cicatrix.*

It is clear, however, that these cardiac effects of adaptation would not themselves be able to ensure its powerful antiarrhythmic effect definitely shown in our experiments.

TABLE 5
Relations Among Histological Structures in the Postinfarct Cicatrix and Adjacent Myocardium (%)

Indices	Control	Adapted
Relative volume of scar tissue	25.2	18.7
Vascularization of border zone	16.5	21.7
Edematous stroma	1.5	0.5
Collagen fibers	56.0	65.2
Fibroblasts	5.1	4.2
Fibrocytes	5.2	8.0
Polymorphonuclear leukocytes	0.5	None
Lymphocytes	11.2	8.1
Plasmacytes	8.6	5.2
Eosinophils	0.7	0.3
Macrophages	10.2	7.5

TABLE 6
Effect of Prior Adaptation to Hypoxia on Brain and Adrenal Beta-Endorphin Contents in Stress

Series	Beta-endorphin (fmol/mg tissue)			
(n = 10 each)	Cortex	Striatum	Cerebellum	Adrenals
Control	2.4 ± 0.7	5.7 ± 1.8	2.1 ± 0.4	1.2 ± 0.3
EPS	0.6 ± 0.1	1.3 ± 0.3	1.4 ± 0.7	0.8 ± 0.3
Adapted	2.8 ± 0.7	7.0 ± 2.2	2.9 ± 0.5	5.1 ± 0.2
Adapted + EPS	2.1 ± 0.8	5.5 ± 2.1	3.0 ± 1.1	0.6 ± 0.1

The fact that adaptation to hypoxia is effective against both ischemic and reperfusion arrhythmias (see above) prompts one to think that its antiarrhythmic action should involve both central and local stress-limiting systems.

To elucidate the role of the central regulatory mechanisms in the antiarrhythmic effect of adaptation, we determined the brain and adrenal contents of the most active opioid peptide, beta-endorphin, in adapted and nonadapted animals in normal conditions and after a severe EPS. Adaptation to hypoxia was carried out in an altitude chamber at 5000 m for 8 weeks, 5 times a week, 6 h a day.

Table 6 shows that EPS decreases the endorphin content in the cortex, striatum, and cerebellum by a factor of 1.5 to 4; adaptation, which itself only slightly increases the endorphin content in the brain structures, at the same time virtually prevents its changes in stress. To understand this remarkable ability of the brain of adapted animals to maintain the normal endorphin concentration despite stress, attention should be paid to the last column in Table 6. There one can see that in the course of adaptation the adrenal concentration of beta-endorphin increases over fourfold. Mobilization of this large surplus in stress proves to be even more complete than in nonadapted animals. As a result, *the stress-induced discharge of beta-endorphin from the adrenal glands of adapted animals exceeds the control one by more than an order of magnitude. Since endorphins check the excitation of the brain adrenergic structures important in arrhythmias and cardiac fibrillation, and also act as analgetics, it is easily conceivable that increased power of the opioid system in adaptation to hypoxia is a factor preventing cardiac fibrillation in acute ischemia.*

It is noteworthy that there is a quantitative correlation between these data and our previous work[37] on the increased adrenal content and stress-induced discharge of catecholamines in

TABLE 7
Effect of Adaptation to Hypoxia on the Neurotransmitter Contents in the Brain Cortex (μg/g tissue)

Compound	Control (n = 5)	Adapted (n = 10)	*p*
Norepinephrine	186 ± 5	150 ± 9	<0.05
Dopamine	132 ± 5	167 ± 5	<0.05
Serotonin	108 ± 4	238 ± 8	<0.01
5-Hydroxyindolyl acetic acid	173 ± 53	270 ± 9	<0.01

adaptation to hypoxia. Thus, adaptation increases the stress discharge of beta-endorphin from 0.44 to 4.49 fmol/mg and that of norepinephrine from 40 to 400 ng/mg of the adrenal gland, i.e., by the same factor of 10. This corresponds to the known fact that catecholamines and opioid peptides checking their effect are synthesized in the same granules, and to our concept of the intimate coupling between the stress-effecting and the stress-limiting systems.

In Chapter 4 it has been shown in detail that the opioid system exerts a many-sided influence on the brain monoaminergic system and, in particular, can activate the serotonergic system involved in attenuation of arrhythmias. Therefore, we suggested that changes in the monoamine metabolism in the brain may also contribute to the antiarrhythmic effect of adaptation to hypoxia.

To check this suggestion, the frontocortical contents of norepinephrine, dopamine, serotonin, and 5-hydroxyindolylacetic acid were determined spectrofluorimetrically after column resolution according to Earley and Leonard.[38] As shown in Table 7, norepinephrine decreased by 35% while dopamine increased by 26%, serotonin by 120%, and its breakdown product by 60%.

A possible explanation of these results stems from the concept of coordination of the opioidergic and the serotonergic systems and their combined action to restrict the arrhythmogenic influence of adrenergic centers on the heart, as detailed in Chapter 4. This tentative explanation pertains mainly to stress-induced and ischemic arrhythmias of central genesis, but is much less applicable to the adaptational protection against reperfusion arrhythmias and impairment of the electric stability in postinfarction cardiosclerosis; in these cases a prominent part is most likely played by the local stress-limiting systems such as the adenosinergic, prostaglandin, and antioxidant ones.

The latter is favored by the recent observation of enhanced resistance to the arrhythmogenic action of a lipid peroxidation (LPO) inducer, H_2O_2, in the isolated auricles from animals adapted to hypoxia (work done by Saltykova and Ustinova). Figure 4 compares the response of 20 control and 20 "adapted" auricles to H_2O_2. As can be seen, in the control occasional auricles stopped contracting already in 1 to 2 min (adapted ones only in 3 to 4 min), and by the 20th min only 2 control, but 12 adapted auricles retained their spontaneous activity. Thus, *adaptation to hypoxia enhances the resistance of cardiac automatism to the arrhythmogenic action of an LPO inducer.* It should be remembered that catecholamines, which injure the heart in stress and acute ischemia, are also LPO inducers and at the same time have a pronounced arrhythmogenic effect.

In the aggregate, the unambiguous evidence available for the powerful cardioprotective (and in particular, antiarrhythmic) effect of adaptation to intermittent hypoxia appears a sound enough basis for using this approach to treat certain types of arrhythmia in man.

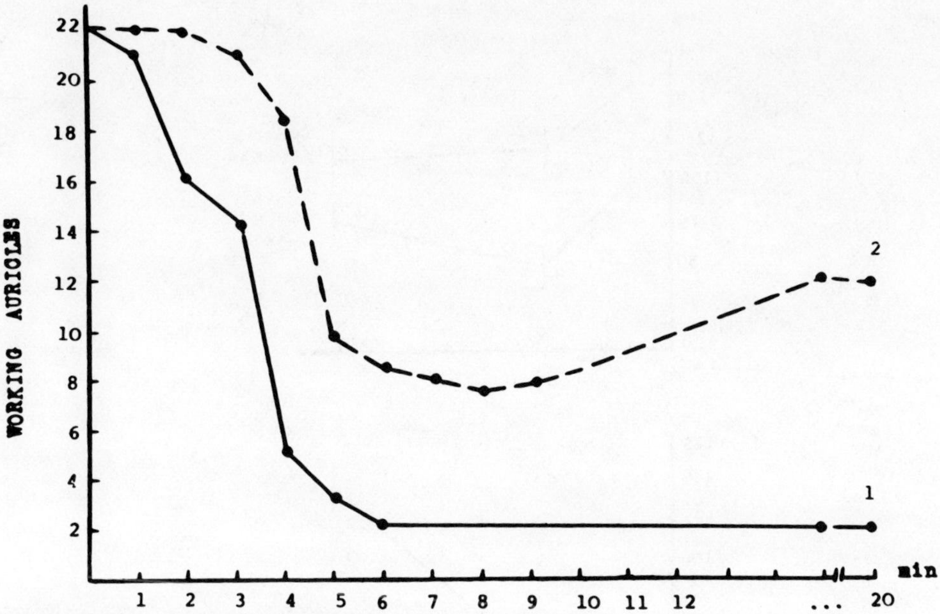

FIGURE 4. Effect of adaptation to hypoxia on the rat atrial resistance to the arrhythmogenic action of hydrogen peroxide. (1) Control, (2) adapted.

III. ADAPTATION TO INTERMITTENT HYPOXIA PREVENTS HEPATIC STRESS DAMAGE AND ATHEROGENIC DYSLIPIDEMIA

The concept of the weighty role of excessive consumption of food cholesterol in the pathogenesis of atherosclerosis[39,40] is now generally recognized. Further studies have shown that central to the development of atherosclerosis (caused by alimentary or any other factors) are the disturbances in lipid turnover in the liver, which is the key organ of cholesterol metabolism. A genetic insufficiency of hepatic receptors that bind the plasma cholesterol in high-density lipoproteins (HDLP)[41] and/or abnormalities in the microsomal system of cholesterol oxidation and elimination,[42,43] and probably some other shifts in the hepatic metabolism ultimately lead to atherogenic dyslipoproteinemia, which is highly conducive to cholesterol deposition in the vascular wall and development of atherosclerosis.

The important part played by hepatic stress damage, and specifically impaired cholesterol oxidation to bile acids, in atherogenic dyslipidemia and atherosclerosis of coronary vessels has already been demonstrated in this book (see Chapters 1 and 2). Here we shall consider our recent results obtained together with Tverdokhlib, which show that hepatic stress damage and atherogenic dyslipidemia can be prevented with prior adaptation to intermittent hypoxia.

As can be seen in Figure 5, adaptation to hypoxia substantially increases the activity of the antioxidant enzyme superoxide dismutase (SOD) and prevents the activation of LPO (as judged by the malonic dialdehyde [MDA] content) in prolonged emotional pain stress (EPS).

Further, it has been found that the adaptation enhances mitochondrial DNA replication in the liver and, what is most important, appreciably attenuates both the decline in nuclear DNA replication and the outburst of DNA repair upon EPS (Table 8), which indicates a lesser degree of DNA damage in stress after adaptation to hypoxia.

The hepatoprotective effect of adaptation to hypoxia is also confirmed by a much smaller extent of stress-induced leakage of the liver-specific enzyme fructose-1-phosphate aldolase into the blood (Figure 5B). Furthermore, such protection against stress also covers the

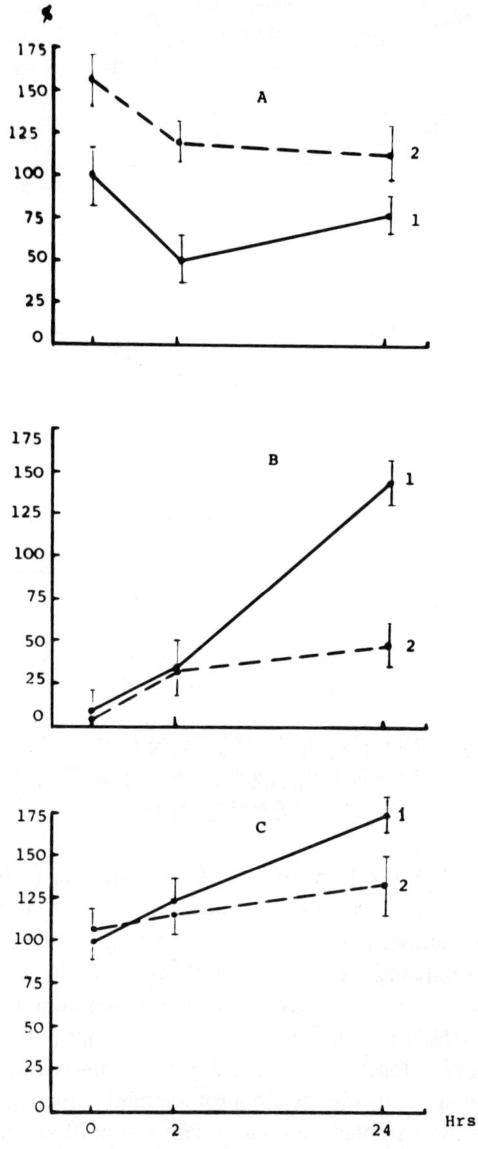

FIGURE 5. Effect of adaptation to hypoxia on (A) superoxide dismutase, (B) fructose-1-phosphate aldolase, and (C) malonic dialdehyde in EPS. (1) Control, (2) adapted. The abscissa is time after EPS; the ordinates are in percent.

microsomal enzyme system. Adaptation to intermittent hypoxia elevates the hepatic cholesterol 7-α-hydroxylase activity and prevents its decline in prolonged stress (Figure 6). Cholesterol hydroxylase plays a key role in cholesterol elimination from the organism; hence, preservation of this enzymic activity in adapted animals allows one to expect attenuation of stress-induced atherogenic dyslipidemia.

The effect of prior adaptation to intermittent hypoxia on the extent of stress-induced atherogenic alterations in plasma lipoproteins is shown in Table 9. As can be seen, such adaptation indeed has a pronounced antiatherogenic effect. First, cholesterol is redistributed among the lipoprotein fractions (increased in HDLP and decreased in low-density lipoproteins [LDLP] and VLDLP) so that the atherogenicity index in adapted animals is markedly lower

TABLE 8
Effect of Adaptation to Hypoxia on Stress-Induced Alterations in Hepatic DNA Replication and Repair Assayed by ^{3}H-Thymidine Incorporation (cpm/mg DNA)

Series	Nuclear DNA repair	DNA replication	
		Nuclear	Mitochondrial
Control	3,700	27,000	38,000
EPS	6,500	16,000	22,100
Adapted	3,950	25,200	52,000
Adapted + EPS	5,000	20,300	40,000

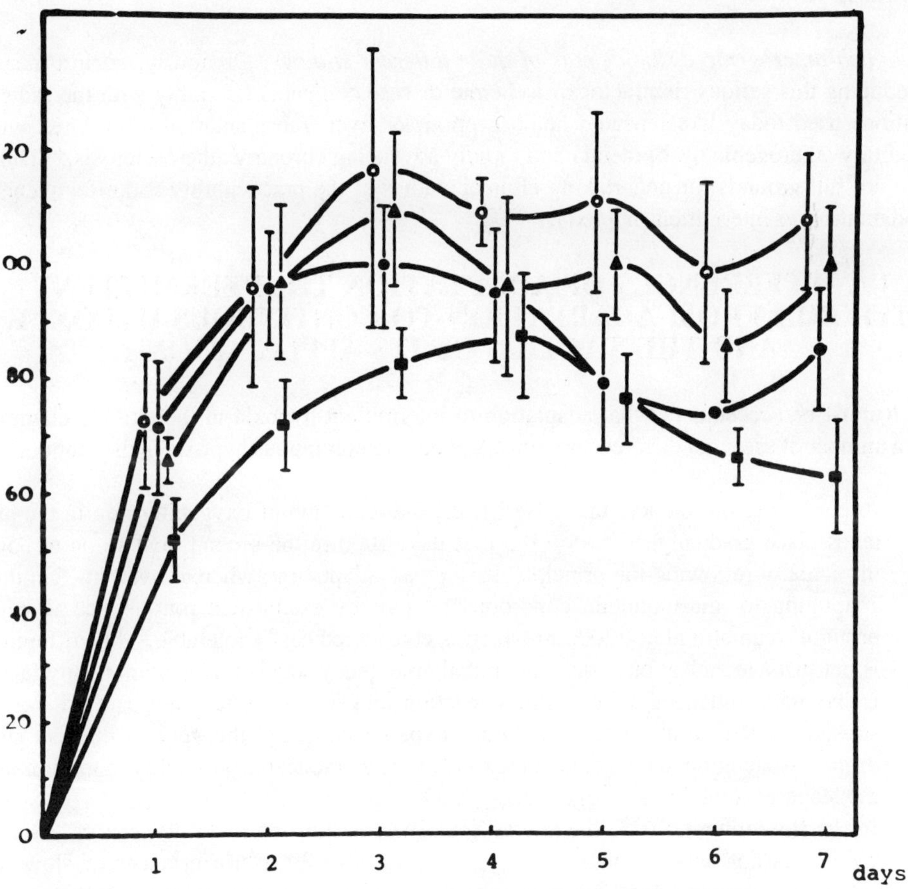

FIGURE 6. Effect of adaptation to hypoxia on ^{3}H-cholesterol oxidation after EPS in rats. (●) Control, (■) EPS, (○) adapted, (▲) EPS in adapted animals.

than in the control. Second, the dyslipoproteinemia caused by severe EPS is much abated by such adaptation, and the atherogenicity index still does not exceed the normal value.

Thus, rather mild adaptation to intermittent dosed hypoxia can be used as an active means of preventing stress-induced atherogenic disturbances.

Taken together with the above data on induction of cholesterol hydroxylase (Figure 6) and P_{450}-linked enzymes (Table 1), all this in essence means that *such adaptation can prevent*

TABLE 9
Indices of Lipid Metabolism in the Serum of Nonadapted and Hypoxia-Adapted Rats

Indices	Control	EPS	Adapted	Adapted + EPS
		(n = 20 each series)		
Total cholesterol	69.5 ± 3.6	58.6 ± 4.5	73.6 ± 2.9	63.8 ± 1.7
Triglycerides	52.8 ± 4.2	40.8 ± 3.2[a]	31.2 ± 3.6[a]	22.9 ± 2.8[a]
HDLP cholesterol	52.6 ± 3.9	22.7 ± 1.7[a]	63.6 ± 2.8[a]	45.9 ± 2.8[a]
VLDLP cholesterol	10.6 ± 0.5	8.1 ± 0.7[a]	6.2 ± 0.7[a]	4.6 ± 0.6[a]
LDLP cholesterol	8.5 ± 1.4	27.3 ± 4.0[a]	4.8 ± 1.6[a]	10.1 ± 1.8[a]
Atherogenicity index	0.4	1.6	0.15	0.35

[a] $p < 0.05$.

or abolish atherogenic dyslipidemias of quite different etiology. Obviously, such a means of reducing this serious risk factor of ischemic disease compares favorably with the radical solutions used today like repeated hemosorption, or liver transplantation to children with hereditary atherogenic dyslipidemia and rapidly advancing coronary atherosclerosis.[44] Thus, there are full grounds for undertaking clinical studies of the practicability and effectiveness of adaptation to intermittent hypoxia.

IV. DIFFERENCES OF ADAPTATION TO INTERMITTENT HYPOXIA FROM ADAPTATION TO CONTINUOUS HYPOXIA, AND THE TACTICS OF ITS APPLICATION

It must be acccentuated that adaptation to intermittent hypoxia in the altitude chamber has a number of essential differences from adaptation to continuous hypoxia in the mountains.

1. According to our tactics, the "rise" (i.e., the reduction of oxygen tension in the air) takes place gradually: to 500 m the first day, 1000 m the second, and so on to 3500 m, actually following the principle of stepwise adaptation, whereas even in "gentle" adaptation to mid-mountain conditions people, by established routine, are directly brought to an altitude of 2000 m which is considered easily tolerable. This difference is not just a technical one, since the initial emergency stage of adaptation to any factor is inevitably attended with a stress reaction and its catabolic effect (i.e., involves substantial structural costs), regulatory hypertension, and the general malaise syndrome. Adaptation to intermittent hypoxia offers a practicable possibility of minimizing the stage or avoiding it altogether.
2. In the intermittent mode, the course usually consisting of 30 to 40 seances actually represents not only adaptation to hypoxia, but also 30 to 40 instances of slow but inevitable reoxygenation, each of which should naturally cause some activation of free-radical lipid oxidation and, accordingly, of the enzymic and nonenzymic antioxidant mechanisms. In full conformity with this, adaptation to intermittent hypoxia has been shown to enhance the activity of the antioxidant enzymes SOD and catalase in the brain and in the liver.[45] Together with Didenko and Arkhipenko we have recently compared the antioxidant enzyme activities in adaptation to intermittent and to continuous hypoxia. In adaptation to intermittent hypoxia in the altitude chamber, the SOD and catalase activities increased by 10 to 12% in the heart, by 38 and 29%, respectively, in the brain, and by 47 and 28% in the liver. In contrast, adaptation to continuous hypoxia (carried out at the Terskol Canyon in the Caucasus, altitude 2100

TABLE 10
Effects of Adaptation to Continuous and Intermittent Hypoxia on the Duration of Grave Arrhythmias and Mortality in Acute Ischemia and Reperfusion

	Ischemia		Reperfusion	
Series, number, and weight of animals	VT + VF[a]	Deaths	VT + VF[a]	Deaths
1. Control I (n = 10, 200—220 g)	21 ± 5	0	42 ± 10	0
2. Acute hypoxia (n = 12, 200—220 g)	130 ± 20	1	142 ± 36	2
3. Continuous, 7d (n = 10, 240—260 g)	117 ± 19	0	259 ± 13	4
4. Continuous, 16 d (n = 11, 280—300 g)	76 ± 36	0	228 ± 25	4
5. Continuous, 30 d (n = 11, 360—380 g)	35 ± 7	0	286 ± 25	5
6. Control II (n = 11, 360—380 g)	96 ± 6	0	184 ± 19	3
7. Intermittent, 30 d (n = 11, 360—380 g)	58 ± 5	0	69 ± 7	0
$p_{1\text{-}2}$	<0.001		<0.001	
$p_{1\text{-}3}$	<0.001		<0.001	
$p_{1\text{-}4}$	<0.05		<0.001	
$p_{5\text{-}6}$	<0.001		<0.05	
$p_{6\text{-}7}$	<0.05		<0.001	

[a] VT, ventricular tachycardia; VF, ventricular fibrillation.

m) caused decreases in these activities: 35% for SOD and 15% for catalase in the heart, 33 and 23%, respectively, in the brain, and 31 and 19% in the liver. Hence, with respect to antioxidant activity, adaptation to intermittent and to continuous hypoxia produce opposite effects. Table 10 shows that such differences prove dramatic for animals tested for cardiac resistance to reperfusion arrhythmias (experiments of Vorontsova and Ustinova). In 30 d, either type of adaptation decreased the total duration of grave ischemic arrhythmias (ventricular tachycardia plus ventricular fibrillation); however, in reperfusion arrhythmias (where LPO is pathogenetically decisive) the situation was essentially different: adaptation to continuous hypoxia increased the duration of reperfusion arrhythmias and raised the mortality to almost 50%, whereas adaptation to intermittent hypoxia significantly shortened the duration of and abolished mortality from reperfusion arrhythmias.

This particular case gives grounds for a more general idea that adaptation to intermittent hypoxia can be protective against both ischemic and reperfusion damage, while adaptation to continuous hypoxia, by lowering the antioxidant potential, aggravates the reperfusion injury and hence all types of reoxygenation damage rather than protects against them. A prolonged stay in the mountains, through a number of mechanisms, appears to make the organism ''unused to the plain''; after coming down, this reveals itself as decreased working ability and general fatigue, which the researchers justly call the ''deadaptation syndrome''. In adaptation to intermittent hypoxia, the subjects spend no more than 3 to 5 h in the altitide chamber and all the rest of their time at normal oxygen tension, whereby the deadaptation syndrome is certainly ruled out.

3. Taking under any conditions only a small part of the day, adaptation to intermittent hypoxia leaves a healthy or a diseased person quite enough time for dosed adaptation to other factors, such as physical load, cold, etc. Under continuous hypoxia in the mountains, such combination of treatments to form harmonious adaptation may prove an excessive burden on the organism.
4. Adaptation to intermittent hypoxia in the altitude chamber allows such strict rationing of the hypoxic exposure as is unrealistic in the mountains. Indeed, roughly defining

the dosage of hypoxic exposure as the product of duration by "intensity" (i.e., altitude), we can say that during a round-the-clock stay even at 1 km the subject gets a hypoxic exposure of 24 arbitrary units, while a 3-h seance at "3.5 km" actually used for adults in this work gives 10.5 units. Regardless of whether or not such calculations are valid, clearly, with the altitude chamber the risk of overdosage is much less than in continuous adaptation in the mountains. This circumstance is quite important, since overexposure to continuous and even intermittent hypoxia may cancel out the beneficial effect of adaptation, e.g., on the cardiac contractile function,[46] and even lead to progressive cardiosclerosis, mainly in the right ventricular myocardium.[31] Further, prolonged hypoxia elevates the pressure in the pulmonary artery;[47,48] therefore, minimization of this adaptive hypertension in the lesser circulation by restricting the duration of hypoxic exposure and with the use of nifedipine is an important feature of the tactics of adaptational therapy and prophylaxis.

5. Finally, unlike adaptation in the mountains, the state of adaptation to intermittent hypoxia can be easily sustained for extended periods with "maintenance visits" to the altitude chamber two to three times a week. In just this way we have succeeded, for example, in stabilizing the antihypertensive effect of adaptation in animals with hereditary hypertension.[23]

As regards the general tactics, it should be borne in mind that just as with any other type of adaptation, this process and especially its initial stage requires maintenance of an optimal vitamin balance in the organism. This first of all applies to the group of precursors and cofactors for nucleic acid and protein synthesis: orotic and folic acids, vitamin B_{12}, methionine, lysine, etc. For instance, it has been shown that in adaptation of animals to hypoxia, besides a rise in blood hemoglobin, there is a release from the bone marrow of immature erythrocytes — reticulocytes. Administration of a complex of B_{12}, folic, and orotic acids during adaptation prevents this reticulocytosis as the bone marrow in this case can ensure complete maturation of all erythrocytes generated.[49] Equally necessary are sufficient amounts of vitamins A, C, and E.

Another quite essential aspect is the great individual variations in tolerance to hypoxia, which most likely have their molecular basis in the functional arrangement of the mitochondrial respiratory chain.[50-53] This makes it necessary to determine the hypoxic tolerance in individuals before using such adaptation with therapeutic or preventive purposes; thus, respiratory and circulatory responses to oxygen-depleted gas mixtures should be recorded, the greater reaction being indicative of the lower tolerance to hypoxia.

In the aggregate, the above provides grounds for applying the experimentally proven great potential of adaptation to dosed intermittent hypoxia in the altitude chamber in prevention and treatment of, first and foremost, those diseases that are difficult or impossible to cure with contemporary pharmacological means.

We have used such adaptation to reduce the risk factors of ischemic disease, to abolish grave neurasthenic syndromes and associated arrhythmias, and to treat some other diseases. This clinicophysiological study has been the subject of a special joint publication.*

V. REGIMEN AND ORGANIZATION OF ADAPTATION TO INTERMITTENT HYPOXIA IN THE "MOUNTAIN CLIMATE HALL"

The medical altitude chamber *Ural-1* has been described in detail elsewhere, and its appearance is shown in Figure 7. It consists of the low-pressure chamber proper (the "hall")

* Meerson, F. Z., Tverdokhlib, V. P., Boev, V. M., and Frolov, B. A., *Adaptation to Intermittent Hypoxia in Therapy and Prophylaxis* (in Russian), Nauka, Moscow, 1989.

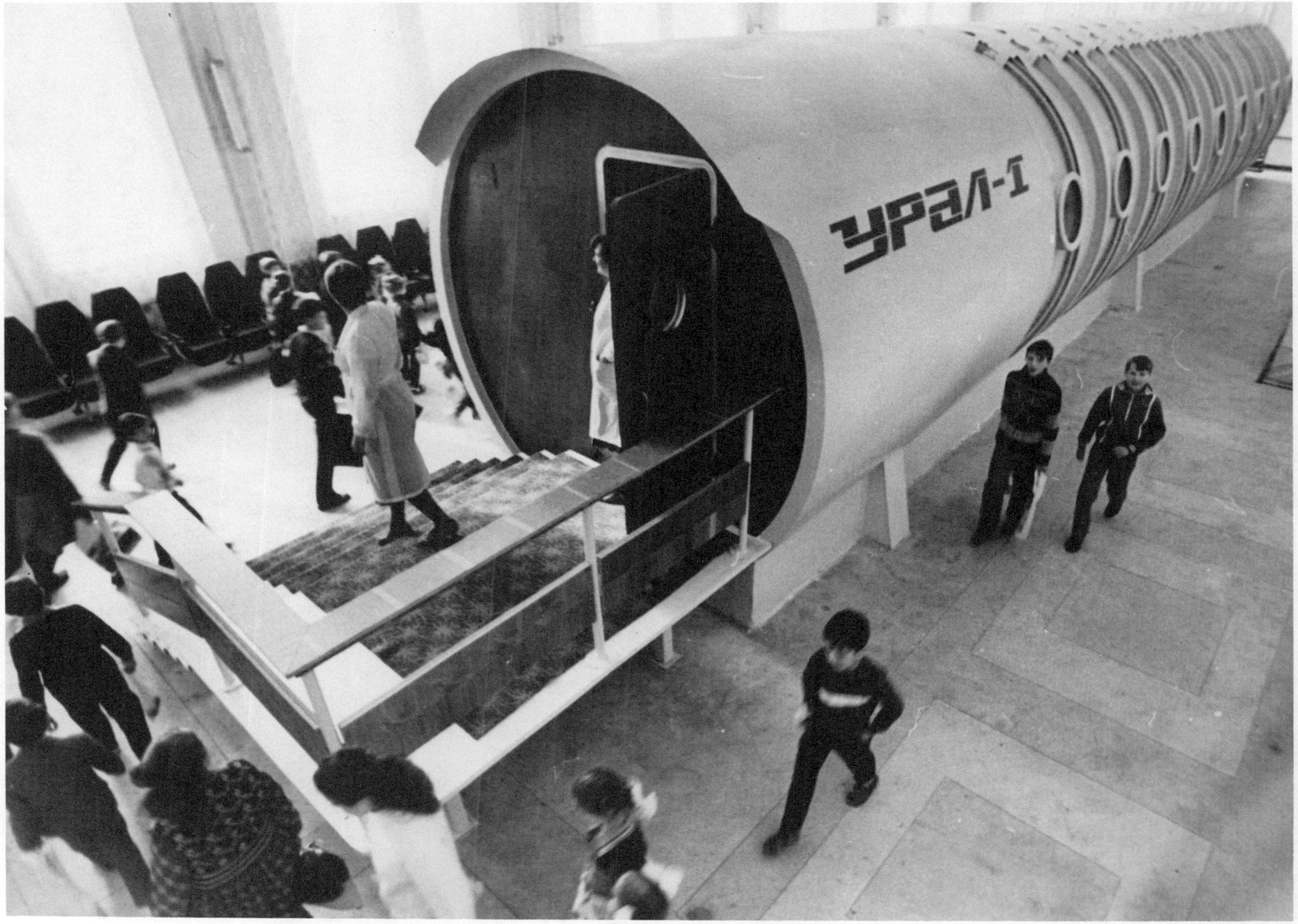

FIGURE 7. The medical multiseater altitude chamber *Ural-1*.

and remote evacuation and conditioning system providing "ascent" and "descent" rates of 2 to 10 m/s. Such altitude chambers should be installed at policlinics, rehabilitation centers, and clinical research institutions.

Prior to, in the course of, and after adaptation the patients were examined in a specialized Hypobaric Therapy Unit, in clinical departments such as cardiological, neurological, etc., and in the functional diagnosis labs — biochemical, immunological, etc. The results of examinations were forwarded to a panel of experts. At the very first stage, the patients were screened for the following contraindications:

1. Ischemic heart disease, III-degree hypertensive disease, valvular defects, and cardiac failure
2. Impaired brain circulation, craniocerebral injury
3. Grave bronchial asthma
4. Exacerbated chronic and acute inflammatory processes in the lungs
5. Diffuse pneumosclerosis, extensive pleural adhesions, pronounced emphysema with symptoms of pulmonary or cardiac insufficiency
6. Active foci of infection; exacerbation of chronic tonsillitis, sinusitis, cholecystitis, etc.
7. Inflammatory lesions of middle ear and accessory nasal sinus
8. Diseases affecting the permeability of eustachian tubes
9. Pregnancy; hemorrhage-prone uterine fibromyoma
10. Decompensated diabetes mellitus
11. Hernia of any localization
12. Manifestations of hepatorenal insufficiency
13. All psychoneurotic diseases associated with improper behavior during treatment
14. Lack of psychoemotional "readiness" and negative attitude to the particular treatment

This very exacting list of contraindications served primarily to avoid complications, and can be made more flexible in the future.

VI. EFFECT OF ADAPTATION TO INTERMITTENT HYPOXIA ON TOLERANCE OF APPARENTLY HEALTHY UNTRAINED SUBJECTS AND ON SOME RISK FACTORS OF ISCHEMIC HEART DISEASE*

The subjects were apparently healthy untrained males aged 35 to 49, total number 22, selected in the outpatient department of a rehabilitation center. All men in this group displayed characteristic signs of the detrained state: decreased tolerance to substantial physical loads, excess weight, headaches, cardialgias, and impaired sleep. Still, they were all working and showed no IHD symptoms in the veloergometric test.

The course of adaptation to hypoxia reduced the mean body weight by 2 kg, which is in line with the observations that such adaptation hypothalamically checks the appetite. The sleep was normalized, blood pressure reduced, and complaints of headaches and heartaches disappeared in all subjects; 5 of 11 smokers dropped the habit.

Table 11 demonstrates the effect of adaptation on the basic circulation parameters at rest and under maximal veloergometric load. Adaptation increased the total amount of work performed by 27% and the maximal output by 15%, with the oxygen consumption at rest decreased by 20% and the maximal consumption remaining the same. The systolic and the diastolic pressure also decreased both at rest and at peak load. As a result, the double product

* Participants in the work: Ya. I. Kots, V. A. Grigor'evskikh, O. I. Tikhomirov, I. A. Aleshin, O. A. Altukhov, S. V. Perepelkin, R. E. Funin, V. B. Volovich, T. V. Krasnova, N. N. Setko, S. M. Shashtineider, and M. M. Pavlova.

TABLE 11
Effect of Adaptation to Intermittent Hypoxia on Circulation and Physical Endurance

Indices	Before adaptation	After adaptation
Heart rate (min^{-1})		
Rest	69.1 ± 1.4	61.2 ± 1.7[a]
Load	152.6 ± 3.9	138.4 ± 6.0[a]
Arterial pressure (mmHg)		
Systolic		
Rest	147.1 ± 1.4	117.6 ± 1.7[a]
Load	205.9 ± 7.2	183.4 ± 5.1[a]
Diastolic		
Rest	93.3 ± 2.1	79.1 ± 2.1[a]
Load	101.6 ± 3.7	87.7 ± 7.6
Double product (AP_s·HR/100) at peak load	314.9 ± 11.4	249.5 ± 13.1[a]
Total work (kJ)	71.5 ± 6.5	93.0 ± 8.6[a]
Maximal power (W)	135.5 ± 8.8	155.5 ± 6.7
Oxygen consumption (ml/min)		
At rest	5.4 ± 0.6	4.4 ± 0.2
Maximal	21.3 ± 1.9	22.4 ± 1.7

[a] $p < 0.05$.

at peak load was 21% lower; with the higher maximal output, the efficiency of cardiac function under load was enhanced almost by a factor of 1.5.

Thus, *adaptation to intermittent hypoxia, without any additional measures, improves the performance of untrained subjects and enhances the efficiency of the heart which often limits the maximal load.*

It is known that in the detrained state decreased tolerance to physical load is usually accompanied by decreased functional capacity of the external respiration. Our studies have shown that adaptation to intermittent hypoxia increases the forced vital capacity and the forced exhaled volume by 20% and the maximal pulmonary ventilation by 40%.

Thus *in adaptation to intermittent hypoxia the enhanced efficiency of circulation combines with the greater functional capacity of external respiration; this apparently must contribute to the improved performance under maximal load.*

One of the criteria for assessing the tolerance to physical load is the extent of enzymemia, i.e., leakage of enzymes into the blood caused by cell membrane damage. Such events in stress[18] and physical loading[54] of untrained persons are in great measure determined by LPO activation; accordingly, such activation is a factor limiting the tolerable load, while administration of antioxidants to suppress LPO increases the tolerated intensity and duration of the load.[55] Table 12 demonstrates that adaptation to hypoxia lowers more than by half the blood serum levels of asparagine aminotransferase (AST) and alanine aminotransferase (ALT) at rest, and appreciably attenuates (AST) or virtually abolishes (ALT) their increase under maximum load; this probably results from the greater stability of cell membranes in the adapted organism. Quite in line with the idea of the cytoprotective role of the antioxidant mechanisms, Table 12 further shows that adaptation increases the serum content of the copper-containing protein ceruloplasmin, which has antioxidant activity,[56] and the SOD activity in the erythrocytes; concomitantly the amount of LPO products — MDA and dienic conjugates — is lowered to roughly the same extent. *Thus, it can be thought that enhanced activity of the natural antioxidant systems of the organism is one of the factors restricting the enzymemia and increasing the physical endurance in adaptation to hypoxia.*

Further analysis of the data obtained has revealed that adaptation to intermittent hypoxia

TABLE 12
Effect of Adaptation to Intermittent Hypoxia on the Blood Biochemical Indices

Indices	Before adaptation	After adaptation
Aspartate aminotransferase (nmol/ml·h)		
Rest	640 ± 12	280 ± 45[a]
Load	1040 ± 110	490 ± 40[a]
Alanine aminotransferase (nmol/ml·h)		
Rest	610 ± 10	320 ± 50[a]
Load	1110 ± 110	390 ± 50[a]
Superoxide dismutase (U)	110 ± 4	122 ± 3[a]
Ceruloplasmin (mg/l)	250 ± 15	315 ± 12[b]
Malonic dialdehyde (nmol/ml)	6.8 ± 0.4	5.6 ± 0.3[c]
Dienic conjugates (OD U/mg lipid)	0.87 ± 0.09	0.66 ± 0.04[c]

[a] $p < 0.01$.
[b] $p < 0.001$.
[c] $p < 0.05$.

TABLE 13
Effect of Adaptation to Intermittent Hypoxia on the Extent of Atherogenic Dyslipoproteinemia in Men (age 34 to 49) with Initial Cholesterol over 230 mg/dl

Indices	Before adaptation	After adaptation	*p*
Total cholesterol (mg/dl)	268 ± 4 (n = 15)	239 ± 7 (n = 15)	<0.05
HDLP cholesterol (mg/dl)	46 ± 2 (n = 15)	50 ± 3 (n = 14)	
LDLP cholesterol (mg/dl)	184 ± 10 (n = 15)	163 ± 10 (n = 14)	<0.05
Triglycerides (mg/dl)	188 ± 24 (n = 15)	129 ± 17 (n = 15)	<0.05
Atherogenicity index	4.6	3.9	

differentially affects the body weight and the serum cholesterol level in untrained persons differing in the initial values of these indices.

In the group taken as a whole, the mean cholesterol level did not exceed normal values and did not change in adaptation. The circulating triglycerides were also normal, and there was only a tendency to their decrease in adaptation. The average body weight reduction was about 2 kg (from 80.2 to 78.1 kg). Thus, in persons without pronounced disturbances of cholesterol metabolism or appreciable obesity, this mode of adaptation does not affect the lipid metabolism and just moderately reduces the body weight. These results are noteworthy because both humans and animals exposed to stress[57-59] develop pronounced hypercholesterolemia observed even with a constant diet. From this viewpoint our adaptation to gradually increasing hypoxia was not apparently stressful for the subjects.

Then we examined a group of 15 subjects with excessive weight and disturbed cholesterol metabolism (Table 13). In this group total cholesterol and circulating triglycerides exceeded the norm, while the cholesterol content in the antiatherogenic HDLP fraction was subnormal; accordingly, the atherogenicity index was elevated to 4.6 (normal values 3 and less).[60] In this case adaptation decreased the total cholesterol and triglyceride contents and did not change the HDLP cholesterol; as a result, the atherogenicity index decreased to 3.9. It is noteworthy that the average body weight reduction in this group was greater (from 95.2 to 91.1 kg). It can therefore be supposed that adaptation to hypoxia (which has been experimentally shown to activate cholesterol oxidation to bile acids in the liver) affects the lipid metabolism and the body weight mostly in those cases when these parameters substantially deviate from the norm.

In the aggregate, it can be stated that *in untrained, apparently healthy subjects adaptation to hypoxia increased the tolerance to physical loads, improved the performance and efficiency of circulation and external respiration, and decreased somewhat the body weight in hypercholesterolemic and obese subjects.*

It was also noted that half of the smokers examined dropped the habit. To appreciate these facts, it should be borne in mind that decreased tolerance to physical load, elevated arterial pressure, excess body weight, smoking, and atherogenic dyslipidemia constitute the major risk factors of ischemic heart disease. The observed reduction of these factors can be a point of departure for a special quantitative study of the effects of adaptation to intermittent hypoxia in these respects.

An interesting facet of the problem is the influence of adaptation on the amount of circulating immune complexes (CIC), which are held to be important in atherogenesis[61] and development of IHD.[62] Thus, examination of a group of 26 enlisted men (yardbirds) experiencing new social conditions, greater physical loads, and hence a certain extent of stress, has revealed markedly higher amounts of CIC (91.0 ± 6.7 U) as compared with a control group of donors of the same sex and age (50.1 ± 4.4 U). This is quite in line with the concept of the aggravating influence of stress on the formation of CIC,[63] which is associated with the poststress enhancement of the humoral immune response[64-65] and appearance of tissue antigens in the circulation.[66,67] A course of adaptation resulted in a pronounced decrease in this index (42.2 ± 4.5 U) which then remained close to normal for at least one month after the end of hypoxic exposure (61.4 ± 3.4 U).

There are at least two ways in which the CIC may be involved in the pathogenesis of IHD: interference with the lipoprotein turnover and damage to the vascular endothelium. Thus, the above data can be regarded as a beneficial effect of adaptation to intermittent hypoxia on an important immune mechanism that may under certain conditions aggravate the risk factors of IHD. On the whole, the influence of adaptation on the IHD risk factors undoubtedly deserves further study.

VII. EFFECT OF ADAPTATION TO INTERMITTENT HYPOXIA ON THE COURSE OF NEURASTHENIA AND THE EXTENT OF ARRHYTHMIAS IN NEUROCIRCULATORY DYSTONIA*

Cardiologists and neuropathologists know patients with the neurasthenic syndrome attended by pronounced arrhythmias that, being pathogenetically vague, are often termed idiopathic. On the one hand, direct clinicophysiological studies of the last decades testify that even in paroxysms of such arrhythmias the coronary flow is adequately enhanced, i.e., there is no ischemia.[68] Moreover, such arrhythmias may progress and even develop into idiopathic heart fibrillation with angiographically intact coronary arteries. On the other hand, quite important in this pathogenetic process are the psychopathic peculiarities of the personality and the occurrence of stressful situations,[21,69] and this is what points to the neurogenic origin of such arrhythmias (Chapter 2).

All this was put forth as a basis for treating neurasthenias and such arrhythmias with the same set of drugs, namely mild tranquilizers, neuroleptics, and antidepressants.[70-71] However, this therapy is far from being always efficacious, but most commonly has more or less pronounced side effects altering the patients' behavior.

* Participants in the work: A.A. Lebedev, Ya. I. Kots, V. I. Kornev, V. B. Volovich, I. A. Aleshin, V. S. Grigor'evskikh, R. E. Funin, O. A. Altukhov, and V. Bobylev.

Since adaptation to intermittent hypoxia activates the central stress-limiting systems and concurrently restricts or abolishes the disturbances to cardiac electric stability, it was reasonable to assess its effect on the course of neurasthenia and mentioned arrhythmias. We have examined two groups of patients:

1. Neurasthenic patients with depressive or phobic disorders — 15 persons aged 16 to 37, selected and examined at the Orenburg psychoneurological dispensary
2. Patients with idiopathic (i.e., neurogenic) arrhythmias — 13 persons aged 19 to 41, selected and examined at the therapeutic clinic of the Orenburg Medical Institute.

Before adaptation, the neurasthenic patients displayed pronounced phobic, depressive, and autonomic disorders (cardiophobia, nosophobia, fear of leaving the house alone, fear of crossing the street, anxiety, tearfulness and fatigue, persisting headaches, impaired attention and working ability, sweating, and cold limbs). The 15 patients with a marked syndrome of this kind were specially selected from a large population to assess the effect of adaptation as definitely as possible. They were also subjected to psychological tests (proofreading test, Krepelin's numerical ability test, and Schulte's table-reading test of attention).

Adaptation resulted in substantial improvement of the patients' condition. The effect was most clearly pronounced in the abatement of phobic reactions; the long-sustained fears disappeared or were emotionally deactualized, resulting in normalized behavior and relief of emotional tension in communication. The patients with depressive disorders developed interest for the surroundings, a more favorable attitude to people, and a brighter outlook for the future. By the end of the adaptation course, radical improvement was observed in seven patients and improvement with clearly reduced symptoms in the other eight.

In the group as a whole, the average number of mistakes in the proofreading test decreased from 22 ± 4 to 11 ± 3, indicating improved attention and concentrating ability. Similar results were obtained in the Krepelin's counting test (inital mean of 48 ± 4 correct additions in 5 min increasing to 62 ± 4 after adaptation) and in the Schulte's test (time needed to find 25 consecutive numbers in the table decreasing from 235 ± 11 s to 194 ± 11 s). In these objective psychological tests for attention and the rate of mental processes, positive shifts were observed in the overwhelming majority of patients: all 15 in the Krepelin's test, and 13 in the proofreading and Schulte's tests; in one case there were no changes in the two latter tests, and there was a single case of some deterioration.

Taking into account the beneficial effect of adaptation on the condition of neurasthenic patients, we then studied its influence on patients with idiopathic nonischemic arrhythmias exhibiting a hypochondriac syndrome. They were complaining of heart intermissions, cardialgias, lack of air, sleep disorders, and were overanxious about their health. In all cases antiarrhythmic drugs were not effective enough. Latent coronary failure or other organic heart diseases were ruled out by standard veloergometric testing, an electrophysiological study with transesophageal cardiac stimulation, ECG in 12 indirect leads, and echoCG. We could therefore be sure that we were dealing with regulatory arrhythmias.

The main means of quantitating these arrhythmias was the 24-h monitoring with a Lenta-MT unit. All 13 patients examined had ventricular extrasystoles and 10 of them had supraventricular extrasystoles as well. By the type of ventricular extrasystoles, six patients belonged to Lown's class 1-2, three to class 3, and four to class 4.

Table 14 lists the cumulative number of extrasystoles in 24 h for each individual case, and demonstrates the effect of adaptation on these rhythm disorders. As can be seen, when the relative changes are averaged, adaptation to intermittent hypoxia decreases the number of both ventricular and supraventricular extrasystoles about threefold. The antiarrhythmic effect is more pronounced in men: ventricular extrasystoles are reduced by 82 ± 4% (p <0.001) vs. 47 ± 15% (p <0.05) in women, and the pattern is much the same with

TABLE 14
Results of 24-h ECG Monitoring Before and After Adaptation to Intermittent Hypoxia

Case no. (sex)	Ventricular ES			Supraventricular ES			Sinoatrial block		Group ventricular ES		Beats in 24 h	
	Before	After	%change	Before	After	%change	Before	After	Before	After	Before	After
1 (F)	11,461	9,214	−20	3	—	−100	—	—	—	—	74,797	71,988
2 (F)	1	—	−100	100	54	−46	95	12	—	—	83,670	86,951
3 (F)	27,479	25,332	−8	—	—		—	—	108	469	82,458	76,013
4 (F)	2,211	1,042	−53	—	—		—	—	184	81	76,864	77,167
5 (F)	111	45	−59	2	—	−100	—	—	—	—	85,596	92,328
6 (M)	24,846	14,503	−42	—	—		—	—	—	—	98,926	110,006
7 (M)	42	2	−95	40	—	−100	—	—	—	—	89,069	90,301
8 (M)	45	—	−100	69	14	−80	22	—	3	—	68,317	64,144
9 (M)	1,525	504	−67	34	25	−24	—	—	82	—	88,868	79,571
10 (M)	881	82	−91	326	42	−87	458	8	78	—	58,333	62,654
11 (M)	39	12	−69	4,083	2,252	−45	—	—	—	—	75,399	75,333
12 (M)	428	107	−75	300	15	−96	—	—	—	—	84,970	78,577
13 (M)	91	19	−79	24	20	−17	—	—	—	—	70,502	71,529
Mean change			67 ± 8 (p <0.001)			69 ± 9 (p <0.001)						

supraventricular extrasystoles. When the day and the night periods are analyzed separately, ventricular extrasystole is more affected during the day (86 ± 8% in men and 63 ± 10% in women); the effect on supraventricular extrasystole is about the same in either period. It is noteworthy that adaptation suppresses group extrasystole, which is the most grave form in this contingent: it was completely abolished in 3 out of 5 patients and reduced more than by half in the fourth. There was a single case when despite some reduction of ventricular extrasystole the number of group extrasystoles increased; this turned out to be due to a marked (more than 10-mm) mitral valve prolapse, which appears to be a contraindication against adaptation to hypoxia in the altitude chamber.

Out of three patients with recorded sinoatrial block, such periods completely disappeared in one case and became much less frequent in the other two.

The antiarrhythmic effects of adaptation appear to be rather selective, as there were no appreciable changes in the diurnal heart rate, sinus node function, sinoatrial conduction, etc.

After adaptation, just as with the neurasthenic patients described above, there was marked improvement of the psychic status, and first of all abatement of the hypochondriac syndrome, normalization of sleep, disappearance of cardialgias, and fewer complaints of intermissions and palpitation. This improvement was more pronounced among men. Thus, adaptation to intermittent hypoxia has a definite therapeutic effect in neurasthenia with phobic and depressive phenomena, and a marked antiarrhythmic effect in so-called idiopathic and in essence regulatory arrhythmias.

The latter effect is quite in line with the earlier experimental works on the antiarrhythmic action of adaptation in stress, acute ischemia and reperfusion, infarction, and postinfarction cardiosclerosis.[19] Most probably it is due to the adaptive activation of the stress-limiting systems — opioidergic, serotonergic, antioxidant ones[11,45]— whose metabolites act as antiarrhythmics.[72] Since in animals adaptation to intermittent hypoxia is also known to reduce the postinfarct scar,[19] the body of data obtained makes promising the use of such adaptation for abolishing arrhythmias in and rehabilitating patients with certain forms of postinfarction cardiosclerosis.

By and large, these data would suffice to demonstrate the potential of adaptation to hypoxia for prevention and treatment of some heart diseases, and, conforming to the framework of this book, we could have restricted ourselves to that. However, the earlier experimental facts that such adaptation causes profound changes in the immune system, suppresses the development of allergic arthritis in animals, and decreases the amount of immune complexes in the blood prompted us to use it in treating some allergic diseases. The positive effects obtained are considered in the next section and, in our opinion, testify that the potentialities of adaptation to intermittent hypoxia go far beyond the frame of cardiology.

VIII. EFFECT OF ADAPTATION TO INTERMITTENT HYPOXIA ON THE INDICES OF THE IMMUNE SYSTEM AND ON THE COURSE OF SOME ALLERGIC DISEASES*

Examination and adaptation to intermittent hypoxia with therapeutic purposes has been carried out with three groups of patients.

The first group was children (6 to 14 years old) with atopic bronchial asthma; the duration of disease was 2 to 6 years, and drug therapy had been at best only briefly effective.

* Participants in the work: M. N. Volyanik, V. K. Bannikov, A. I. Smolyagin, S. N. Afonina, N. M. Lifshits, M. A. Frolova, I. N. Chainikova, V. K. Fillipov, I. Yu. Kil'divatov, A. A. Nikonorov, O. P. Pavlovskaya, and O. G. Kislova.

Adaptation to hypoxia in the *Ural-1* multiseater altitude chamber was carried out according to a modified technique[73] successfully used for several years.[18] The adaptation course consisted of 20 to 25 seances; in the first 5, the patients were gradually "taken up" to 3.5 km above sea level. The "ascent" and "descent" rate in each seance was 2 to 3 m/s and each exposure lasted 1 h.

The second group was adult patients with allergic dermatoses. The total number was 21 (12 men and 9 women); the duration of diseases was 4 to 30 years; in all cases drug therapy was poorly effective.

The third group consisted of six women aged 30 to 40, with autoimmune thyroiditis (Hashimoto's disease) of 1- to 10-year duration; in all cases conventional treatment had poor results.

The adults in the second and third groups were adapted similarly to the children, with one essential difference that each hypoxic exposure lasted 3.5 h.

All patients before and after adaptation were examined for the major indices of the immune status: the number of B and T lymphocytes in rosette tests,[74] the serum contents of C3 (complement factor) and immunoglobulins by radial immunodiffusion,[75] and CIC by polyethylene glycol precipitation.[76] For patients with thyroiditis, the titer of autoantibodies to thyroid water-salt extracts was determined by passive hemagglutination according to Boyden.[77] Patients with allergic dermatoses were tested for the intensity of cell response in the phytohemagglutinin test and histamine induction of T suppressors.[78] Asthmatic children were also tested for several indices of neurohumoral regulation: plasma 11-oxycorticosterole content[79] including its free and protein-bound fractions,[80] blood histamine[81] and serotonin,[82] and catecholamine excretion with urine.[83]

It has been found that children with atopic bronchial asthma display no pronounced deviations from the norm in the total amount of lymphocytes and circulating T cells, though the relative amount of B cells is somewhat increased. At the same time, the serum IgG and IgM contents are appreciably reduced (36 and 17%, respectively), while the CIC are elevated 2.5-fold. This suggests that such disbalance between the higher B count and the lower Ig content reflects not just a functional failure of the B system, but rather a pathogenetic link of the disease associated with enhanced formation of immune complexes which are important triggers of allergic disorders in this kind of pathology.[84]

Adaptation of the asthmatic children to intermittent hypoxia caused some further increase in the relative content of B lymphocytes, but, most importantly, completely normalized the serum Ig and CIC levels. It is noteworthy that the decline in CIC had a corollary in the enhanced C3 content, which is likely to reflect the reinforced organismic defense against immune-complex pathology since activated C3 is know to disperse the CIC.[85] Of especial practical importance is the fact that such normalization of the humoral immune indices was observed in an overwhelming majority of children with bronchial asthma: CIC reduction in 86% of cases, enhanced C3 in 91%, restored Ig in 70% (IgA) to 83% (IgM).

This beneficial effect of adaptation on the immune system in bronchial asthma appears to be associated with certain changes in neurohumoral regulation. Indeed, there was an increase in the blood 11-oxycorticosterone content and especially in its free physiologically active fraction, an increase in the sympathoadrenal activity revealed as enhanced catecholamine excretion with urine (epinephrine by 69%, norepinephrine by 117%), and a substantial decrease in blood histamine, which is a major mediator of allergic reactions.[86]

All this makes understandable why the curative effect of adaptation, which is due to natural regulatory readjustment of the immune system, is incomparably more stable than that of many drug-based approaches, and obviates the use of such extreme and often dangerous means as stress hormones.[87]

In the second group, 21 patients with allergic dermatoses (18 with atopic neurodermatitis and 3 with true eczema) were evaluated with respect to their clinical status, the above-

TABLE 15
Effect of Adaptation to Intermittent Hypoxia on the Indices of Cell and Humoral Immune Status of Patients with Allergic Dermatoses

Indices	Healthy controls	Patients	
		Before	After
Leukocytes (count per mm³)	6100 ± 205	6430 ± 144	6600 ± 151
Lymphocytes (per mm³)	1719 ± 41	1736 ± 65	1718 ± 62
(% leuk.)	28.2 ± 1.4	27.0 ± 0.7	27.3 ± 0.9
T cells (per mm³)	1258 ± 43	1128 ± 60	984 ± 77[a]
(% lymph.)	69.9 ± 1.5	64.8 ± 2.7	56.0 ± 3.9[a]
B cells (per mm³)	337 ± 27	425 ± 53	409 ± 51
(% lymph.)	19.4 ± 2.3	24.5 ± 2.8	20.9 ± 2.2
Phytohemagglutinin test (mm)			
PHA	26.1 ± 1.7	15.5 ± 2.2[a]	15.9 ± 2.8[a]
PHA + histamine	27.6 ± 1.9	5.2 ± 1.1[a]	13.7 ± 1.9[a]
Difference	+1.5 ± 0.4	−10.3 ± 2.3[a]	−2.6 ± 2.6
Immunoglobulins (mg %)			
A	254 ± 19	109 ± 12[a]	233 ± 40
M	151 ± 14	87 ± 11[a]	127 ± 20
G	1847 ± 287	991 ± 59[a]	1658 ± 183
E	—	460 ± 106	339 ± 123
CIC (U)	50 ± 4	68 ± 7	33 ± 4
Histamine (ng/ml)	40 ± 3	75 ± 3[a]	37 ± 7

[a] $p < 0.05$.

mentioned immunological parameters, and blood histamine. The clinical evaluation included the total afflicted skin area, the area of continuous lesion (percent), and the extent of pruritus on a five-point scale.

Directly after the course of adaptation to intermittent hypoxia in the altitude chamber, improvement was observed in 9.6% of patients, marked improvement in 80.9%, and clinical reconvalescence in 9.5%. The total afflicted area was reduced from 44 ± 6% to 16 ± 5%, continuous lesion area from 29 ± 6% to 8 ± 5%, and pruritus from 3.7 to 0.2 points on the average. Concurrently, the immunological indices determined in ten patients were also normalized as shown in Table 15: the contents of IgA, G, and M in the serum increased while that of IgE decreased, and CIC fell more than by half. The T suppressors became less sensitive to histamine as evidenced by the considerably smaller effect of histamine in the intracutaneous phytohemagglutinin test, and the blood histamine became normal.

There were no changes in the leukocyte count, absolute and relative number of lymphocytes or T and B populations, i.e., the adaptation had no immunodepressive effect.

At 1 month after the course, 18 patients could be re-examined; clinical reconvalescence was documented for 50%, marked improvement for 39%, and only 11% showed re-exacerbation by that moment. The total afflicted skin area in 1 month was 14 ± 5%, and pruritus (1.0 point) still remained much abated.

In assessing the positive result of the adaptational treatment of allergic dermatoses, attention should be paid to two issues.

1. In allergic dermatoses, just as in the allergically originating bronchial asthma, besides other alterations in the immune system there is a substantial rise in the circulating immune complexes, and in both cases this is abolished with adaptation.
2. Treatment of allergic dermatoses with drugs — tranquilizers,[89] antihistamine agents,[90] vitamins,[91] immunomodulators[92,93] — in many cases has no appreciable result. This

has led to the use of agents that certainly have adverse side effects, such as glucocorticoids,[94,95] or of invasive techniques like hemosorption[96] and plasmapheresis,[97] which are fraught with complications.[98,99] Much better results are obtained with mountain-climate therapy,[100,101] which is also safe enough, but for most patients this inevitably involves quite long and repeated journeys. Adaptation to intermittent hypoxia in the altitude chamber is devoid of all these shortcomings, and is an efficient and convenient means of treating this pathology. To make a note, there is much in evidence that the duration of the course ought to be extended.

In the third group, the six patients with case histories of 1 to 10 years initially had complaints fitting into the picture of a pronounced autonomic asthenic syndrome. Autoimmune thyroiditis was diagnosed after immunological examination that revealed high titers of antithyroid antibodies in the blood (1:640 to 1:24,800).

After adaptation to intermittent hypoxia, the patients' condition improved and the high erythrocyte sedimentation rate was attenuated.

Quite demonstrative results were obtained in the immunological examination. Before adaptation, the patients with autoimmune thyroiditis had lower counts of blood lymphocytes, mainly at the expense of T cells; the number of B cells did not appreciably change so that their relative content increased. Such changes in the lymphocyte subpopulations may reflect not only the peculiarities of the disease, but also those of the previous treatment, which included (not less than a year before) short courses of glucocorticoid hormones. However, the most significant alterations were observed in the humoral immune status: a twofold increase in CIC with a high level of antithyroid antibodies and lowered content of IgA and IgG.

Adaptation to hypoxia did not normalize the lymphocyte composition, causing some further decline in the portion of T cells, but markedly decreased the contents of CIC (1.6-fold) and antithyroid autoantibodies (titers from 0 to 1:1,280), and restored to normal the IgA and IgG levels. Though it is premature to claim a definite therapeutic effect of adaptation to intermittent hypoxia in Hashimoto's disease, the objective changes in the immune status are clearly much the same as in the allergic diseases considered above.

Thus, formation of a structural trace in the immune system in the course of adaptation to intermittent hypoxia, manifesting itself as an increasing portion of B cells and some reduction of T cells, favors normalization of the humoral defense in allergic (bronchial asthma and eczema) and autoimmune (thyroiditis) diseases. Such adaptation also markedly attenuates, through a mechanism that is still to be elucidated, the amount of circulating immune complexes in these disorders.

IX. PROSPECTS OF THE USE OF ADAPTATION TO INTERMITTENT HYPOXIA

We have seen that adaptation to hypoxia alleviates the detrained state, reduces some IHD risk factors, and hence may be used as an efficient means of preparing the people burdened with such risk factors to physical exercise, i.e., as an element of combined prevention of IHD. Adaptation to intermittent hypoxia is a promising approach to drug-free prevention and therapy in cardiology, neuropathology, pediatrics, and allergology. Still, collation of the positive clinical results with the experimental data gives rise to an impression that the potentialities of this approach are far greater than the present-day achievements.

1. With healthy individuals, adaptation to intermittent hypoxia should be used not just to prepare them for frequent or prolonged stays at high altitudes, flight work, etc., but first and foremost to enhance their resistance to stress, in particular occupational

stress. Adaptation is also a practical means of rehabilitating people prone to stress-linked diseases. With the power of modern analytical methods, such works will also contribute much to elucidation of the role of central and local stress-limiting systems in the adaptation of the organism to the environment.

2. No less important is the influence of adaptation to hypoxia on the circulation and neuroendocrine regulation in selected contingents with hereditary hazards and manifest risk factors of IHD and hypertension. Attended with caution, adaptation may be used even in the postinfarction stage to prevent recurrences of infarction, arrhythmias, and impairment of cardiac contractility, i.e., to attain the goals already documented in the experiment.
3. There seems to be much promise in the use of adaptation to hypoxia to treat the major endogenous psychoses, in particular some forms of schizophrenia. In this context, a marked intrinsic similarity must be accentuated between the insulin-shock treatment and adaptation to hypoxia. Indeed, with increasing doses of insulin the brain has to adapt to a deficiency of the main energy source, glucose, whereas with repeated hypoxia it adapts to a deficiency of the ultimate electron acceptor, oxygen. At the same time it is obvious that adaptation to hypoxia is incomparably more sparing than insulin shocks or massive doses of psychotropic drugs used nowadays to treat schizophrenia. Provided strict observance of the contraindications mainly related to the state of circulation, and rational use of sedatives during the actual hypoxic exposure, this method appears undebatably safe, and assessment of its efficacy highly expedient.
4. Another aspect of the influence of adaptation on the higher divisions of the human nervous system is that it promotes accumulation of large amounts of opioid peptides in the adrenals and mobilization of this reserve in stress, and prevents not only stress damage, but also the decline in the opioid peptide content in the brain. Since it is known that the craving for opiates may be related to their endogenous deficit, a question of considerable practical import arises as to how adaptation to intermittent hypoxia would affect the addiction to morphine.
5. The most currently tangible line of development is further and expanded use of adaptation to hypoxia for treating allergic and autoimmune disorders such as rheumatic arthritis, autoimmune hemolytic anemias, autoimmune juvenile diabetes, autoimmune nephropathies, myasthenias, and others.
6. With certain reserve, another trend stems from a number of experimental observations that adaptation of animals in the altitude chamber impedes growth of tumors.[103-106] The most recent data[107] show that this line of research has at least two different aspects: first, the impeding effect of adaptation on tumor growth through the antitumor immunity system, and second, the application of adaptation to hypoxia in combined tumor treatment with drugs, radiation, and surgery. In this case advantage can be taken, among other things, of the ability of adaptation to enhance the organismic resistance to surgical stress and ionizing radiation[108] as well as to chemical agents; thus, adaptation may be helpful at the rehabilitation stage after the radical modern measures of tumor treatment.
7. Finally and unavoidably, notwithstanding all the commendable features of the *Ural-1* chamber, the novel and differentiated applications of adaptation to hypoxia would call for new specialized and optimized designs of altitude chambers.

All new trends have one thing in common: their development is unpredictable. Therefore, today it is hardly possible and really needless to guess which of the above-listed aspects will yield the most notable results. Obviously, these and other potentialities of adaptational therapy can only be actualized provided faithful participation of clinicians and high standards of general and specialized examination. In any case, it must be underscored again that this painstaking work on the develoment of the novel method of drug-free therapy and prophylaxis follows the same path that the organism usually takes itself by adapting to the mileu and in just this way protecting itself from damage. In other words, adaptation is the cornerstone of the natural prevention of diesease. Relying upon the general principle ''do as Nature does'', it may in future be possible to check the inflationary dependence of mankind on assorted drugs, and to learn to cure some now refractory maladies.

REFERENCES

1. **Meerson, F. Z.,** *Adaptation, Stress and Prophylaxis,* Springer-Verlag, Berlin, 1984.
2. **Meerson, F. Z., Pomoinitskii, V. D., and Yampol'skaya, B. A.,** Dynamics of DNA, RNA, and protein synthesis in cardiac-muscle mitochondria and nuclei in adaptation to altitude hypoxia (in Russian), *Vopr. Med. Khim.,* 5, 538, 1972.
3. **Blagovestova, N. P., Loginova, E. V., and Simonov, E. E.,** Duration of the reaction of bone marrow to acclimation to hypoxia (in Russian), *Probl. Kosm. Biol.,* 8, 198, 1968.
4. **Pavlov, A. D.,** On the adaptation of macromolecular synthesis in bone marrow cells to ''altitude'' (in Russian), in *Geographical Environment and Population Health,* Nal'chik, 1970, 84.
5. **Meerson, F. Z.,** *Common Mechanism of Adaptation and Prophylaxis* (in Russian), Nauka, Moscow, 1973.
6. **Pshennikova, M. G.,** Protein synthesis in neurons and glial cells of the rat stellate ganglia in adaptation to altitude hypoxia (in Russian), *Fiziol. Zh. SSSR im. I.M. Sechenova,* 3, 421, 1973.
7. **Meerson, F. Z., Pshennikova, M. G., Kapel'ko, V. I., Radzievskii, S. A., and Novikova, N. A.,** Heart neural regulation in adaptation to altitude hypoxia (in Russian), *Kardiologiya,* 12, 50, 1975.
8. **Meerson, F. Z., Gomazkov, O. A., and Shimkovich, M. V.,** Adaptation to high altitude hypoxia as factor preventing development of myocardial ischemic necrosis, *Am. J. Cardiol.,* 31, 31, 1973.
9. **Meerson, F. Z., Maizelis, M. Ya., Malkin, A. B., Leikina, E. M., Kruglikov, R. I., and Popko, N. A.,** Activation of protein and RNA synthesis in the brain as a factor of adaptation to high altitude hypoxia (in Russian), *Dokl. Akad. Nauk SSSR,* 227, 1969, 1987.
10. **Meerson, F. Z., Krants, D., and Sadyraliev, G. S.,** Dynamics of protein synthesis in rat brain neurons and glia in adaptation to high altitude hypoxia (in Russian), *Tsitologiya,* 15, 324, 1973.
11. **Meerson, F. Z., Ustinova, E. E., and Manukhina, E. B.,** Prevention of cardiac arrhythmias by adaptation to hypoxia: regulatory mechanisms and cardiotropic effect, *Biomed. Biochem. Acta,* 48, 83, 1989.
12. **Meerson, F. Z., Frolov, B. A., and Afonina, S. N.,** Mechanism of the protective action of adaptation to hypoxia on the development of allergic arthritis (in Russian), *Byull. Eksp. Biol. Med.,* 10, 403, 1985.
13. **Meerson, F. Z., Isabaeva, V. A., and Ivanshina, A. Z.,** Enhanced development and preservation of conditioned reflexes in animals adapted to hypoxia (in Russian), *Dokl. Akad. Nauk SSSR,* 202, 982, 1972.
14. **Meerson, F. Z., Solomatina, E. S., Vikhlyaev, Yu. I., and Klygul', T. A.,** Effect of adaptation to altitude hypoxia on animal behavior in a conflict situation (in Russian), *Zh. Vyssh. Nervn. Deyat. im. I. P. Pavlova,* 23, 751, 1973.
15. **Meerson, F. Z., Maizelis, M. Ya., Leikina, E. M., Popko, N. A., and Gvirtsman, A. I.,** Effect of training to altitude hypoxia on the intensity of protein synthesis in the brain and the resistance of animals to a convulsive factor (in Russian), *Byull. Eksp. Biol. Med.,* 1, 280, 1970.
16. **Meerson, F. Z., Ugolev, A. A., and Golubeva, L. Yu.,** Prevention of cardiac stress damage with adaptation to altitude hypoxia (in Russian), *Kardiologiya,* 11, 91, 1980.
17. **Meerson, F. Z., Tverdokhlib, V. P., and Nikonorov, A. A.,** Prevention of atherogenic dyslipoproteinemias and complex metabolic disturbances in the liver in emotional pain stress (in Russian), *Vopr. Med. Khim.* 6, 104, 1988.
18. **Meerson, F. Z.,** *Pathogenesis and Prevention of Stress-Induced and Ischemic Damage to the Heart* (in Russian), Meditsina, Moscow, 1984.
19. **Meerson, F. Z., Ustinova, E. E., and Orlova, E. H.,** Prevention and elimination of heart arrhythmias by adaptation to intermittent high altitude hypoxia, *Clin. Cardiol.,* 12, 783, 1987.
20. **Skinner, J. E.,** Psychological stress and sudden cardiac death: brain mechanisms, in *Stress and Heart Disease,* Beamish, R. E., Singal, P. K., and Dhalla, N. S., Eds., Martinus Nijhoff, Boston, 1985, 44.
21. **Lown, B.,** Sudden cardiac death: biobehavioral perspectives, *Circulation,* 76 (Suppl.), 1, 1987.
22. **Slater, I. D. H., Tuffley, R. E., and Willaims, E. S.,** Control of aldosterone secretion during acclimation to hypoxia in man, *Clin. Sci.,* 37, 327, 1969.

23. **Meerson, F. Z., Barbarash, N. A., and Dvurechenskaya, G. Ya.,** Hindering effect of adaptation to hypoxia on the advance of hereditary hypertension in rats (in Russian), *Dokl. Akad. Nauk SSSR,* 241, 14, 1978.
24. **Meerson, F. Z., Barbarash, N. A., and Davydova, T. M.,** On the preventive effect of prior adaptation to high altitude hypoxia on the development of deoxycorticosterone-salt hypertension in rats (in Russian), *Kardiologiya,* 7, 14, 1971.
25. **Meerson, F. Z., Sukhikh, G. T., and Frolov, B. A.,** Effect of adaptation to intermittent hypoxia on some indices of immunoresponsiveness (in Russian), *Patol. Fiziol. Eksp. Ter.,* 4, 73, 1981.
26. **Frolov, B. A.,** Stress Impairment of the Function of the Immune System and Its Prevention (in Russian), D.Sc. thesis, Leningrad, 1987.
27. **Meerson, F. Z., Evseev, V. A., Davydova, T. V., and Giber, L. M.,** Effect of adaptation to high altitude hypoxia on the indices of nonspecific resistance, hemagglutinin production, and development of adjuvant arthritis in rats (in Russian), *Byull. Eksp. Biol. Med.,* 1, 12, 1980.
28. **Meerson, F. Z., Frolov, B. A., Smolyagin, A. I., and Filipov, V. K.,** Effect of adaptation to hypoxia on immediate and delayed-type allergic reactions (in Russian), in *Adaptation and Resistance of the Organism in Mountain Conditions,* Naukova Dumka, Kiev, 1986, 56.
29. **Sukhikh, G. T. and Meerson, F. Z.,** Prevention of the depression of normal killer activity in stress with adaptation to intermittent hypoxia (in Russian), *Byull. Eksp. Biol. Med.,* 4, 458, 1985.
30. **Boev, V. M., Setko, N. P., and Perepelkin, S. V.,** Correction of lipid peroxidation in chemical stress with prior adaptation to hypoxia (in Russian), in *Biochemistry for Medicine,* Abstr. Sci. Conf., Yakovlev, G. M., Ed., Nauka, Leningrad, 1988, 42.
31. **Poupa, O., Krofta, K., and Prochazka, J.,** Acclimation to simulated high altitude and acute cardiac necrosis, *Fed. Proc., Fed. Am. Soc. Exp. Biol.,* 25, 1243, 1966.
32. **Rasmussen, M. M., Reimer, K. A., Kloner, R. A., and Jennings, R. B.,** Infarct size reduction by propranolol before and after coronary ligation in dogs, *Circulation,* 56, 794, 1977.
33. **Lown, B., Verrier, R. L., and Corbalan, R.,** Psychological stress and threshold for repetitive ventricular response, *Science,* 132, 834, 1973.
34. **Avtandilov, G. G. and Salbiev, K. D.,** Morphometric and pathohistological characteristics of myocardial infarction (in Russian), *Arkh. Patol.,* 9, 62, 1974.
35. **Nepomnyashchikh, L. M.,** *Pathological Anatomy and Ultrastructure of the Heart* (in Russian), Nauka, Novosibirsk, 1981.
36. **Meerson, F. Z., Ustinova, E. E., Orlova, É. Kh., Rozhitskaya, I. I., and Evsev'eva, M. E.,** Protective action of adaptation to high altitude hypoxia in cardiac arrhythmias and fibrillation (in Russian), *Fiziol. Zh.,* 34, 71, 1988.
37. **Meerson, F. Z., Pshennikova, M. G., and Matlina, É. Sh.,** Effect of prior adaptation to high altitude hypoxia on the catecholamine content in the hypothalamus, adrenals, and heart under great physical load (in Russian), *Vopr. Med. Khim.,* 2, 172, 1977.
38. **Earley, C. J. and Leonard, B. E.,** Isolation and assay of noradrenaline, dopamine, 5-hydroxytryptamine and several metabolites from brain tissue using disposable Bio-Rad columns packed with Sephadex G 10, *J. Pharm. Methods,* 1, 67, 1978.
39. **Anichkov, N. N.,** Main results of research conducted in the Department of Pathological Anatomy, Institute of Experimental Medicine of the USSR Academy of Medical Sciences, on the problem of atherosclerosis (in Russian), *Vestn. Akad. Med. Nauk SSSR,* 11, 29, 1961.
40. **Khalatov, S. S.,** *Cholesterol Disease in its Pathophysiological and Clinical Sense* (in Russian), Nauka, Moscow, 1946.
41. **Goldstein, J. L. and Brown, M. S.,** Familial hypercholesterolemia, in *The Metabolic Basis of Inherited Disease,* Stanbury, J., Wyngaarden, J., and Frederickson, D., Eds., McGraw-Hill, New York, 1983.
42. **Archakov, A. I.,** *Microsomal Oxidation* (in Russian), Nauka, Moscow, 1975.
43. **Salganik, R. I., Manankova, N. M., and Semenova, L. A.,** Hypercholesterolemic effect of microsomal enzyme induction in rat liver (in Russian), *Vopr. Med. Khim.,* 4, 468, 1977.
44. **Brown, M. S. and Goldstein, J. L.,** How low-density lipoprotein receptors affect cholesterol metabolism and development of atherosclerosis, *In the World of Science* (Russ. trans. from *Scientific American,* 1, 27, 1985.
45. **Gerasimov, A. M., Kovalenko, E. A., Kasatkina, N. V., Amelina, D. Sh., Balashova, T. C., and Budennaya, T. Yu.,** Paradoxical reaction of some intracellular mechanisms for protection from oxygen in the adaptation of the organism to hypoxia (in Russian), *Dokl. Akad. Nauk SSSR,* 244, 492, 1979.
46. **Meerson, F. Z., Pshennikova, M. G., Kapel'ko, V. I., Radzievskii, S. A., and Novikova, N. A.,** Neural regulation of the heart in adaptation to high altitude hypoxia (in Russian), *Kardiologiya,* 12, 50, 1975.
47. **Ostadal, B. and Widimsky, J.,** *Intermittent Hypoxia and Cardiopulmonary System,* Academia, Prague, 1985.

48. **Liljestrand, G.**, Regulation of pulmonary arterial blood pressure, *Arch. Intern. Med.*, 81, 162, 1943.
49. **Meerson, F. Z. and Ananurova, L. A.**, Effect of inhibitors and activators of nucleic acid and protein synthesis on adaptation to high altitude hypoxia (in Russian), *Izv. Akad. Nauk Turkm. SSR, Ser. Biol.*, 5, 24, 1973.
50. **Korneev, L. A. and Luk'yanova, L. D.**, Peculiarities of myocardial energy metabolism and contractility in rats with different sensitivity (in Russian), *Patol. Fiziol. Eksp. Ter.*, 3, 53, 1987.
51. **Luk'yanova, L. D.**, Mechanisms of regulation of oxygen-dependent processes in the cells in animals with different sensitivity to hypoxia (in Russian), in *Abstr. IV All-Union Symp. on Physiological Problems on Adaptation,* Tartu, 1984, 128.
52. **Luk'yanova, L. D., Ugolev, A. T., Kharadurov, S. V., Popova, O. A., Romanova, V. E., and Balmukhanov, B. S.**, Role of succinic acid in the interaction of the respiratory chain and the microsomal system for oxidation of xenobiotics at different pO_2 values (in Russian), in *Mitochondrial Processes in the Temporal Patterns of Life Activity,* Pushchino, 1978, 14.
53. **Luk'yanova, L. D.**, Oxidative Metabolism and Nerve-Tissue Reactivity in Surviving Preparations and in the Whole Organism (in Russian), D.Sc. thesis, Moscow, 1971.
54. **Meerson, F. Z., Krasikov, S. I., Boev, V. M., and Kagan, V. E.**, Effect of antioxidant on the resistance of the untrained organism to maximal load (in Russian), *Byull. Eksp. Biol. Med.*, 7, 17, 1982.
55. **Meerson, F. Z., Kagan, V. E., Beresneva, Z. V., Boev, V. M., and Prilipko, L. L.**, Effect of antioxidant on human cardiac contractile function and endurance to physical load (in Russian), *Teor. Prakt. Fiz. Kul't.*, 8, 53, 1983.
56. **Yaropolov, A. I., Sergeev, A. G., and Basevich, V. V.**, Mechanism of the antioxidant action of ceruloplasmin (in Russian), *Dokl. Akad. Nauk SSSR,* 291, 237, 1986.
57. **Wolf, S. L.**, History of the study of stress and heart disease, on *Stress and Heart Disease,* Beamish, R. E., Singal, P. K., and Dhalla, N. S., Eds., Martinus Nijhoff, Boston, 1985, 3.
58. **Polozhentsev, S. D. and Rudnev, D. A.**, Dynamics of some indices of lipid metabolism in young men in the course of adaptation to prolonged physical and psychoemotional loads (in Russian), *Fiziol. Cheloveka,* 12, 151, 1986.
59. **Tverdokhlib, V. P., Lobanova, G. T., and Meerson, F. Z.**, Prevention of stress dyslipidemia with adaptation of animals to intermittent hypoxia (in Russian), *Byull. Eksp. Biol. Med.*, 2, 681, 1986.
60. **Klimov, A. N.**, Causes and conditions of the development of atherosclerosis (in Russian), in *Preventive Cardiology,* Kositskii, G. I., Ed., Meditsina, Moscow, 1977, 260.
61. **Klimov, A. N., Denisenko, A. D., and Nagornev, V. A.**, Lipoprotein-antibody immune complexes (in Russian), in *Immunoresponsiveness and Atherosclerosis,* Meditsina, Leningrad, 1986, 107.
62. **Osipov, S. G., Bakhov, N. I., and Sidorenko, B. A**, Immune complexes in the blood serum of patients with ischemic heart disease (in Russian), *Ter. Arkh.*, 53, 31, 1981.
63. **Isenberg, D. A., Cris, A. J., and Morrow, W.**, Variations in circulating immune complex levels with diet, exercise and sleep: a comparison between normal controls and patients with systemic lupus erythematosus, *Ann. Rheum. Dis.*, 40, 466, 1981.
64. **Sukhikh, G. T. and Frolov, B. A.**, Activating effect of stress exposure on the primary immune response in rats (in Russian), *Byull. Eksp. Biol. Med.*, 2, 127, 1982.
65. **Di Padova, F., Di Padova, G., and Rovagnati, P.**, Appearance of spontaneously Ig-secreting B-cells in human peripheral blood after surgery, *Clin. Exp. Immunol.*, 65, 582, 1986.
66. **Bogdanova, E. D., Kagan, V. E., and Kuliev, I. Ya.**, Activation of lipid peroxidation in the brain and appearance of antibodies to brain antigens in stress (in Russian), *Immunologiya,* 2, 65, 1981.
67. **Evseev, V. A. and Magaeva, S. V.**, Stress in the mechanisms of development of secondary immunodeficient states (in Russian), *Vestn. Akad. Med. Nauk SSSR,* 8, 18, 1985.
68. **Smetnev, A. S., Firstova, M. M., Bunin, Yu. A., Malyshev, Yu. M., Klimbovskii, A. A., Nargizyan, A. B., and Asymbekova, É. U.**, The state of myocardial blood flow in patients with different forms of supraventricular cardiac rhythm disorders (in Russian), *Kardiologiya,* 3, 39, 1985.
69. **Verrier, R. L. and Lown, B.**, Behavioral stress and cardiac arrhythmias, *Annu. Rev. Physiol.*, 46, 155, 1984.
70. **Raiskii, V. A.**, *Psychotropic Drugs in the Clinics of Internal Diseases* (in Russian), Meditsina, Moscow, 1983.
71. **Skibitskii, V. V.**, Differentiated psychopharmacotherapy in cardiac rhythm disorders (in Russian), *Kardiologiya,* 5, 48, 1987.
72. **Meerson, F. Z.**, Stress-limiting systems of the organism and protection against arrhythmias (in Russian), *Kardiologiya,* 7, 5, 1987.
73. **Uspenskaya, E. P.**, Treatment of patients with bronchial asthma under reduced barometric pressure (in Russian), in *Methodical Recommendations for Clinicians,* Ukhalovskii, I. N. and Fedoseev, G. F., Eds., Leningrad, 1977.
74. **Petrov, R. V., Stenina, M. A., and Lebedev, K. A.**, Peculiarities of quantitation of T lymphocytes and other rosette-forming cells in the blood of healthy and diseased people (in Russian), *Byull. Eksp. Biol. Med.*, 1, 197, 1976.

75. **Mancini, C., Carbonara, A., and Heremans, J.,** Immunochemical quantitation of antigens by single radical immunodiffusion, *Immunochemistry,* 2, 235, 1965.
76. **Haskova, V., Kaslik, V., and Riha, I.,** Simple method of circulating immune complex detection in human sera by polyethylene glycol precipitation, *Z. Immun. Forsch.,* 154, 399, 1978.
77. **Boyden, S. V.,** The absorption of protein on erythrocytes treated with tannic acid and subsequent hemagglutination by antiprotein sera, *J. Exp. Med.,* 93, 107, 1951.
78. **Zhukov, V. I., Usenko, R. S., and Veksler, Kh. M.,** Assay of immunoresponsiveness in patients with chronic dermatoses by an endermal phytohemagglutinin and histamine test (in Russian), *Vestn. Dermatol. Venerol.,* 3, 12, 1984.
79. **Pankov, Yu. A. and Usvatova, I. Ya.,** Assay of 11-oxycorticosteroids in blood plasma by their fluorescence in a sulfuric acid-alcohol reagent (in Russian), in *Methods of Study of Some Hormones and Mediators,* Meditsina, Moscow, 1965, 137.
80. **Pavlikhina, L. V., Usvatova, I. Ya., and Bunatyan, A. F.,** Fluorimetric method of separate determination of free and protein-bound 11-oxycorticosteroids in peripheral blood plasma (in Russian), in *Methods of Study of Some Humoral Regulation Systems,* Meditsina, Moscow, 1967, 50.
81. **Proshina, L. Ya.,** Assay of histamine and serotonin in one blood sample (in Russian), *Lab. Delo,* 2, 90, 1981.
82. **Kulinskii, V. I. and Kostyukovskaya, L. S.,** A modified method of serotonin assay in human blood (in Russian), *Lab. Delo,* 7, 390, 1969.
83. **Matlina, É. Zh., Kiseleva, Z. M., and Safieva, I. Z.,** Assay of epinephrine, norepinephrine, dopa and dopamine in one sample of urine (in Russian), in *Clinical Biochemistry,* Belarus', Minsk, 1976, 256.
84. **Bakulin, M. P., Sil'vestrov, V. P., and Karaulov, A. V.,** Preasthma and bronchial asthma: questions of clinical immunology (in Russian), *Ter. Arkh.,* 12, 33, 1987.
85. **Kul'berg, A. Ya.,** *Regulation of the Immune Response* (in Russian), Meditsina, Moscow, 1986, 148.
86. **Ado, A. D.,** *General Allergology* (in Russian), Meditsina, Moscow, 1978.
87. **Sergeeva, K. M. and Uspenskaya, E. P.,** *Bronchial Asthma in Children* (in Russian), Meditsina, Leningrad, 1984, 180.
88. **Wallace, A.,** The exposure treatment of burns, *Lancet,* 1, 501, 1951.
89. **Pototskii, I. I.,** *Neurodermatitis* (in Russian), Naukova Dumka, Kiev, 1986.
90. **Sergeev, Yu. V. and Potekaev, N. S.,** Clinical effectiveness and prospects for the use of zaditen (ketotifen) in therapy of allergic dermatoses (in Russian), *Vestn. Dermatol. Venerol.,* 4, 52, 1987.
91. **Tishchenko, L. D.,** A New Method of Antirecurrence Treatment of Eczema and Psoriasis with Phytovitamin Preparations (in Russian), D.Sc. thesis, Moscow, 1980.
92. **Skripkin, Yu. K.,** *Neurodermatitis* (in Russian), Moscow, 1967.
93. **Shaposhnikov, O. K., Gorbunov, V. P., and Shchedrin, V. I.,** Effect of thymic cytomedins (thymalin) on the course of some skin diseases (in Russian), *Vestn. Dermatol. Venerol.,* 4, 4, 1987.
94. **Agakishev, D. D.,** Effectiveness of nonspecific desensitizing therapy of patients with neurodermatitis and the dynamics of immunological indices (in Russian), *Vestn. Dermatol. Venerol.,* 3, 51, 1984.
95. **Shakhtmeister, I. Ya.,** *Pathogenesis and Treatment of Eczema and Neurodermatitis* (in Russian), Meditsina, Moscow, 1970.
96. **Lopukhin, Yu. M.,** Neurodermatitis disseminata as a dermatosis of autoimmune genesis and the results of its treatment by hemosorption (in Russian), *Abstr. II All-Union Congress of Dermatologists and Venerologists,* Vladimir, 1983, 160.
97. **Bazyka, A. P. and Zhunusova, A. K.,** Treatment of patients with neurodermatitis using exchange plasmaphoresis (in Russian), *Vestn. Dermatol. Venerol.,* 10, 50, 1984.
98. **Dmitriev, A. A.,** Modern notion of hemoperfusion through activated charcoal in the internal disease clinics (in Russian), *Ter. Arkh.,* 55, 140, 1983.
99. **Ryzhko, V. V., Gorodetskii, V. M., and Borisov, B. A.,** Intensive plasmaphoresis, probable difficulties and complications (in Russian), *Ter. Arkh.,* 59, 70, 1987.
100. **Zoirov, P. G.,** Eczema, neurodermatitis, and psoriasis among children in Tadzhikistan (in Russian), *Vestn. Dermatol. Venerol.,* 5, 56, 1986.
101. **Isaeva, E. T.,** Treatment of Patients with Psoriasis, Eczema, and Neurodermatitis Using Mineral-Water Baths from the Garm Chashma Spring in Pamir (in Russian), Ph.D. thesis, Dushanbe, 1970, 16.
102. **MeLaran, C. J., Gersh, B. J., Surgue, D. D., Hammill, S. C., Zinsmeister, A. R., Wood, D. L., Holmes, D. R., and Osborn, M. J.,** Out of hospital cardiac arrest in patients without clinically significant coronary artery disease: comparison of clinical, electrophysiological and survival characteristics with those in similar patients who have clinically significant coronary artery disease, *Br. Heart J.,* 58, 583, 1987.
103. **Heston, W. E. and Pratt, A. W.,** Effect of concentration of oxygen on occurrence of pulmonary tumors in strain A mice, *J. Natl. Cancer Inst.,* 22, 707, 1956.
104. **Arkhipov, G. N.,** Growth of transplantable tumor (M-1 sarcoma) in the process of hypoxic training of rats in the altitude chamber (in Russian), *Byull. Eksp. Biol. Med.,* 6, 73, 1961.

105. **Tannok, I. F. and Steel, G. G.,** Tumor growth and cell kinetics in chronically hypoxic animals, *J. Natl. Cancer Inst.,* 45, 123, 1970.
106. **Herndon, B. L., Lally, J. J., and Hacker, M.,** Atmospheric pressure effects on tumor growth: hypobaric anoxia and growth of a murine transplantable tumor, *J. Natl. Cancer Inst.,* 70, 738, 1983.
107. **Kulish, O. P.,** Effect of high-mountain conditions on the antitumor activity of cyclophosphane and its action on the lymphoid tissue cells (in Russian), *Eksp. Onkologiya,* 3, 60, 1985.
108. **Barbashova, Z. I.,** Some results of a study of a nature of organismic resistance and mechanisms of its changes (in Russian), *Kosm. Biol.,* 6, 13, 1969.

Chapter 8

CONCLUSION

In this book, with the heart as a vivid example, we have considered three types of mechanisms that have not been discussed heretofore and that help the organism to prevent or abolish stress-induced, ischemic, reperfusion, allergic, chemical, and even radiation damage.

The first type of such defense forms as the organism adapts to repetitive action of one particular environmental factor, for instance, hypoxia. As it does so, the adaptation has its material basis in a systemic structural trace; the latter has quite ramified architectonics, with elements ensuring enhanced resistance not to a single factor, but to many environmental factors. The scheme in Figure 1 demonstrates this cross-protective effect of adaptation to intermittent hypoxia, which we could have seen to be quite useful not only in experimental prophylaxis and therapy, but also in the treatment of several rather diverse human diseases. In our opinion, such cross protection is the most important principle of drug-free prophylaxis and therapy, and shows much promise, in particular in preventive cardiology.

The second type of defense, which we have considered in Chapters 3 through 5, relates to the concept of stress-limiting systems; these systems are coupled with the stress reaction and check it at both central and cellular levels, preventing thereby the stress-induced damage. In this mechanism, the organism adapts not to any particular and specific factor, but rather to unavoidable physiologically stressful situations. A course of such brief and mild enough, noninjurious exposures to stress gradually enhances the power or the efficiency of central and local stress-limiting systems: from the opioidergic and the GABA-ergic ones in the brain to the prostaglandin and the antioxidant ones in the cells and organs.

Thus, in this case the systemic structural trace of such adaptation also proves rather ramified, and there is also a broad cross-protective effect manifesting itself as not just enhanced resistance to severe emotional pain stress (EPS) or other kinds of stress, but also protection of the heart from ischemic and reperfusion damage and arrhythmias, and of the whole organism from direct chemical or radiation injury, etc. As depicted in Figure 2, in the organism adapted to totally nonspecific hard situations, the greater physiological power of the panoply of stress-limiting systems really protects it against stress-linked injury in exposure to diverse external influences. This attempt at a physiological interpretation of the ''university of hard knocks'' still covers only part of the issue, since rigorous experiments of this decade have shown that activation of the stress-limiting systems, besides protecting the animals' internal organs from damage, profoundly alters their behavior in a biologically advantageous direction. Such data are available for the GABA-ergic,[1] the opioidergic,[2] the serotonergic,[3] the antioxidant,[4] and other systems.

The contents of this book show that there are at least four ways in which the stress-limiting systems can be activated with preventive purposes in cardiology and other fields of clinical medicine.

1. Repetitive dosed exposure to moderate stress. As shown recently, this can be achieved not only by immobilization or EPS, but equally well by means quite applicable to man, such as electroacupuncture or exposure to cold. Such treatment is consistently accompanied with activation of the opioidergic and other stress-limiting systems; an experimental course of transauricular electroacupuncture prevents the stress-induced drop in the cardiac fibrillation threshold and abates the ischemic arrhythmias. Thus, the contemporary physiotherapeutic and reflexotherapeutic means offer a practicable way of enhancing the efficiency of the stress-limiting systems and consequently the resistance of the heart to stress, ischemic, and other kinds of damage.

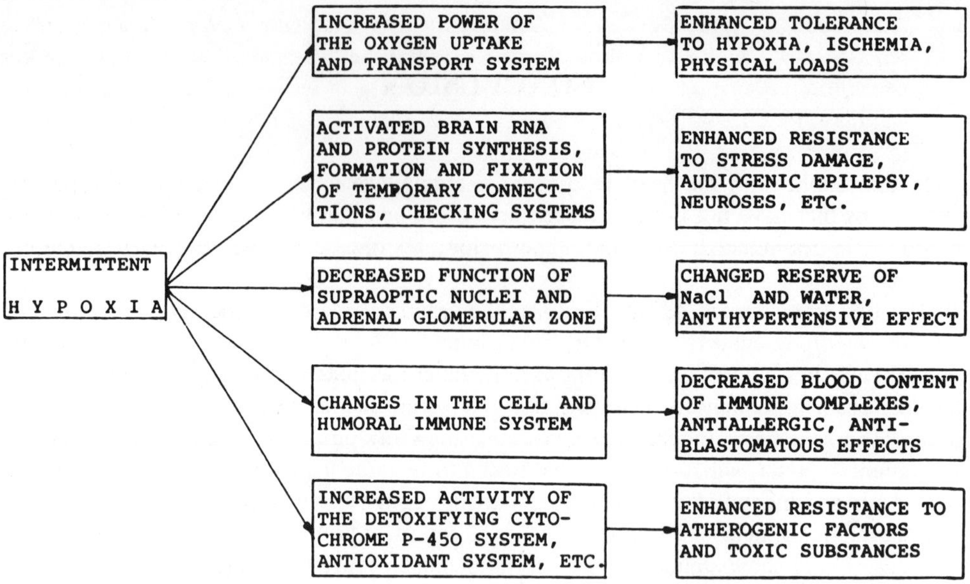

FIGURE 1. The systemic structural trace and the protective effects of long-term adaptation to hypoxia.

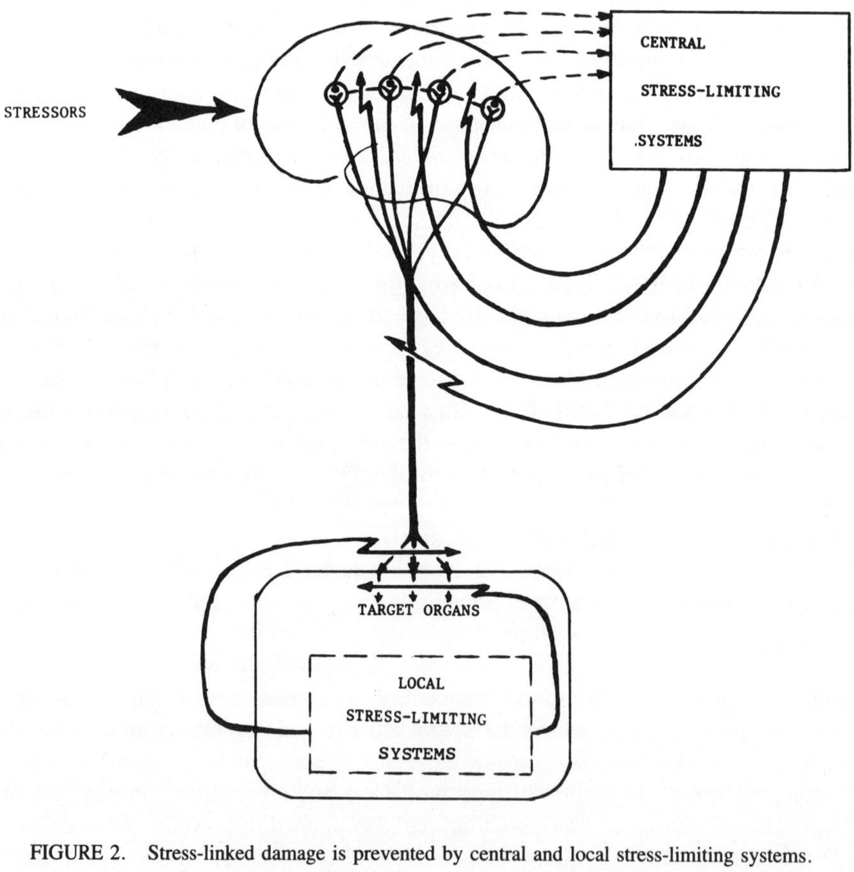

FIGURE 2. Stress-linked damage is prevented by central and local stress-limiting systems.

2. Adaptation to moderate exposure to various environmental factors. Since a stress reaction is evoked by the most diverse external factors acting on the organism, the stress-limiting systems are also naturally activated. Thus we have seen that in adaptation to intermittent high altitude hypoxia there are increases in the opioid peptide content in the adrenals, serotonin in the brain, antioxidant enzymes in the cardiac muscle, etc. These and other important adaptive changes have allowed the use of adaptation to intermittent hypoxia in the altitude chamber to reduce the risk factors of ischemic heart disease, to abolish grave forms of neurasthenia and the so-called idiopathic (neurogenic) arrhythmias.
3. Use of pharmacological activators of stress-limiting systems, which enhance the content of their mediators or the activity of their receptors. Such effects on the GABA-ergic system are exhibited by sodium valproate, which raises the blood and brain GABA levels, and by agonists of benzodiazepine receptors potentiating the GABA effects; stimulatory for the serotonergic system are opioid peptides and serotonin precursors, and so on.
4. Administration of natural mediators of the stress-limiting systems, or synthetic analogs thereof, to directly make up for the insufficiency of these systems. Examples of these are GABA, GHBA, opioid peptides and their synthetic analogs, serotonin, α-tocopherol, synthetic antioxidants, coenzyme Q, and adenosine derivatives.

The third type of defense built up by the organism in the course of adaptation (to stress and probably other factors) reveals itself in that the cell structures and systems become "hardier", i.e., can better withstand the action of the natural degrading agents involved in autolysis. A putative mechanism of this stabilization phenomenon has been considered in Chapter 6 (Figure 13), and implies an important role of "stress proteins" discovered in the last decade. Regardless of how valid this hypothesis, the phenomenon as such is an irrefutable fact. *In vitro,* autolysis and inactivation of SR membranes, mitochondria, and creatine phosphokinase are markedly retarded in preparations from stress-adapted animals. *In vivo,* prior adaptation to stress diminishes by 40% the infarct size despite the same ischemic zone in coronary ligation, i.e., enables the cells to withstand ischemia. Of course, to make practical use of such mechanisms is a quite appealing, albeit in many aspects debatable, goal.

By and large, the drug-free adaptational protection of the organism, and first of all the heart, follows the most natural way that the organism normally takes itself as it adapts to the environment to avoid damage. Clearly, active control over this process, rational dosing, and combination of the factors to which adaptation takes place will make such protection more efficient. At the same time the knowledge of the basic molecular mechanisms of adaptation will allow the use of metabolites that naturally take part in this process, and thus speed up the development of unorthodox approaches to pharmacological protection of the heart. In the end, it should be stressed that all this is but one example from the now rapidly emerging field of *adaptational medicine*. This is indeed the medicine of the nearest future.

REFERENCES

1. **Petty, F. and Sherman, A.,** GABA-ergic modulation of learned helplessness, *Pharmacol. Biochem. Behav.*, 15, 567, 1981.
2. **Puglisi-Allegra, S. and Oliverio, A.,** Naloxone potentiates shock-induced aggressive behavior in mice, *Pharmacol. Biochem. Behav.*, 15, 513, 1981.
3. **File, S., James, T., and MacLeod, N.,** Depletion in amygdaloid serotonin concentration and changes in social and aggressive behavior, *J. Neurol. Transm.*, 50, 1, 1981.

4. **Voronina, T. A., Smirnov, L. D., Tilekeeva, U. M., and Dyumaev, K. M.,** Role of the GABA-benzodiazepine-receptor complex in the anxiolytic action of 3-hydroxypyridines, new tranquilizers of non-benzodiazepine structure (in Russian), *Byull. Eksp. Biol. Med.*, 5, 571, 1986.

INDEX

A

B

C

D

T

U

V

W

X